Handbook of Applied Health Economics in Vaccines

HANDBOOKS IN HEALTH ECONOMICS
EVALUATION SERIES

Series editors: Alastair Gray and Andrew Briggs

Existing volumes in the series:

Decision Modelling for Health Economic Evaluation
Andrew Briggs, Mark Sculpher, and Karl Claxton

Applied Methods of Cost-effectiveness Analysis in Healthcare
Alastair M. Gray, Philip M. Clarke, Jane L. Wolstenholme,
and Sarah Wordsworth

Applied Methods of Cost-Benefit Analysis in Health Care
Emma McIntosh, Philip Clarke, Emma Frew, and Jordan Louviere

Economic Evaluation in Clinical Trials 2e
Henry A. Glick, Jalpa A. Doshi, Seema S. Sonnad, and Daniel Polsky

Applied Health Economics for Public Health Practice and Research
Rhiannon Tudor Edwards and Emma McIntosh

Distributional Cost-Effectiveness Analysis
Richard Cookson, Susan Griffin, Ole F. Norheim, and Anthony J. Culyer

Handbook of Applied Health Economics in Vaccines

Edited by

David Bishai, MD, MPH, PhD
Logan Brenzel, PhD

and

William V. Padula, PhD

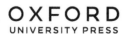

OXFORD
UNIVERSITY PRESS

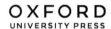

OXFORD
UNIVERSITY PRESS

Great Clarendon Street, Oxford, OX2 6DP,
United Kingdom

Oxford University Press is a department of the University of Oxford.
It furthers the University's objective of excellence in research, scholarship,
and education by publishing worldwide. Oxford is a registered trade mark of
Oxford University Press in the UK and in certain other countries

© Oxford University Press 2023

The moral rights of the authors have been asserted

First Edition published in 2023

Published in the United States of America by Oxford University Press
198 Madison Avenue, New York, NY 10016, United States of America

British Library Cataloguing in Publication Data
Data available

Library of Congress Control Number: 2022936459

ISBN 978-0-19-289608-7

DOI: 10.1093/oso/9780192896087.001.0001

Printed in the UK by
Ashford Colour Press Ltd, Gosport, Hampshire

Series preface

Economic evaluation in healthcare is a thriving international activity that is increasingly used to allocate scarce health resources, and within which applied and methodological research, teaching, and publication are flourishing. Several widely respected texts are already well established in the market, so what is the rationale for not just one more book, but for a series? We believe that the books in the series Handbooks in Health Economic Evaluation share a strong distinguishing feature, which is to cover as much as possible of this broad field with a much stronger practical flavor than existing texts, using plenty of illustrative material and worked examples. We hope that readers will use this series not only for authoritative views on the current practice of economic evaluation and likely future developments, but for practical and detailed guidance on how to undertake an analysis. The books in the series are textbooks, but first and foremost they are handbooks.

Our conviction that there is a place for the series has been nurtured by the continuing success of two short courses we helped develop—Advanced Methods of Cost-Effectiveness Analysis, and Advanced Modelling Methods for Economic Evaluation. Advanced Methods was developed in Oxford in 1999 and has run several times a year ever since, in Oxford, Canberra, and Hong Kong. Advanced Modelling was developed in York and Oxford in 2002 and has also run several times a year ever since, in Oxford, York, Glasgow, and Toronto. Both courses were explicitly designed to provide computer-based teaching that would take participants through the theory but also the methods and practical steps required to undertake a robust economic evaluation or construct a decision-analytic model to current standards. The proof-of-concept was the strong international demand for the courses—from academic researchers, government agencies, and the pharmaceutical industry—and the very positive feedback on their practical orientation.

So the original concept of the Handbooks series, as well as many of the specific ideas and illustrative material, can be traced to these courses. The Advanced Modelling course is in the phenotype of the first book in the series, *Decision Modelling for Health Economic Evaluation*, which focuses on the role and methods of decision analysis in economic evaluation. The Advanced Methods course has been an equally important influence on *Applied Methods of*

Cost-Effectiveness, the third book in the series which sets out the key elements of analyzing costs and outcomes, calculating cost-effectiveness, and reporting results. The concept was then extended to cover several other important topic areas. First, the design, conduct, and analysis of economic evaluations alongside clinical trials have become a specialized area of activity with distinctive methodological and practical issues, and its own debates and controversies. It seemed worthy of a dedicated volume, hence the second book in the series, *Economic Evaluation in Clinical Trials*. Next, while the use of cost–benefit analysis in healthcare has spawned a substantial literature, this is mostly theoretical, polemical, or focused on specific issues such as willingness to pay. We believe the fourth book in the series, *Applied Methods of Cost-Benefit Analysis in Health Care*, fills an important gap in the literature by providing a comprehensive guide to the theory but also the practical conduct of cost–benefit analysis, again with copious illustrative material and worked out examples.

Each book in the series is an integrated text prepared by several contributing authors, widely drawn from academic centers in the United Kingdom, the United States, Australia, and elsewhere. Part of our role as editors has been to foster a consistent style, but not to try to impose any particular line: that would have been unwelcome and also unwise amidst the diversity of an evolving field. News and information about the series, as well as supplementary material for each book, can be found at the series website: <http://www.herc.ox.ac.uk/books>.

Alastair Gray
Oxford
Andrew Briggs
Glasgow

Foreword

Vaccination to prevent contagious diseases resulted from a happy accident—the observation by British physician and scientist Edward Jenner that milkmaids were essentially immune from smallpox, and (subsequently) that being infected by the (relatively mild) cowpox disease conferred immunity against smallpox. Our word "vaccination" derives from the Latin word for "cow" (*vacca*). Smallpox was an incredibly deadly disease, killing 300 million people in the 20th century, and 400 million in the last 100 years before it was eradicated near the end of the 20th century. By inventing vaccines, Jenner is said to have saved more lives than any other person in human history.

Since then, the science of vaccines has moved through numerous important steps. For over a century, vaccines were made by creating weakened or inactivated pathogens. The famous Salk and Sabin polio vaccines used this same basic approach in the 1950s. Addition of adjuvants strengthened the immune response created by vaccines. New coronavirus disease 2019 (COVID-19) vaccines—developed at an unprecedented speed and with outstanding protection from the disease—instead use "messenger RNA" (mRNA) to teach a body's cells how to make a protein (or even a piece of one) to create an immune response without actually infecting the subject. This technique offers considerable promise for future vaccines.

A key feature of vaccines is their role in creating "herd immunity." In simple terms, herd immunity arises when the percent of the population who become immune (either from vaccines or by surviving an infection) exceeds $(R_0 - 1) / R_0$, where R_0 (called the "reproduction rate") is the number of persons naturally infected by a newly infected person. Some pathogens have a very low R_0 so vaccination is often not necessary to limit outbreaks. Others have very high contagion levels. Measles, for example, has $R_0 = 12$ to 18, so to prevent spreading of measles requires (using the midpoint) that 14/15/=93.3% of the population must either become immunized by vaccination or survive a natural infection to prevent the disease from spreading. COVID-19 has an R_0 of about 2.0–3.0 depending on the variant, thus requiring effective vaccination coverage (combined with disease-based immunity) of about two-thirds of any self-contained population. The number needed to be vaccinated interacts with the vaccine efficacy (the rate of protection provided) in obvious ways.

This raises another key feature of vaccines—they are "public goods" in the sense that all people receiving a vaccination not only protect themselves but also confer a small benefit on the entire remaining population. This benefit is obviously larger as the R_0 of the pathogen increases. Standard economic analysis (Phelps, 2017) shows that private incentives to become vaccinated lead to vaccination rates that are too low, so public policy interventions can become necessary to reach optimal levels of vaccination coverage in any given population.[1]

Multiple issues can reduce vaccine uptake. Things that deter vaccination coverage include painful or health-risking side effects, the necessity of multiple shots to achieve full immunity, and the mode of administration (in descending order of preference, oral, intramuscular injection, and intravenous injection). Apparently simple issues can also confound distribution through the supply chain, including the "cold chain" requirements for storage from manufacturing up to the point of final administration (both temperature and volume of space), and even requisite shelf space for storage of supplies.

In the production process itself, supply chain availability of key components can rate-limit production, as can the simple issue of availability of glass vials of appropriate size and characteristics, and even the availability of needles to give injections. Complete consideration of these issues requires a comprehensive systems analysis review of all facets of vaccine production, distribution, financial, and logistics issues that can deter patients' access to vaccines, and information campaigns (Madhavan, Phelps, Rouse, & Rappuoli, 2018).

In addition to their primary health effects, vaccines can have profound economic implications that extend far beyond avoided healthcare costs. Worker productivity rises when contagious diseases are suppressed. Particularly in areas where endemic diseases such as malaria exist, school participation and final educational attainment suffer, so vaccines that either prevent the disease or reduce disease severity can lead to long-term economic gains from improved education and higher final attainment levels. These will increase future worker productivity, make for a more informed electorate, and even reduce the rate at which people undertake harmful consumption choices (tobacco, alcohol abuse, lack of exercise, and obesity) (Phelps, 2010).

---

[1] The "cost" of vaccination can be monetary, physical, or psychological, and may be based on misinformation. In rural and lower-income areas, travel costs to receive second and third shots may reduce vaccination rates in a way similar to the effect of monetary fees. Fear of physical pain or other adverse reaction also inhibits vaccination acceptance. Sometimes, misinformation deters vaccination acceptance, such as in individuals who believe the now-refuted concept that vaccine adjuvants lead to autism in children.

The worldwide COVID-19 pandemic highlighted another important economic consequence of vaccine development. The economies of most nations of the world came to a near standstill when the only available public interventions were "shelter in place" and quarantine of those either actually or potentially affected. Only the emerging hope of vaccination success brought these economies back toward full employment, which can only be achieved when worldwide vaccination rates reach necessary levels.

The first chapter of this handbook explores these and other related issues relating to vaccine production and use. Chapter 2 goes into detail about methods to evaluate vaccines using appropriate methods of estimating costs, while Chapters 3 and 4 provide important details about proper methods of evaluation using up-to-date methods of cost-effectiveness analysis. An application of these methods to evaluate the cost-effectiveness of the vaccines against COVID-19 is presented in Chapter 4. Chapter 5 covers the global landscape for immunization financing, providing insights about the structure of key global initiatives to expand and sustain immunization programs and on how the different actors within them interact.

Vaccines are some of the greatest miracles of medical science. Those who invent them, finance them, distribute them, promote them, administer them, and, yes, those who receive them are advancing human well-being. This handbook aims at assisting those undertaking economic evaluation of various vaccine programs to sharpen their skills, increase their credibility, and through their work, hopefully, help to focus vaccine development and administration on those diseases where vaccines matter most.

Charles E. Phelps

References

Madhavan, G., Phelps, C. E., Rouse, W. B., & Rappuoli, R. (2018). Vision for a systems architecture to integrate and transform population health. *Proceedings of the National Academy of Sciences of the United States of America*, 115(50), 12595–12602. doi:10.1073/pnas.1809919115

Phelps, C. E. (2010). *Eight questions you should ask about our health care system (even if the answers make you sick)*. Stanford, CA: Hoover Institution Press.

Phelps, C. E. (2017). Externalities in health and medical care. In *Health economics* (6th ed., pp. 387–411). New York, NY: Routledge Press.

Contents

Introduction to the handbook

David Bishai

Complexity surrounding the development, production, distribution, storage, injection, and surveillance of vaccines has fascinated economists for good reason. Much can go wrong. Much can go right. Triumph can save millions of lives and billions of dollars. But failures can multiply out of control and cost jobs, reputations, and set back progress for decades.

Economists are also drawn to the study of vaccines because they are exquisite economic products. They are supremely valuable to societies yet often scarce and neglected except in a crisis. Because they prevent something from happening, their invisibility creates a constant need to create and spread information about their value. The invisibility demands transparent and meticulous models of the value of vaccines so that the right choices can be made by myriad stakeholders.

Vaccine stakeholders include literally every human being. From the day of birth until the end of life, there is always a choice to be made about whether to receive a vaccine and how valuable it will be. From newborns getting BCG shots in the nursery to hospice patients deciding on a COVID-19 vaccine, these products are inescapable. Most choices about vaccines occur in an information-scarce environment. Price signals that could guide an efficient choice are seldom functional because public subsidies abound. Information about the benefits and risks of a shot change over time as epidemics wax and wane and safety data emerge. The stakeholders responsible for financing the subsidies or setting prices are forced to make vital decisions that proxy what fully informed people would pay, but there are never any fully informed people anywhere. The authors and editors of this handbook were drawn to vaccine economics because of both its importance and the appeal of connecting models of economic value to life-saving decisions.

Many of the chapters in this handbook had their genesis in classroom sessions with policymakers and practitioners who needed to apply economic tools to their work in immunization programs and health systems. In 2017,

David Bishai, *Introduction to the handbook* In: *Handbook of Applied Health Economics in Vaccines*. Edited by: David Bishai, Logan Brenzel and William V. Padula, Oxford University Press. © Oxford University Press 2023. DOI: 10.1093/oso/9780192896087.001.0001 with a grant from the Bill & Melinda Gates Foundation, a consortium known as Teaching Vaccine Economics Everywhere (TVEE) started with faculty from Johns Hopkins University, Aga Khan University, Indian Institute of Hospital Management Research University, Makerere University, and Witwatersrand University. (The University of Ouagadougou and Mahidol University joined in 2019.) The goal of TVEE was to prepare and deliver a curriculum in vaccine economics that stretched from introductory material to advanced methods with an audience ranging from policymakers and practitioners to economics graduate students. After several workshops to develop outlines of the necessary fundamentals in the field, the curriculum was organized around modules on economic principles, costing, economic evaluation, financing, and resource tracking. Courses were co-taught live in university settings and online with slides and videos available in French and English. Many of the participants in these courses were practitioners so there was a focus on immediately applying principles to problems. The exercises accompanying this handbook have undergone extensive classroom-based refinement.

This handbook goes beyond the original classroom material by including material from leaders in the field to fill in essential areas and connect readers to emerging consensus in the areas of vaccine costing, evaluation, and guidance. The economics lessons learned during the COVID-19 pandemic are still emerging, but the authors have incorporated them whenever possible.

If nothing else, the ongoing struggle to solve the economic problems surrounding the deployment of COVID-19 vaccines will stimulate many more readers and practitioners to consider the economics of vaccines. This is a beautiful field and promises life-changing rewards.

Acknowledgments

Bishai, Brenzel, and Padula wish to thank the countless individuals who have studied vaccine economics through the Teaching Vaccine Economics Everywhere (TVEE) program. Faculty and workshop participants in Burkina Faso, India, Pakistan, South Africa, Thailand, and Uganda spent weeks discussing the elements of vaccine economics that were central to both research and policymaking. Their support of TVEE, and feedback, instilled a sense of confidence that the content in this handbook could deliver change in vaccine capacity building throughout countries and communities worldwide.

We would like to acknowledge the supporting roles of Shreena Malaviya, Gatien de Broucker, and Mandy Chen, whose efforts to manage elements of the manuscript development from start to finish were critical in its success.

The editors and authors also wish to thank their families, whose daily support of efforts to develop this manuscript during the midst of the COVID-19 pandemic was instrumental to completing this work.

Financial support was provided through a grant to the Johns Hopkins University (INV-009627). This funding source has made this handbook openly accessible to individuals seeking to learn more about excellence in vaccine economics.

Acknowledgments

List of abbreviations

AMC	Advance Market Commitment
BCR	benefit–cost ratio
BIA	budget impact analysis
BMGF	Bill & Melinda Gates Foundation
CBA	cost–benefit analysis
CCA	cost–consequence analysis
CEA	cost-effectiveness analysis
CET	cost-effectiveness threshold
CFA	cost-finding analysis
CHEERS	Consolidated Health Economic Evaluation Reporting Standards
CI	confidence interval
CIA	cost-identification analysis
CMA	cost-minimization analysis
cMYP	Comprehensive Multi-Year Plan
COI	cost of illness
COVAX	COVID-19 Vaccines Global Access
COVID-19	coronavirus disease 2019
CUA	cost–utility analysis
DALY	disability-adjusted life year
DCVM	Developing Country Vaccine Manufacturer
DOF	Department of Finance
DOH	Department of Health
ED-5Q	EuroQol five-dimensions
EPI	Expanded Program on Immunization
EVPI	expected value of perfect information
EVPPI	expected value of perfect parameter information
EVSI	expected value of sample information
FDI	Federation Dentaire Internationale
GDP	gross domestic product
GNI	gross national income
HALY	health-adjusted life year
hib	*Haemophilus influenzae* type b
HPV	human papillomavirus
HRQoL	health-related quality of life
HSIS	health system and immunization strengthening
ICER	incremental cost-effectiveness ratio
IFFIm	International Finance Facility for Immunization
JCVI	Joint Committee on Vaccination and Immunisation

JRF	Joint Reporting Form
LMICs	low- and middle-income countries
MDP	Markov decision process
MI4A	Market Information for Access to Vaccines
MNC	multinational corporation
mRNA	messenger RNA
MVP	Meningitis Vaccine Project
NHA	National Health Accounts
NHB	net health benefit
NHI	national health insurance
NHIS	National Health Insurance Scheme
NIP	national immunization program
NITAG	National Immunisation Technical Advisory Group
NMB	net monetary benefit
NUVI	new and underutilized vaccine introduction
OOP	out of pocket
PAHO	Pan American Health Organization
PCV	pneumococcal conjugate vaccine
PFM	public financial management
PFP	private for-profit
PNFP	private not-for-profit
PPS	post-polio syndrome
PSA	probabilistic sensitivity analysis
QALY	quality-adjusted life year
QHES	Quality of Health Economic Studies
R&D	research and development
RCT	randomized controlled trial
ROI	return on investment
SE	standard error
SEIR	Susceptible–Exposed–Infected–Recovered
SG	standard gamble
SIA	supplementary immunization activity
SIR	Susceptible–Infected–Recovered
SIRV	Susceptible–Infected–Recovered–Vaccinated
TTO	time trade-off
UK	United Kingdom
UNICEF SD	UNICEF Supply Division
US	United States
VAS	visual analog scale
VFC	Vaccines for Children
VPD	vaccine-preventable disease
WHO	World Health Organization

Contributors

Editors

David Bishai, MD, MPH, PhD, is Adjunct Professor of Population, Family and Reproductive Health in the Bloomberg School of Public Health at Johns Hopkins University in Baltimore, Maryland, USA.

Logan Brenzel, PhD, is Senior Program Officer at the Bill & Melinda Gates Foundation in the District of Columbia, USA.

William V. Padula, PhD, is Assistant Professor of Pharmaceutical & Health Economics in the School of Pharmacy at the University of Southern California, Los Angeles, and Fellow in the Leonard D. Schaeffer Center for Health Policy & Economics in Los Angeles, California, USA.

Contributors

Onaopemipo Abiodun
PhD Candidate
International Health
Johns Hopkins Bloomberg School of Public Health
Baltimore, MD, USA

G. Caleb Alexander
Professor of Epidemiology and Medicine
Johns Hopkins Bloomberg School of Public Health
Baltimore, MD, USA

Y. Natalia Alfonso
Health Economist, PhD Candidate
International Health
Johns Hopkins Bloomberg School of Public Health
Baltimore, MD, USA

David Bishai
Adjunct Professor
Population Family and Reproductive Health
Johns Hopkins Bloomberg School of Public Health
Baltimore, MD, USA

David Bloom
Professor
Global Health & Population
Harvard T.H. Chan School of Public Health
Boston, MA, USA

Logan Brenzel
Senior Program Officer
Bill & Melinda Gates Foundation
Seattle, WA, USA

Gatien de Broucker
Senior Health Economist
International Vaccine Access Center, Department of International Health
Johns Hopkins Bloomberg School of Public Health
Baltimore, MD, USA

Colleen Burgess
Principal Consultant
Ramboll Health Sciences
Phoenix, AZ, USA

Susmita Chatterjee
Senior Health Economist
George Institute for Global Health
New Delhi, India

Grace Chee
Project Director
MOMENTUM Routine Immunization Transformation and Equity
JSI Research & Training Institute, Inc.
Arlington, VA, USA

Clarke B. Cole
Manager
Non-Communicable Diseases
Clinton Health Access Initiative
Accra, GH

David W. Dowdy
Associate Professor
Department of Epidemiology
Johns Hopkins Bloomberg School of Public Health
Baltimore, MD, USA

Emmanuel F. Drabo
Assistant Professor
Health Policy and Management
Johns Hopkins University
Baltimore, MD, USA

Ijeoma Edoka
Health Economics and Epidemiology Research Office
Department of Internal Medicine, School of Clinical Medicine,
Faculty of Health Sciences
University of the Witwatersrand
Johannesburg, South Africa
School of Public Health, Faculty of Health Sciences
University of the Witwatersrand
Johannesburg, South Africa

Beth Evans
Program Manager
Global Vaccines Team
Clinton Health Access Initiative
Boston, MA, USA

Ciaran N. Kohli-Lynch
Research Fellow
Center for Health Services & Outcomes Research
Northwestern University
Chicago, IL, USA

Carleigh Krubiner
Bioethics Lead
Research Environment
Wellcome Trust
London, GB

Ann Levin
President
Levin & Morgan LLC
Bethesda, MD, USA

Joseph F. Levy
Assistant Professor
Department of Health Policy and Management
Johns Hopkins Bloomberg School of Public Health
Baltimore, MD, USA

Shreena Malaviya
Senior Health Economist
Purple Squirrel Economics
Toronto, ON, CA

Chrispus Mayora
Lecturer
Health Policy Planning and Management
Makerere University School of Public Health
Kampala, UG

R. Brett McQueen
Assistant Professor
Skaggs School of Pharmacy and Pharmaceutical Sciences
University of Colorado Anschutz Medical Campus
Aurora, CO, USA

Andrew Mirelman
Technical Officer
Health Systems Governance and Financing
World Health Organization
Geneva, CH

William V. Padula
Assistant Professor
Department of Pharmaceutical & Health Economics
University of Southern California
Los Angeles, CA, USA

Ankur Pandya
Associate Professor of Health Decision Science
Health Policy and Management
Harvard T.H. Chan School of Public Health
Boston, MA, USA

George Pariyo
Chief of Operations
Senior Management Team
Serum Africa Medical Research Institute (SAMRI)
Kampala, UG

Charles E. Phelps
Professor and Provost Emeritus
University Professor and Provost Emeritus
Economics and Public Health Sciences
University of Rochester
Rochester, NY, USA

Siriporn Pooripussarakul
Independent Researcher
Bangkok, Thailand

Natalie M. Reid
Director
Monument Analytics
Baltimore, MD, USA

Stephen Resch
Lecturer
Department of Health Policy and Management
Harvard T.H. Chan School of Public Health
Boston, MA, USA

Dan Salmon
Professor
Department of International Health
Johns Hopkins Bloomberg School of Public Health
Baltimore, MD, USA

Soleine Scotney
Country Director
Clinton Health Access Initiative (CHAI) Cambodia
Phnom Penh, KH

Mark Sculpher
Professor and Director
Centre for Health Economics
University of York
York, GB

J. P. Sevilla
Research Associate
Global Health and Population
Harvard T.H. Chan School of Public Health
Boston, MA, USA

Julia F. Slejko
Associate Professor
Department of Pharmaceutical Health Services Research
University of Maryland School of Pharmacy
Baltimore, MD, USA

Jonothan Tierce
Principal
Monument Analytics, Inc.
Baltimore, MD, USA

Stéphane Verguet
Associate Professor of Global Health
Global Health and Population
Harvard T.H. Chan School of Public Health
Boston, MA, USA

Elizabeth Watts
Doctoral Researcher
Health Policy & Management
University of Minnesota
Minneapolis, MN, USA

Tommy Wilkinson
Senior Researcher
Health Economics Unit, School of Public Health
University of Cape Town
Cape Town, ZA

1

PRINCIPLES OF VACCINE ECONOMICS

Edited by David Bishai and Chrispus Mayora

1.0

Section introduction: principles of vaccine economics

David Bishai and Chrispus Mayora

Fundamentals matter. Vaccines are some of the most complex molecules ever invented and the social systems that deploy, monitor, and finance them are equally complex. Much of the peculiarities of vaccine economics arises from the peculiarities of vaccines. The most eccentric thing about vaccines is that many of them can benefit the person who gets the shot as well as the people around them. Furthermore, not everyone will obtain the same amount of benefit because of varying risk levels in the population. Coronavirus disease 2019 (COVID-19) vaccines illustrate these points well. The massive public investments to subsidize supply of and stimulate demand for COVID-19 vaccines were predicated on a sure forecast that without public investment the free market was doomed to fail. In many countries, even with the public sector investments, a COVID-19 vaccine at a price of $0 was not attractive to many who were at lower risk and did not appreciate the benefits their shot would offer their community.

There are also many technical peculiarities of vaccines such as their production and delivery that have economic policy implications, which will be the focus of Chapter 1.1. The need to closely monitor storage, delivery practices, and wastage as well as the methods of reaching children either through routine pediatric visits or supplemental immunization activities and campaigns are key special features of vaccines with implications for costs and financing.

The fundamental elements of economics such as price, demand, and supply take on a new meaning in the world of vaccines, which are often "free" to most consumers. Chapter 1.2 adapts these fundamental tools of economics to highly subsidized goods like vaccines. By increasing supply and demand while keeping prices low, these tools will be fundamental in understanding policies to achieve better coverage. With the extensive role of public sector

David Bishai and Chrispus Mayora, *Section introduction: principles of vaccine economics* In: *Handbook of Applied Health Economics in Vaccines*. Edited by: David Bishai, Logan Brenzel and William V. Padula, Oxford University Press.
© Oxford University Press 2023. DOI: 10.1093/oso/9780192896087.003.0001

subsidies and regulations, the prices charged for vaccines also deviate substantially from the marginal cost per dose. Chapter 1.3 describes how costs of vaccines are determined, highlighting the cost differences between newer vaccines where companies must recover their substantial outlay required for discovery and traditional older vaccines whose production costs resemble undifferentiated commodities produced in competitive markets. Specifically, approaches to procurement of vaccines that keep prices affordable for low-income countries, but preserve a robust supply environment will be discussed.

On the demand side of vaccine economics lies the perennial problem of substantial social benefits in terms of herd immunity that might remain elusive if consumers choose to free ride. This topic is raised in Chapter 1.4 where the foundations of vaccine hesitancy are rooted in the behavioral economics violations of rational perception of risks. Fear and dread of the unknowns surrounding either a new vaccine or a new disease can sway rational choices away from the cold calculation of expected health risks and health benefits. Finally, we close the chapter with an economic look at how vaccines are delivered to patients and the potential economies and diseconomies of reaching people in outreach programs versus in routine clinics (Chapter 1.5).

1.1
Introduction to global vaccine systems

Gatien de Broucker

Developing vaccines requires balancing different characteristics to ensure effectiveness and safety, from the choice of biotechnology (vaccine type) to its delivery system(s) to users. This handbook will discuss how these characteristics all factor into costs, from research and development to manufacturing and distribution.

The biotechnology must trigger an immune response associated with a specific pathogen that will persist beyond taking the vaccine. This immune response must be able to recognize subsequent exposure to the infectious agent quickly and curb its replication and pathology. Additionally, the immune response upon vaccination must be harmless to the vaccinated individual and impose negligible risk of adverse effects in the long term.

Beyond provoking an immune response in clinical settings, vaccines must work effectively in the real world—in combination with other vaccines and treatments, and in a variety of climates and settings. Standards are set for transporting and storing vaccines from production to use using a cold chain, and for the use of each vaccine in specific populations through vaccination schedules and recommendations based on medical status. Vaccines are sensitive to environmental and biological factors: variations in temperature, delay between production and usage, as well as deviations from the vaccination schedule are known shortcomings to their protective effect (Babirye et al., 2012).

In addition to upholding these standards, immunization programs are designed to maximize vaccine coverage, with the goal of achieving herd immunity where everyone in the population benefits either directly or indirectly from the protective effect of vaccines. People who do not benefit directly from vaccine protection for a variety of reasons (e.g., being unvaccinated, having a weakened immune system, vaccine protection has lost its potency) can still benefit from others being directly protected and not transmitting the disease.

Gatien de Broucker, *Introduction to global vaccine systems* In: *Handbook of Applied Health Economics in Vaccines.*
Edited by: David Bishai, Logan Brenzel and William V. Padula, Oxford University Press. © Oxford University Press 2023.
DOI: 10.1093/oso/9780192896087.003.0002

In this chapter, we briefly introduce the biotechnology behind vaccines along with the different vaccine types and discuss the strategy and logistics of immunization programs. Regulatory and monitoring systems are discussed in Chapter 1.3 of this handbook.

1.1.1 Vaccine types

The vaccine technology encompasses the molecular make-up of the vaccine, most often referred to as the vaccine type, and aims to ensure an appropriate immune response to different pathogens, and their viability beyond the clinical settings. We distinguish three types of vaccines based on the biological unit used: vaccines containing the whole pathogen, or a subunit of it, or based on nucleic acid (either DNA or RNA). All types aim to stimulate an immune response to a specific pathogen. Their development and production costs differ greatly.

Whole pathogen vaccines include live-attenuated and inactivated vaccines, which present, respectively, a weakened or dead pathogen to the immune system. Recent advances in genetic engineering introduced chimeric vaccines, where the genes or proteins of the pathogen of interest are mounted on a different pathogen. Vaccines against the following pathogens or disease use this technology: cholera, coronavirus disease 2019 (COVID-19), Ebola, hepatitis A, influenza, Japanese encephalitis, measles, mumps, pertussis (whooping cough), poliomyelitis, rabies, rotavirus, rubella, smallpox, tuberculosis, typhoid, varicella (chickenpox), varicella (zoster), and yellow fever.

Subunit vaccines present only the antigen, that is, the part of the pathogen used to identify it by the immune system. They include polysaccharide, conjugate, and recombinant vaccines, using either polysaccharides or proteins often combined with adjuvants to stimulate an immune response. Other subunit vaccines present products related to the pathogen, such as toxoid vaccines, which present the (inactivated) toxin generated by the bacterium rather than the bacterium itself, and virus-like particle vaccines. Vaccines against the following pathogens or disease are subunit vaccines: dengue, diphtheria, hepatitis B, *Haemophilus influenzae* type b, human papillomavirus (HPV), meningococcal meningitis, pertussis, pneumococcal disease, rotavirus, shingles, tetanus, and typhoid.

Developed more recently, *nucleic acid vaccines* supply the genetic code for the body's cells to produce the antigen and provoke an immune response using DNA plasmids, messenger RNA (mRNA), or a viral vector. Nucleic acid vaccines, particularly those using a viral vector, promise to be faster and easier to develop and produce on a large scale (Pardi, Hogan, Porter, & Weissman, 2018; Siegrist, 2018). The vaccines against COVID-19 manufactured by Pfizer and Moderna are the first vaccines using the mRNA technology to be approved by regulatory agencies. Merck's vaccine against Ebola uses the viral vector technology and is approved for use in several countries, including the US (Centers for Disease Control and Prevention, 2021a; Dolzhikova et al., 2017).

1.1.2 The strategy and logistics of immunization programs

After manufacturing, vaccines have a finite lifespan, subject to environmental factors. To minimize wastage and optimize vaccination coverage, governments manage a large procurement, storage, and delivery system which is part of the Expanded Program on Immunization (EPI) or National Program on Immunization, built to sustain routine immunization and any supplemental immunization activities.

The inclusion/exclusion of each vaccine in a country's EPI is determined partly by the country's disease burden, but also by a vaccine's cost to the government, safety, shelf life, and the duration of protective effect. Several vaccines prevent diseases that are common to most regions of the world, such as measles, tetanus, diphtheria, or pertussis. Others are more relevant to specific areas, such as yellow fever and dengue in equatorial and tropical countries, and influenza in colder climates. Finally, some vaccines are most useful to prevent outbreaks caused by a combination of environmental and human factors often brought forward in humanitarian crises, such as the cholera vaccine. Alternatively, vaccines excluded from the EPI can still be used in a country, for instance, as a traveler's vaccine: rabies, yellow fever (in countries where it is not endemic), and typhoid fever can be provided to travelers visiting countries where the risk of contracting these diseases is increased.

1.1.2.1 Routine vaccination and supplemental immunization activities

The choice of strategy for each vaccine, either to vaccinate systematically or punctually, depends on several factors both endogenous and exogenous to a country's EPI.

Ongoing, planned, and contingent on population growth, the systematic immunization of newborns and infants through *routine immunization* constitutes the main share of immunization activities in a country. Routine immunization tends to be the most efficient at increasing vaccine coverage, although inequities persist (Chopra et al., 2020). Routine immunization can leverage (or strengthen) postnatal medical visits for infants, in synergy with the public health effort in maternal and child health. In high-income countries, where older adults are also a target population, routine immunization further strengthens regular medical check-ups. However, sustaining adequate vaccine coverage through routine immunization is subject to supply- and demand-side constraints and is challenging to do. Known constraints include vaccine dose stockouts and wastage, which often constrict the supply of vaccines to specific areas in a country. Deficient vaccine confidence (or increased vaccine hesitancy) and missing facility visits for neonatal care are common factors that influence the demand for vaccines (discussed further in Chapter 1.4).

In situations when the vaccine coverage falls short either nationally or subnationally, increasing the risk of, or causing, outbreaks, governments may organize vaccination campaigns or child health days and child health weeks known as *supplementary immunization activities* (SIAs), often with the support of international health agencies. A large amount of healthcare resources can be redirected towards an SIA for specific vaccines (e.g., measles), aiming to "catch-up" and reach those children who are unimmunized. In recent years, the term "zero-dose" child was coined to define inequalities in immunization and assess the impact of SIAs more accurately (Portnoy, Jit, Helleringer, & Verguet, 2018). While they can be a cost-effective intervention to prevent major outbreaks, as is the case for measles (Bishai et al., 2011), SIAs are resource intensive and, in some circumstances, can undermine the delivery of routine immunization in resource-constrained settings (Chakrabarti, Grépin, & Helleringer, 2019).

The international effort to vaccinate against COVID-19 using vaccines from different manufacturers qualifies as an SIA. If vaccination continues beyond the current crisis caused by the pandemic and is added to the vaccine schedules, it would become part of routine immunization in a similar pathway as for the influenza vaccine in the aftermath of the 2009 H1N1 pandemic (Centers for Disease Control and Prevention, 2010).

1.1.2.2 Target population

For optimal and lasting immunogenicity, and to account for the age-specific morbidity and mortality of diseases, vaccines are typically associated with a target population.

Newborns and infants are the primary target population for all routine immunization schedules as vaccines effectively prevent deadly or debilitating diseases, which not only would affect the child's life, but also that of their caregivers. The routine immunization of children globally provides a very high value of return-on-investment: $21 saved in healthcare cost and productivity loss averted for every dollar invested in immunization in countries eligible for Gavi support over two decades (Sim, Watts, Constenla, Brenzel, & Patenaude, 2020). Furthermore, infants are also the target population of many other public health interventions under the scope of neonatal care and hence more accustomed to regular medical visits. Conversely, conducting SIAs and strengthening routine immunization for zero-dose children may also provide them with these other healthcare services they would not otherwise be exposed to.

Comparatively, adults tend to interact less often with the healthcare system than children, and to be less inclined to follow their vaccination schedule for a variety of reasons. The general adult population is a target population for specific vaccines such as the influenza vaccine (recommended annually), for boosters (e.g., Td or Tdap booster), and for traveler's vaccines (when relevant). There are three groups within the adult population more specifically targeted for routine immunization: immunocompromised adults, older adults (65 years and above), and pregnant women. Immunocompromised adults, older adults, and pregnant women may receive additional doses of the vaccines provided during childhood (e.g., pneumococcal, meningococcal, and hepatitis vaccines), subject to clinical advice (Centers for Disease Control and Prevention, 2021b).

1.1.2.3 Vaccine selection

National Immunization Technical Advisory Groups (NITAGs) provide recommendations on new vaccine introductions, the choice of product, the vaccine schedule, and priorities within the country (Gavi, 2021b; Howard, Walls, Bell, & Mounier-Jack, 2018; Steffen et al., 2021). Examples of national level NITAGs in high-income countries include the Advisory Committee on Immunization Practices (ACIP) in the US and Joint Committee on Vaccination and Immunisation (JCVI) in the UK. There are over 170 NITAGs in countries around the world listed at https://www.nitag-resource.org/. At the global level, a group called the Strategic Advisory Group of Experts on Immunization (SAGE) meets to advise the World Health Organization (WHO). The WHO then compiles a list of prequalified vaccines to guide UN agencies' procurement of vaccines and national governments. Countries use NITAG recommendations (Howard et al., 2018), or those from the their Ministry of Health and other agencies when these is no NITAG in place, to prioritize vaccines that can alleviate the most disease cases—and, thus, related healthcare costs—and deaths, based on their budget and on the availability of external funding (Steffen et al., 2021). The WHO and Gavi (officially, Gavi, the Vaccine Alliance, formerly known as the Global Alliance for Vaccines and Immunization) guide the vaccine selection process in low- and middle-income countries with severe budget constraints, providing them with technical assistance and a financing plan to afford their introduction and sustain their use. With shared funding and negotiated vaccine dose prices, Gavi facilitates the procurement of 12 vaccines for routine immunization and SIAs ("catch-up campaigns"): pentavalent, rotavirus, pneumococcal, HPV, inactivated polio, Japanese encephalitis, measles, measles–rubella, meningitis A, typhoid, cholera, and yellow fever vaccines (Gavi, 2019, 2021a). These policy and financing mechanisms are discussed in Chapter 5 of this handbook.

In the last decades, countries (in particular, high-income countries) also considered population demand for vaccines, or lack thereof, when making decisions about vaccine selection. In 2013, the Japanese government introduced the HPV vaccine in its routine immunization program, targeting girls aged 12–16 years, aiming to prevent HPV infection and cervical cancer. This introduction was met with considerable negative news coverage in the Japanese media, and a growing, but unfounded, reticence from parents for their daughters to get the vaccine. While the HPV vaccine still technically appears in the Japanese vaccine schedule, the Ministry of Health suspended its use indefinitely (Ikeda et al., 2019). In Denmark, the HPV vaccine introduction also met with adverse public opinion. However, while the uptake of the HPV vaccine significantly decreased, it was still offered through the routine immunization program (Suppli et al., 2018).

1.1.2.4 Vaccine schedules

Each country's EPI plans its routine immunization program using a vaccine schedule. The schedule aligns every vaccine procured by the government for the EPI with their target population, defined by age and health status (e.g., healthy, immunocompromised). As an essential part of primary healthcare, pediatricians and general physicians use this schedule at every medical visit to assess the need to vaccinate and plan with patients and caregivers for follow-up visits.

Timely vaccination is essential for optimal immunogenicity and protection, particularly in infants, and to manage supply-side constraints efficiently. Late vaccination for specific vaccines, such as the measles vaccine,
is considered as a risk factor for outbreaks (Babirye et al., 2012). To manage
such risk, vaccine schedules can also include recommendations on catch-up
vaccination for missed doses.

Detailed vaccine schedules are available through national and regional
health agencies. Selected examples of vaccine schedules are listed below:

- WHO recommendations for routine immunization (global): http://www.
  who.int/immunization/policy/immunization_tables/en/.
- US Centers for Disease Control and Prevention: https://www.cdc.gov/
  vaccines/schedules/index.html.
- European Center for Disease Prevention and Control: https://vaccine-
  schedule.ecdc.europa.eu/.
- National Health Mission of India: http://www.nrhmhp.gov.in/content/
  immunization.
- Immunization schedules for Africa: http://www.vacfa.uct.ac.za/immun
  ization-schedules-africa (hosted by the University of Cape Town, South
  Africa).

1.1.2.5 Delivery vehicle and logistics

Among environmental factors, vaccines are most sensitive to changes in
temperature and exposure to sunlight and air. Vaccine packaging, delivery,
and handling are, therefore, carefully planned and monitored. Vaccine
doses are packaged in vials, tubes, or ampoules. Vials typically contain multiple doses of vaccines, which are meant for several people. Once a vial is
opened, vaccine doses must be used rapidly: within 6 hours or up to 28 days
for select vaccines. Healthcare workers refer to the WHO Multi-Dose Vial
Policy and description of each vaccine to manage the use of multi-dose vials
(WHO, 2014).

Before and between uses, vials are stored and transported in temperature-
controlled containers or refrigerators, shaping the vaccine "cold chain." Most
vaccines are sensitive to warmer temperatures, hence the need for constant
refrigeration. Malfunctioning or mishandled refrigerators can bring the temperature below the freezing point, which also affects vaccines in liquid form.
Several vaccines can be freeze dried to prevent freeze damage. Vaccine vials

usually feature a vaccine vial monitor, a heat-sensitive label, which indicates whether they were exposed to excessive heat (WHO, 2020).

Such constraints lead to wastage, where doses issued to a healthcare facility or outreach team were not administered to patients (Equation 1.1.1 and Table 1.1.1) (WHO, 2005). Wastage costs are distinct from waste management costs. The latter refers to the costs associated with the management of used disposable items, such as syringes and gloves. Wastage is inextricable to vaccine programming: efficient vaccine program management reduces, but never eliminates, wastage. Wastage rates vary significantly between vaccines, regions, and immunization programs, and must be appraised to cost and plan immunization programs properly. For instance, vaccine wastage rates in India varied between 13.2% (pentavalent vaccine; Pune district) and 50.8% (oral polio vaccine; Kangra district) in one study (Das et al., 2020).

Equation 1.1.1. Vaccine wastage rate:

$$Vaccine\ wastage\ rate = 1 - \frac{Number\ of\ doses\ administered}{Number\ of\ doses\ issued}$$

Assumptions and methods to integrate the wastage rate into economic models are discussed in Chapter 2.5. Common reasons for wastage are listed in Table 1.1.1.

Maintaining and operating cold chains and assuming some level of wastage ensure that the available vaccine doses are in optimal condition to stimulate an immune response. Using doses subjected to inadequate storage risks affecting the effectiveness of the vaccine. For instance, recognized shortcomings in the measles vaccine effectiveness in Uganda include settings where the cold chain does not perform adequately (Mupere et al., 2006).

Table 1.1.1 Types of vaccine wastage

Vaccine wastage in unopened vials	Vaccine wastage in opened vials

• Expiry
• Vaccine vial monitor indication and heat exposure
• Freezing
• Breakage
• Missing inventory
• Theft
• Discarding unused vials returned from an outreach session
	In addition to the types listed in the previous column:
	  • Discarding remaining doses at the end of session
	  • Not being able to draw the number of doses indicated on the label of a vial
	  • Poor reconstitution practices
	  • Submergence of opened vials in water
	  • Suspected contamination
	  • Patient reaction requiring more than one dose

1.1.3 Conclusion

In this chapter, we introduced several considerations associated with developing and using vaccines. This web of actors, programs, regulations, and conventions connecting global and local policies and constraints form the global vaccine systems.

Vaccine research and implementation appear as distinct steps enacted in a strict sequence, separated only, yet firmly, by regulatory approval processes. However, the considerations to implementation we highlighted hint to the contrary. Whereas vaccine rollout is guided by the clinicians who created and tested it, vaccine research is sensitive to rollout constraints and can prioritize the development of vaccines that can accommodate different "real-world" applications beyond the clinical settings. Companies and researchers may favor different biotechnologies and vaccine platforms to make the vaccine highly effective after only one dose was inoculated, or transportable and storable in resource-constrained settings with a deficient cold chain. For instance, the Johnson & Johnson COVID-19 vaccine marketed in 2021 distinguishes itself from the others as a one-dose (rather than two-dose) vaccine—a strong advantage for implementation in low-income settings (in both high- and low-income countries).

Economic evaluations play an essential role in providing evidence of affordability, sustainability, and relevance to NITAGs and governments, but also in suggesting research priorities for pharmaceutical companies seeking to expand their product portfolio. Furthermore, more fundamental research led by economists, and behavioral and social scientists also provides insights on factors influencing demand, such as vaccine hesitancy.

The study of vaccine economics, in both its applied and fundamental forms, must accompany progress in vaccine development and rollout so we do not spoil this effective protection against humanity's microscopic foe.

References

Babirye, J. N., Engebretsen, I. M. S., Makumbi, F., Fadnes, L. T., Wamani, H., Tylleskar, T., & Nuwaha, F. (2012). Timeliness of childhood vaccinations in Kampala Uganda: A community-based cross-sectional study. *PloS One, 7*(4), e35432–e35432. doi:10.1371/journal.pone.0035432

Bishai, D., Johns, B., Nair, D., Nabyonga-Orem, J., Fiona-Makmot, B., Simons, E., & Dabbagh, A. (2011). The cost-effectiveness of supplementary immunization activities for measles: A stochastic model for Uganda. *Journal of Infectious Diseases, 204*(Suppl 1), S107–S115. doi:10.1093/infdis/jir131

Centers for Disease Control and Prevention. (2010). Prevention and control of influenza with vaccines: Recommendations of the Advisory Committee on Immunization Practices (ACIP), 2010. *Morbidity and Mortality Weekly Report, 59*(RR08), 1–62.

Centers for Disease Control and Prevention. (2021a). *Ebola vaccine: Information about Ervebo˚.* https://www.cdc.gov/vhf/ebola/clinicians/vaccine/index.html

Centers for Disease Control and Prevention. (2021b). *Recommended adult immunization schedule for ages 19 years or older, United States, 2021.* https://www.cdc.gov/vaccines/schedules/hcp/imz/adult.html

Chakrabarti, A., Grépin, K. A., & Helleringer, S. (2019). The impact of supplementary immunization activities on routine vaccination coverage: An instrumental variable analysis in five low-income countries. *PloS One, 14*(2), e0212049. doi:10.1371/journal.pone.0212049

Chopra, M., Bhutta, Z., Blanc, D. C., Checchi, F., Gupta, A., Lemango, E. T., . . . Victora, C. G. (2020). Addressing the persistent inequities in immunization coverage. *Bulletin of the World Health Organization, 98*(2), 146–148. doi:10.2471/BLT.19.241620

Das, M. K., Sood, M., Tambe, M. P., Sharma, T. D., Parande, M. A. G., Surwade, J. B., . . . Sindhu, M. (2020). Documentation of vaccine wastage in two different geographic contexts under the universal immunization program in India. *BMC Public Health, 20*(1), 556. doi:10.1186/s12889-020-08637-1

Dolzhikova, I. V., Tokarskaya, E. A., Dzharullaeva, A. S., Tukhvatulin, A. I., Shcheblyakov, D. V., Voronina, O. L., . . . Gintsburg, A. L. (2017). Virus-vectored Ebola vaccines. *Acta Naturae, 9*(3), 4–11.

Gavi. (2019). *Annual program report.* https://www.gavi.org/sites/default/files/programmes-impact/our-impact/apr/Gavi-Progress-Report-2019_1.pdf

Gavi. (2021a). *Detailed product profiles.* https://www.gavi.org/news/document-library/detailed-product-profiles

Gavi. (2021b). *Gavi vaccine funding guidelines.* https://www.gavi.org/sites/default/files/support/Vaccine_FundingGuidelines.pdf

Howard, N., Walls, H., Bell, S., & Mounier-Jack, S. (2018). The role of National Immunisation Technical Advisory Groups (NITAGs) in strengthening national vaccine decision-making: A comparative case study of Armenia, Ghana, Indonesia, Nigeria, Senegal and Uganda. *Vaccine, 36*(37), 5536–5543. doi:10.1016/j.vaccine.2018.07.063

Ikeda, S., Ueda, Y., Yagi, A., Matsuzaki, S., Kobayashi, E., Kimura, T., . . . Kudoh, K. (2019). HPV vaccination in Japan: What is happening in Japan? *Expert Review of Vaccines, 18*(4), 323–325. doi:10.1080/14760584.2019.1584040

Mupere, E., Karamagi, C., Zirembuzi, G., Grabowsky, M., de Swart, R. L., Nanyunja, M., & Mayanja, H. (2006). Measles vaccination effectiveness among children under 5 years of age in Kampala, Uganda. *Vaccine, 24*(19), 4111–4115. doi:10.1016/j.vaccine.2006.02.038

Pardi, N., Hogan, M. J., Porter, F. W., & Weissman, D. (2018). mRNA vaccines—a new era in vaccinology. *Nature Reviews. Drug Discovery, 17*(4), 261–279. doi:10.1038/nrd.2017.243

Portnoy, A., Jit, M., Helleringer, S., & Verguet, S. (2018). Impact of measles supplementary immunization activities on reaching children missed by routine programs. *Vaccine, 36*(1), 170–178. doi:10.1016/j.vaccine.2017.10.080

Siegrist, C.-A. (2018). Vaccine immunology. In S. A. Plotkin, W. A. Orenstein, & P. A. Offit (Eds.), *Plotkin's vaccines* (7th ed., pp. 16–34). Philadelphia, PA: Elsevier.

Sim, S. Y., Watts, E., Constenla, D., Brenzel, L., & Patenaude, B. N. (2020). Return on investment from immunization against 10 pathogens in 94 low- and middle-income countries, 2011–30. *Health Affairs, 39*(8), 1343–1353.

Steffen, C. A., Henaff, L., Durupt, A., Omeiri, N. E., Ndiaye, S., Batmunkh, N., . . . Hombach, J. (2021). Evidence-informed vaccination decision-making in countries: Progress, challenges and opportunities. *Vaccine, 39*(15), 2146–2152. doi:10.1016/j.vaccine.2021.02.055

Suppli, C. H., Hansen, N. D., Rasmussen, M., Valentiner-Branth, P., Krause, T. G., & Mølbak, K. (2018). Decline in HPV-vaccination uptake in Denmark—the association between HPV-related media coverage and HPV-vaccination. *BMC Public Health, 18*(1), 1360. doi:10.1186/s12889-018-6268-x

World Health Organization. (2005). *Monitoring vaccine wastage at country level: Guidelines for programme managers* (WHO/V&B/03.18/Rev.1). https://apps.who.int/iris/bitstream/handle/10665/68463/WHO_VB_03.18.Rev.1_eng.pdf

World Health Organization. (2014). *WHO policy statement: Multi-dose vial policy (MDVP).* https://apps.who.int/iris/bitstream/handle/10665/135972/WHO_IVB_14.07_eng.pdf

World Health Organization. (2020). *What is VVM and how does it work?* https://www.who.int/immunization_standards/vaccine_quality/What%20is%20VVM%20and%20how%20does%20it%20work.pdf

1.2

Relevance of health economics to vaccines

David Bishai and Chrispus Mayora

Economics informs problems of choice and allocation when there is uncertainty and scarcity. The world of vaccines and vaccinations abounds with these dilemmas. There are many choices, few resources, and never enough information. Enter vaccine economics.

This chapter offers an introduction to the multiple ways that economics can be applied to systems tasked with discovering, financing, distributing, tracking, and administering the world's vaccines. It sets the stage for deeper coverage of these topics in subsequent chapters.

The case of vaccines for coronavirus disease 2019 (COVID-19) starkly illustrates the many applications of vaccine economics. As the epidemic emerged, securing safe and effective vaccines became a priority for politicians, business leaders, and public health officials. Speed was paramount. The past pace of vaccine discovery based on private pharmaceutical companies financed mostly by private investors would be too slow. Relying solely on private revenue streams to incentivize research and pay for production would be too inequitable. Scientific uncertainty clouded whether a safe and effective vaccine against SARS-CoV-2 virus could even be developed.

Even after safe and effective vaccines emerged, the world's systems for allocation of vaccines between countries and people in countries faced challenges in overcoming inequalities, misinformation, and misallocation. Guidelines for prioritization of vaccine allocation to countries and subpopulations in countries appropriately stressed a combination of moral considerations besides just economic efficiency. However, the human systems tasked with following these guidelines when they clashed with economic self-interest broke down. Data systems to track gaps in vaccine distribution and available human and physical resources relevant to vaccines were wanting.

David Bishai and Chrispus Mayora, *Relevance of health economics to vaccines* In: *Handbook of Applied Health Economics in Vaccines*. Edited by: David Bishai, Logan Brenzel and William V. Padula, Oxford University Press. © Oxford University Press 2023. DOI: 10.1093/oso/9780192896087.003.0003

One answer to the predictable barriers to efficient and fair vaccine al-location is to create institutions designed to break through these barriers. Governments instituted COVID-19 vaccine priority groupings internally and the World Health Organization (WHO) developed global guidelines to support countries in their allocation of COVID-19 vaccines (WHO, 2020, 2021). One example is the COVID-19 Vaccines Global Access (COVAX) Facility, led by WHO, the Coalition for Epidemic Preparedness Innovations (CEPI), Gavi, and UNICEF. Within COVAX, the global collaboration of the Access to COVID Tools Accelerator (ACT) includes government and global health and civil society organizations such as CEPI, Gavi, the Global Fund, WHO, UNICEF, the Pan American Health Organization (PAHO), and the World Bank. COVAX maintains a pooled fund for an advance market commitment wing where donor countries can support access to COVID-19 vaccines on be-half of low-income countries.

Vaccine economics was able to shed light and offer guidance in many of the areas highlighted in the case of COVID-19 vaccines. In the area of finance for vaccine discovery, years of work in developing alternative financial incentives for pharmaceutical discovery were at hand (Kickbusch, Krech, Franz, & Wells, 2018; Kremer, Levin, & Snyder, 2020; Yamey et al., 2020). Advance market commitments are public sector promises to guarantee future demand and help assure private companies that a successful product will generate the revenue to pay off prior investments and maintain production. In addi-tion, governments and groups of governments became the largest investors in private firms seeking to discover COVID-19 vaccines. As investors, govern-ments had to manage various types of uncertainty in assembling a portfolio of candidate vaccines to invest in (McDonnell et al., 2020; Shnaydman, 2020). Multigovernmental purchasing cooperatives helped to pool buying power of middle- and lower-income countries through COVAX (Kuehn, 2020). Frameworks for how to distribute the vaccine fairly while achieving goals of controlling morbidity, mortality, and negative societal impact were ap-proached by applying both ethical and economic principles (Grauer, Löwen, & Liebchen, 2020; National Academies of Sciences, Engineering, & Medicine, 2020). The logistics for getting COVID-19 vaccines from factories to ware-houses to vaccination sites disclosed long-standing weaknesses in vaccine distribution systems. In the public–private partnerships tasked to distribute and deliver vaccine, bottlenecks emerged and economic principles that high-lighted information flows helped to solve them (Lee, Mueller, & Tilchin, 2017).

The COVID-19 vaccines case highlights the importance of uncertainty and information as key factors that can create inefficiency. Vaccine makers faced uncertainty about the odds of successful discovery and changes in demand, revenue, and liability. Vaccination systems faced uncertainty about the delivery schedules and the role of vaccine hesitancy. The economic principles used to manage uncertainty required measures to pool risks into larger and larger groups and ultimately required both national governments and multigovernmental entities to share and manage risk.

The role of scarcity loomed even larger in the roll-out of COVID-19 vaccines. The traditional market-driven approach to handle scarcity through prices set by supply and demand could not be used because of equity concerns and the large footprint of government investments and advance purchase commitments. The large role of government and multigovernmental agencies in vaccine procurement has always been a major feature of vaccine economics. Government involvement in vaccine markets does not mean that market economics is of no use in understanding vaccine distribution. Instead, it implies the need to appreciate the function of heavily regulated markets instead of free markets. For many in public health, vaccines are "free," so the price of a free thing seems strange. This chapter will outline why the price of a vaccine—even a "free" one—is extremely useful to manage and minimize the burden of scarcity.

The first part of this chapter will develop the relevance of health economics to vaccines by describing the system responsible for vaccines and vaccination. This approach makes sure we cover all the elements and highlight the many areas where economic principles apply. The second part of this chapter develops the foundational microeconomics of vaccine supply and demand, highlighting the role of scarcity and public goods.

1.2.1 Vaccines and the immunization system

An economic system is composed of organizational units of human agents who abide by norms, rules, and cultural expectations called "institutions" in order to adjust and adapt to a changing environment (Grossman, 1967). The WHO Building Blocks Framework (WHO, 2010) has identified the typical units that one will find in a health system. The building blocks of medical products, financing, information, service delivery, governance, and workforce are all at work in the system responsible for vaccines and vaccination (Fig. 1.2.1). As shown in the figure, changes in the institutions governing financing for discovery, procurement, distribution, and delivery will create actions and reactions by the units responsible for

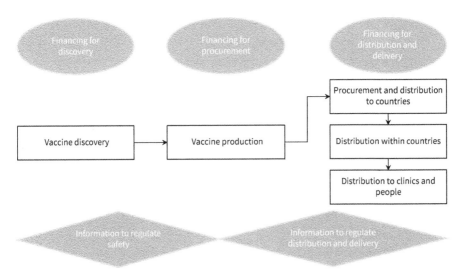

Fig. 1.2.1 Vaccines and vaccination system.

vaccine discovery, production, and distribution. For example, if institutional changes provide investments for vaccine discovery out of public funds instead of private capital markets, then vaccine discovery can be prioritized by what governments say is important (e.g., COVID-19 vaccines) as opposed to what financial investors think will generate the most revenue. The informational state shown by the diamonds at the bottom of the figure can also affect the system. If new information arises about social disparities in vaccine distribution, then institutional reforms can be crafted to make new incentives for the vaccine to be distributed to unreached priority populations.

1.2.1.1 The role of financing

There are financial reasons limiting private investment in vaccines for the world's most needed vaccines: HIV, tuberculosis, and malaria (Bishai, Lin, & Kiyonga, 2001; Bishai & Mercer, 2001; Kremer, 2002). A financing system for vaccine discovery that relies heavily on private capital markets will undervalue diseases that affect people who cannot pay high prices. With privately financed vaccine discovery, firms are motivated to discover new products so they can obtain a patent that awards them monopoly rights to produce and sell it. The investments they make in discovery will be paid back after the product is approved because the patent allows them to mark up the price without fear

Table 1.2.1 The range of vaccine prices negotiated by the Pan American Health Organization's Revolving Fund

Vaccine	Weighted average price per dose
DTaP/IPV/Hep B/Hib (hexavalent acellular)	$21.12
Meningococcal ACYW135	$20.30
Varicella	$15.85
Inactivated polio (IPV)	$3.10
DPT Hib lyophilized (pediatric)	$3.00
Measles/mumps (Zagreb)/rubella	$2.75
BCG	$0.23
DPT (pediatric)	$0.18
Oral polio bivalent (bOPV)	$0.17

DTaP/IPV/Hep B/Hib, diphtheria, tetanus, pertussis, polio, hepatitis B, and *Haemophilus influenzae* type b.

of direct competition. Higher prices will lead to less demand as poorer consumers are priced out of the market. These high prices build in financial inequity in who will receive new vaccines which skews decisions about what products to produce towards vaccines for diseases of affluent countries and not low- and middle-income countries.

Because newer vaccines are covered by patents or have not yet garnered competition, their prices are higher. Table 1.2.1 shows the price variation between newer vaccines like hexavalent, meningococcal, and varicella as opposed to the older generic vaccines like bacillus Calmette–Guérin (BCG), diphtheria, pertussis, and tetanus (DPT), and oral polio. Table 1.2.1 is presenting prices that have been negotiated by PAHO (2020). These prices are much lower than any one individual could obtain because PAHO represents the purchasing power of 41 countries. Firms can offer reduced prices because PAHO purchases in bulk and can offer reliable forecasts of future demand. Pooled purchasing to achieve lower prices is a basic principle of vaccine economics.

Once vaccines are procured, the financing and economic choices for their distribution and delivery inside a country play a large role in determining success. Most countries have both public and private systems for distribution of vaccines to venues and to pay the staff to store, schedule, and administer vaccines. The advantages of the public sector include the ability to maintain a focus on the most vulnerable populations and to occasionally deploy campaigns and door-to-door delivery strategies. However, the public sector requires taxation or foreign assistance to secure public finances. The private sector can deliver vaccines with finances raised by fees, but private providers will seldom focus on the most vulnerable groups. Costs per fully immunized child vary widely depending on the delivery strategy selected (Vaughan et al., 2019).

1.2.1.2 The role of information

Removing barriers to the flow of information emerges as an important area to improve system function. Scientific data on technologies to enhance safety, and efficacy, as well as credible data on the burden of vaccine-preventable disease can help spur rapid vaccine development. For example, when members of the Meningitis Vaccine Project (MVP) began to develop a vaccine for meningitis A in sub-Saharan Africa, they searched for a way to bind the bacterial antigen to a carrier molecule that would incite immunity. When they approached pharmaceutical companies who kept their technology licenses behind a paywall, they found their way blocked by licensing fees that would make the vaccine price out of range for most African countries. But MVP kept searching and found an appropriate chemical pathway that had been developed by a scientist at the Food and Drug Administration with a license owned by the US government. This offered a low-cost and effective method to conjugate polysaccharides to a carrier protein. This small snippet of information kept the final price of the Menafrivac vaccine well below $1.00 and shaved off years of product development (Bishai, Champion, Steele, & Thompson, 2011).

Information about the cost-effectiveness of various antigens has had a dramatic effect on scaling up vaccine programs and new vaccine introduction (Hutubessy, Henao, Namgyal, Moorthy, & Hombach, 2011). Estimates of the cost per life saved or disability-adjusted life year averted is a critical element among many criteria used to assess whether or not to introduce a new vaccine (Pooripussarakul, Riewpaiboon, Bishai, Muangchana, & Tantivess, 2016). Studies comparing the cost of vaccination to the cost of vaccine-preventable disease in low- and middle-income countries routinely find that money spent on vaccines generates financial savings. If one includes the dollar value of a death averted, one dollar spent on vaccines in low- to middle-income countries would return $19.80 in averted cost of illness or $52.20 based on a value-of-statistical-life approach from 2021 to 2030 (Sim, Watts, Constenla, Brenzel, & Patenaude, 2020).

1.2.2 The price of free things

From the perspective of consumers, vaccines often appear to have a zero price. The absence of prices that would ordinarily signal value, scarcity, and abundance to consumers increases the importance of economic analysis to determine the efficient level of supply. Furthermore, even when vaccines' monetary price to a consumer is $0, there will still be costs that the individual must bear in the form of transportation, lost work time, and minor or major side effects. These private disincentives to vaccination face off against the public interests to achieve herd immunity.

Vaccines are dual public and private goods. They offer private benefits by helping protect the vaccine recipient, but they also provide public benefits to the community by lowering rates of contagious disease. They are neither a wholly pure public good nor a wholly pure private good. The duality is the root of an eternal policy dilemma in the economics of vaccines. The perspective of an individual trying to know how much cost to bear to get the private benefits of vaccination clashes with the perspective of a health planner trying to invest in procurement and subsidies to drive up the vaccine coverage rates to offer the public benefit. The public investments can crowd out reliance on the private willingness to pay for vaccination. Furthermore, as the coverage rates get higher and higher, the disease prevalence goes lower and lower. The personal benefit from vaccination becomes smaller (Geoffard & Philipson, 1997).

Ordinarily, consumers' demand curve and industry's supply curve would meet at a point of equilibrium and efficiency. However, for vaccines, the money price to the consumer is zero and the demand curve (Fig. 1.2.2) is driven by out-of-pocket costs required for transportation and waiting time. Meanwhile, the supply curve is driven by public procurement of vaccines. Total market supply and total market demand are not running off of the same price point. Furthermore, the private demand expressed by consumers is based on their own private calculation of benefit. In contrast, the public supply secured by the public procurement is based on a calculation of public benefit that includes benefits of herd immunity, future labor productivity, and avoidance of publicly financed losses due to vaccine-preventable disease.

The demand curve (Fig. 1.2.2) is a graph relating prices on the vertical axis to the number of units sold on the horizontal axis. The downward slope is common sense: fewer people want and can afford a thing with a high price and more people want and can afford a thing with a low price. Trying to minimize both monetary and non-monetary costs of obtaining vaccinations is a basic policy to improve uptake.

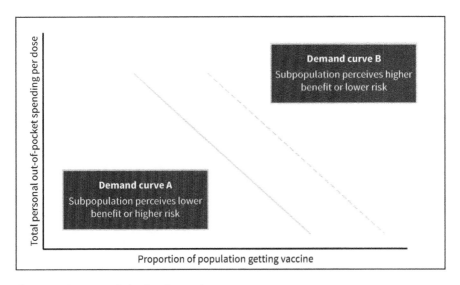

Fig. 1.2.2 Downward-sloping demand curves.

Implied in the downward-sloping demand curve is an inherent disparity. Those who access something with a high price have social and economic advantages compared to those who have to wait for lower prices. Even when monetary prices are zero, disparities in vaccine uptake can be seen because the out-of-pocket costs for transportation and waiting are more easily borne by those with more means. Vaccine hesitancy (discussed further in Chapter 1.4) can also create disparities if misinformation about vaccine benefits or risks is more concentrated in a particular subpopulation. Fig. 1.2.2 shows two demand curves. The solid demand curve on the left might be a subgroup with an information set making them think that vaccine benefits are lower/vaccine risks are higher compared to the subpopulation on the right with the dotted line. Interventions that improve information, beliefs, and trust can shift demand curves to the right and improve vaccine uptake.

The upward-sloping supply curves (Fig. 1.2.3) also reflect common sense. Holding all else equal, there are fewer firms who are able to make a profit when the price per dose is low. Thus, the number of doses supplied is lower at low prices and higher at high prices. The supply curves in Fig. 1.2.3 can be shifted from curve A on the left to curve B on the right if there are innovations that lower production costs. Pooled purchasing helps lower companies' unit cost of marketing and contracting and lowers their future risk by offering reliable demand forecasts backed up by larger numbers of buyers. Other ways to lower production costs are to scale up the production process. Larger production facilities based on larger orders are able to cut costs and shift the supply curve

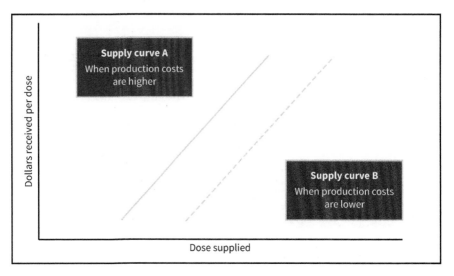

Fig. 1.2.3 Upward-sloping supply curves.

to the right. Public subsidies to scientific and engineering progress can also lower firms' production costs and generate more vaccines at lower costs as long as these innovations remain in the public domain. To the extent that companies find a way to patent technology that was made possible by publicly funded scientists, they will use their monopolistic advantage to raise prices without expanding supply.

The disjunction between vaccine supply and demand is what makes vaccine economics exquisite. In markets for pizza, the social goal of getting every pizza-eater the optimal amount of pizza is achieved by letting the market work things out on its own. Pizza-eating might have unrecognized spillover benefits, but they are nothing like what can be achieved by vaccine uptake.

The public benefits of vaccines have led to massive subsidies of their monetary prices and efforts to improve the information that helps the vaccine system work. Vaccine economists recognize the rationale for this government involvement in the vaccine system and the need to stay deeply involved in a market that can never work things out on its own to achieve the optimal result for society.

1.2.3 Conclusion

Choices with uncertainty and scarcity typify the work of vaccination systems. These are areas where economic analysis can be extremely helpful. The chapter put forth a systems framework showing a reliance on information and finance to chip away uncertainty and scarcity. This is a complex system: action breeds reaction. Setting up one source of finance (e.g., public) crowds out another (e.g., private). Opening up one information flow offers advantages to some and not others. A policy to fix one problem creates another.

The basic tenets of market economics that celebrate a happy equilibrium where supply meets demand cannot be applied because the private demand for vaccines will not automatically align with the demand necessary to produce the public good of herd immunity. However, on vaccine demand, there is plenty of rich economic work to do in measuring factors that affect the response of people to the non-monetary obstacles to vaccination. There is plenty to understand about what makes some subgroups experience rightward and leftward shifts in their demand for vaccines. On vaccine supply, there is much left to uncover about the forces governing the pace of vaccine discovery: the entry of firms and efficiency improvements in vaccine production. Economic research has only begun to develop better insights into the information flows that can improve the vaccine system. The perpetual challenges of financing discovery, production, and distribution of vaccines will remain rich areas for study.

In the wake of the COVID-19 pandemic, access to a safe and effective COVID-19 vaccine became the most important issue in health, politics, and economics. Vaccine economics justly deserves more attention in the wake of COVID-19. However, beyond this one vaccine, there lie horizons where millions more lives can be saved in the 21st century with improvements in the world's vaccine systems.

References

Bishai, D., Champion, C., Steele, M. E., & Thompson, L. (2011). Product development partnerships hit their stride: Lessons from developing a meningitis vaccine for Africa. *Health Affairs*, *30*(6), 1058–1064. doi.org/10.1377/hlthaff.2011.0295

Bishai, D., Lin, M. K., & Kiyonga, C. (2001). Modeling the economic benefits of an AIDS vaccine. *Vaccine*, *20*(3–4), 526–531. doi.org/10.1016/s0264-410x(01)00335-8

Bishai, D., & Mercer, D. (2001). Modeling the economic benefits of better TB vaccines. *International Journal of Tuberculosis and Lung Disease*, *5*(11), 984–993.

Geoffard, P.-Y., & Philipson, T. (1997). Disease eradication: Private versus public vaccination. *American Economic Review*, *87*(1), 222–230.

Grauer, J., Löwen, H., & Liebchen, B. (2020). Strategic spatiotemporal vaccine distribution increases the survival rate in an infectious disease like Covid-19. *Scientific Reports*, *10*(1), 1–10. doi.org/10.1038/s41598-020-78447-3

Grossman, G. (1967). *Economic systems*. Englewood Cliffs, NJ: Prentice-Hall.

Hutubessy, R., Henao, A. M., Namgyal, P., Moorthy, V., & Hombach, J. (2011). Results from evaluations of models and cost-effectiveness tools to support introduction decisions for new vaccines need critical appraisal. *BMC Medicine, 9*(1), 1–4. doi.org/10.1186/1741-7015-9-55

Kickbusch, I., Krech, R., Franz, C., & Wells, N. (2018). Banking for health: Opportunities in cooperation between banking and health applying innovation from other sectors. *BMJ Global Health, 3*(Suppl 1), e000598. doi.org/10.1136/bmjgh-2017-000598

Kremer, M. (2002). Pharmaceuticals and the developing world. *Journal of Economic Perspectives, 16*(4), 67–90. doi.org/10.1257/089533002320950984

Kremer, M., Levin, J., & Snyder, C. M. (2020). Advance market commitments: Insights from theory and experience. *AEA Papers and Proceedings, 110*, 269–273. https://doi.org/10.1257/pandp.20201017

Kuehn, B. M. (2020). Interest in global COVID-19 vaccine alliance grows. *JAMA, 324*(11), 1025–1025. doi.org/10.1001/jama.2020.16966

Lee, B. Y., Mueller, L. E., & Tilchin, C. G. (2017). A systems approach to vaccine decision making. *Vaccine, 35*, A36–A42. doi.org/10.1016/j.vaccine.2016.11.033

McDonnell, A., Van Exan, R., Lloyd, S., Subramanian, L., Chalkidou, K., La Porta, A., . . . Rosenberg, J. (2020). *COVID-19 vaccine predictions: Using mathematical modelling and expert opinions to estimate timelines and probabilities of success of COVID-19 vaccines.* Washington, DC: Center for Global Development.

National Academies of Sciences, Engineering, & Medicine. (2020). *Framework for equitable allocation of COVID-19 vaccine.* Washington, DC: National Academies Press.

Pan American Health Organization. (2020). *PAHO revolving fund vaccine prices for 2020.* https://www.paho.org/en/documents/paho-revolving-fund-vaccine-prices-2020

Pooripussarakul, S., Riewpaiboon, A., Bishai, D., Muangchana, C., & Tantivess, S. (2016). What criteria do decision makers in Thailand use to set priorities for vaccine introduction? *BMC Public Health, 16*(1), 684. doi.org/10.1186/s12889-016-3382-5

Shnaydman, V. (2020). Simulation model for productivity, risk and GDP impact forecasting of the COVID-19 portfolio vaccines. *medRxiv.* doi.org/10.1101/2020.11.01.20214122

Sim, S. Y., Watts, E., Constenla, D., Brenzel, L., & Patenaude, B. N. (2020). Return on investment from immunization against 10 pathogens in 94 low-and middle-income countries, 2011–30. *Health Affairs, 39*(8), 1343–1353. doi.org/10.1377/hlthaff.2020.00103

Vaughan, K., Ozaltin, A., Mallow, M., Moi, F., Wilkason, C., Stone, J., & Brenzel, L. (2019). The costs of delivering vaccines in low- and middle-income countries: Findings from a systematic review. *Vaccine: X, 2*, 100034. doi:10.1016/j.jvacx.2019.100034

World Health Organization. (2010). *Monitoring the building blocks of health systems: A handbook of indicators and their measurement strategies.* https://apps.who.int/iris/bitstream/handle/10665/258734/9789241564052-eng.pdf

World Health Organization. (2020). *WHO SAGE values framework for the allocation and prioritization of COVID-19 vaccination.* https://www.who.int/publications/i/item/who-sage-values-framework-for-the-allocation-and-prioritization-of-covid-19-vaccination

World Health Organization. (2021). *Guidance on developing a national deployment and vaccination plan for COVID-19 vaccines.* https://www.who.int/publications/i/item/WHO-2019-nCoV-Vaccine-deployment-2021.1-eng

Yamey, G., Schäferhoff, M., Hatchett, R., Pate, M., Zhao, F., & McDade, K. K. (2020). Ensuring global access to COVID-19 vaccines. *Lancet, 395*(10234), 1405–1406. doi.org/10.1016/S0140-6736(20)30763-7

1.3

Cost of finding and making vaccines

Implications for immunization programs

Clarke B. Cole, Beth Evans, and Soleine Scotney

1.3.1 Problem statement

Ensuring access to affordable vaccines is a critical function of public health systems. To achieve this, two questions need to be answered: What vaccines are available? Which vaccines are more affordable? This chapter provides an overview of the vaccine market landscape and then discusses the strategies used by decision makers and policymakers to help improve affordability of and sustainable access to vaccines.

The first part of this chapter covers the costs and risks of vaccine development and production and how this influences which vaccines are developed and how much they cost to produce and buy. The second part provides an overview of the vaccine supply landscape to provide an understanding of the range of vaccine companies and products and the ways in which market dynamics incentivize company behaviors. The third part details how procurement modalities and mechanisms impact a country's level of access to vaccines. By the end of this chapter, readers will have an improved understanding of how different decisions and actions can influence access to sustainable supply of affordable vaccines.

1.3.2 Introduction to vaccine costs and pricing

What drives the pricing of vaccines? In highly competitive markets, prices are tied closely to production costs, and in perfect markets, price theoretically

Clarke B. Cole, Beth Evans, and Soleine Scotney, *Cost of finding and making vaccines* In: *Handbook of Applied Health Economics in Vaccines*. Edited by: David Bishai, Logan Brenzel and William V. Padula, Oxford University Press.
© Oxford University Press 2023. DOI: 10.1093/oso/9780192896087.003.0004

equals marginal cost. However, many vaccines markets are oligopolies with a small number of firms holding the greatest market share. As a result, cost plus pricing (i.e., pricing vaccines at cost plus a given margin) is rarely used in vaccines markets. Understanding the costs of vaccine development and production are crucial for recognizing the theoretical floor price of vaccines, particularly given the high costs typically associated with vaccine research and development (R&D). This section explores the components that contribute to the cost of developing and producing vaccines, and how these costs link to prices charged on the market. This is followed by a discussion on different approaches used to set vaccine prices.

1.3.2.1 Vaccine research and development costs

R&D is expensive and risky. Typically, taking a candidate from discovery and preclinical testing through clinical trials and to licensure, including regulatory approvals, is estimated to take between 5 and 18 years (Médecins Sans Frontières, 2010) and cost between US $200 million and US $500 million (André, 2002). The key categories of R&D costs include costs incurred to discover, develop, and bring a vaccine to market (e.g., clinical trials, regulatory approval including World Health Organization (WHO) prequalification of medicines). In some cases, vaccine R&D costs can include costs to in-license product-related intellectual property to further develop a product in-house. Further third-party contributions (e.g., grants, loans, subsidies) are common to support R&D; these should be included in product cost calculations to offset costs.

R&D spending can be considered a fixed cost. R&D costs vary by supplier and product based on scientific hurdles associated with different product types, the size and complexity of clinical trials required, and the developer's operational costs, among other factors.

If development is successful, vaccine developers have significant costs to recoup through sales (unless development funding has been secured externally, e.g., via a grant). Due to the continuous nature of innovation, suppliers may expect to face a roughly normally distributed curve in terms of sales over time—with a period of ramp-up when products become licensed and introduced, a period of steady sales, and then a period of ramp-down as technology is replaced by new, innovative, or competitor products. Thus, not only must developers recoup initial development investments, but they also face a limited period in which they may be able to recoup those costs.

Sometimes, vaccine development is unsuccessful. Analysis of vaccine development data from 1998 to 2009 found that there was just a 6% probability of market entry (i.e., 94% chance of failure) for vaccine candidates from the preclinical phase (Pronker, Weenen, Commandeur, Claassen, & Osterhaus, 2013). When failures occur, the developer no longer has prospects of direct returns on the investments. It has sunk into a failed vaccine candidate. Most suppliers will aim to recover such investments, at least partially, through sales of successful products.

1.3.2.2 Vaccine production costs

Costs of production vary by supplier, product, and geography. In general, costs incurred by vaccine companies throughout the production cycle of a vaccine can be grouped into the following categories (Bill & Melinda Gates Foundation, 2016):

- *Facilities and equipment*: costs associated with fixed assets, including capitalized costs that depreciate over time (e.g., land, buildings, machinery) as well as ongoing costs of upkeep (e.g., repairs and maintenance, utilities).
- *Direct labor*: employee costs (e.g., wages, benefits) directly attributable to a specific vaccine.
- *Consumables*: raw materials used as inputs in production of a specific vaccine such as biological and chemical agents; fill/finish consumables such as vials, stoppers, and seals; packaging consumables such as labels and vaccine vial monitors; and quality control consumables such as inputs for testing kits.
- *Overheads*: operational costs not directly attributable to a specific vaccine such as salaries, training, back-office functions, and insurance.
- *Commercialization*: expenses incurred post regulatory approval associated with selling and marketing the product in the relevant market (e.g., advertising, marketing, distribution, etc.).
- *Licensing*: expenses paid for licensing the right to use product-related intellectual property in order to develop, produce, and/or sell a vaccine.
- *Interest costs*: interest payments as a result of company financing, such as interest costs for working capital (inventories plus receivables minus payables) and interest for capital investments.

- *Third-party contributions*: all contributions (e.g., grants, loans, subsidies) from governments and other organizations should be included in product cost calculations to offset costs.

1.3.2.3 Accounting for vaccine development and production costs

Cost categories can be broadly classified into four groups: fixed, variable, semi-variable, and mixed. The relative contribution of each cost classification determines how changes in volume impact production economics (Bill & Melinda Gates Foundation, 2016).

- *Fixed costs* are costs that do not change as output increases or decreases. Thus, increasing sales volume can spread fixed costs across more doses. Examples include product development costs, facilities, equipment, and third-party financing costs.
- *Variable costs* increase directly with additional output, for example, consumables such as vaccine vials.
- *Semi-variable costs* are correlated with output in aggregate, but not as directly as variable costs. Direct labor costs do not materially increase with each additional vaccine unit produced, but do increase in aggregate proportional to total output, for example, in a stepwise manner as additional shifts are required.
- *Mixed costs* refer to groupings of costs that include both fixed and variable components, for example, commercialization and licensing. In order to understand, model, and plan for the effects of volume on price, it is best to separate mixed costs into their component fixed and variable subcomponents.

1.3.2.4 Impact of vaccine cost structure on vaccine economics

The types of costs faced when developing and producing vaccines are not static; they vary based on several factors. The cost structure of vaccines influences the lower bound of pricing possible for a given vaccine product (presuming suppliers will not sell below fully loaded cost of goods). It is important for procurers to understand the dynamics that influence costs and determine what levers are available to access lower prices.

Costs vary depending on the following factors (Bill & Melinda Gates Foundation, 2016):

- *Production volume.* As production volume increases (up until capacity constraints are reached), the fixed production costs per dose decrease— allowing price to decrease.
- *Predictability.* Predictability of output volumes over time benefits suppliers through:
  - Enabling appropriate amortization of fixed costs.
  - Appropriate sizing of the workforce and efficient operations—for example, purchasing the correct volume of (perishable) consumables.
  - Enabling supply to meet demand: it can take up to 3 years to produce a batch of vaccines due to the complexity of manufacturing (Vidor & Soubeyrand, 2016), meaning that production needs to be well planned in advance to meet target output in the future.
- *Product complexity.* Development of novel vaccines that target areas of unmet health need where there are no existing vaccines may be more expensive and complex than development of vaccine products where a product already exists (Heaton, 2020). This is driven, for example, by the need to generate completely new data and navigate new pathways to licensure. Partnerships with donor agencies or public procurers that help to spread risks (either in terms of upfront funding for R&D costs (an example of push funding) or increased demand certainty (an example of pull funding)) can help to overcome such barriers.
- *Product packaging requirements.* Consumables, including the primary and secondary packages and labels for vaccines, are variable costs, which increase as production increases. Packaging costs can become further compounded with rising production when multiple different vial presentations, secondary packages, and labels are required to serve international markets due to country-specific product preferences and language requirements. Smaller production runs impose additional direct labor costs associated with process management. Furthermore, formulation of both multidose and single-dose vials adds new costs related to additional clinical testing.
- *Regulatory requirements.* Country-specific regulatory approval processes place an administrative burden on suppliers, which increases

resource requirements and costs. When countries simplify or harmonize regulatory requirements, this can speed up time to market entry (Wolf et al., 2020).

- *Fixed and indirect cost allocation possibilities.* The allocation of fixed and indirect costs is a decision that depends on feasible options influenced by the number of products, markets, and time that costs can be split over. While some of these factors are primarily within the suppliers' control, others can be influenced by governments and other purchasers. For example, procurers can improve predictability of demand for suppliers by structuring tenders over longer-term periods or they can signal an intention to introduce particular vaccines in the future, clearly indicating preferred product characteristics. Countries purchasing vaccines can also harmonize regulatory approval processes with international norms, increasing ease of market entry for suppliers and potentially facilitating access to lower prices.

1.3.2.5 Vaccine pricing

Vaccine prices vary from country to country depending on a range of factors, particularly supplier-specific targets for returns on investment, supply-side and demand-side impacts on cost of goods sold, and the extent of uncertainty or predictability in supply forecasts. This section focuses on pricing models used by firms in vaccine markets; however, it is worth noting that the pricing models used by firms are also influenced by purchaser levers (e.g., procurement mechanisms, negotiating power, and ability- or willingness-to-pay). In perfectly competitive markets, firms theoretically use *marginal cost pricing*, which is the practice of setting a price equal to the extra cost of producing an extra unit of output (e.g., vial) including normal profit. This pricing model is not typically used in vaccine markets because few have close to perfect market conditions.

Given high market entry barriers, most vaccine markets are typically oligopolistic with a small number of firms gaining the greatest market share. As a result, firms can be price setters, rather than price takers and alternative pricing models are often used, for example:

- *Reference or competitive pricing*: the practice of setting a price by comparing prices set by competitors in similar markets. This may include external price-setting—in which firms set prices achieved in similar countries matched by geography and/or income level. This is often seen in middle-income countries to inform negotiations or decision-making on product selection.

- *Value-based pricing*: pricing based on the value a product brings to the market or health system can be measured in various ways (e.g., incremental benefit compared to incumbent product, costs averted to a health system by preventing a disease compared to treating it). This method could be used by firms as the basis for setting vaccine prices. Health technology assessment is increasingly being conducted by high-income countries to help make evidence-based decisions on reimbursement and funding based on the value of new product options over existing ones.

- *Tiered pricing*: tiered pricing or price differentiation is the practice of offering different prices to different markets based on ability to pay. This strategy can enable revenue growth through enabling nationwide vaccine introductions at a price affordable to a given government, thus increasing volumes of sales—and potentially in turn spreading fixed production costs over more doses. For example, GlaxoSmithKline uses World Bank gross national income per capita groupings to tier prices of vaccines, in addition to other factors. (GlaxoSmithKline, 2019). While GlaxoSmithKline does not publish prices by tier, review of anonymized vaccine purchase data provided by WHO Market Information for Access to Vaccines (MI4A) shows that prices (e.g., for pneumococcal conjugate vaccine (PCV)) may vary by a factor of up to 25 times between low-income countries and high-income countries (WHO: Immunization Vaccines and Biologicals, 2019). If tiered pricing only consists of one high price for high-income countries and one low price set near marginal costs for low- and middle-income countries (LMICs) then it will not lead to higher profit than simply having one high price for high-income countries. It is the use of multiple middle tiers with mid-level prices above marginal cost that offers firms the ability to capture revenue in excess of costs that would otherwise be lost.

1.3.3 Vaccine supply landscape

This section of the chapter describes the range of vaccine companies developing and manufacturing vaccines. It describes how suppliers perceive and respond to market signals, thus influencing product development.

1.3.3.1 Vaccine suppliers

The landscape of vaccine suppliers has important implications for the availability of affordable vaccines that meet population health needs. The global vaccine market is highly consolidated on the supply side, with four *multinational corporations* (MNCs) accounting for approximately 80% of global vaccine revenues: GlaxoSmithKline plc (which acquired Novartis' vaccines business in 2015), Merck & Co., Inc. (known as Merck, Sharp & Dohme outside the US and Canada), Pfizer Inc., and Sanofi (Access to Medicine Foundation, 2017). Such multinational companies have historically been responsible for bringing high-impact, innovative vaccines (such as Pfizer Inc.'s PCV and Merck & Co., Inc.'s HPV vaccine) to market for the first time. Typically, products are developed in response to high-income country demand and first launched there, before rolling out to lower-income countries (this time lag has decreased in recent years).

There is also a growing number of vaccine companies based in emerging markets, organized as members of the *Developing Countries Vaccine Manufacturers Network* (DCVMN). This network of over 40 manufacturers typically supplies lower-priced, traditional vaccines to the global market (such as pentavalent, measles and rubella, and typhoid vaccines). These products have traditionally been either biosimilar vaccines developed in-house or in-licensed products from innovating companies. While they do not account for a large portion of global vaccine revenues, DCVMN members' contributions to the vaccine market are substantial: in combination, they supply vaccines for approximately 84% of the world's birth cohort each year and represent 64 out of 147 WHO prequalified vaccines (Batson, 2016). In recent years, some DCVMN members have increased their focus on vaccine R&D, including both adapting existing vaccines to meet the specific needs of LMICs and developing novel first-generation products. Provided they adhere to globally accepted quality and safety standards such as WHO prequalification, they should be considered comparable to MNC products.

Adding to the complexity of the vaccine supply landscape are smaller *biotechnology firms*, which are increasingly responsible for conducting early-stage vaccines R&D. When their research shows promise, these vaccine products are usually out licensed to or acquired (sometimes in the form of the entire biotech firm) by larger companies like MNCs or members of the DCVMN for phase II clinical testing onwards and commercialization.

1.3.3.2 Competition in vaccines markets

Markets for newer vaccines are not competitive; they usually include a limited number of suppliers, typically MNCs. The lack of price competition has contributed to high prices in vaccine markets. Because products are usually heterogeneous with regard to product presentation (e.g., different number of doses, cold-chain requirements, or efficacy), it is difficult for buyers to compare products, which further impedes competition. For example, transparency on prices paid by different countries for the same product is relatively low. However, the WHO MI4A vaccine purchase database has helped to increase transparency in this area by publishing anonymized data on prices paid by countries for different vaccine products, which can be viewed based on characteristics such as purchase order volume, procurement mechanism, and country income level.

There are high barriers to entry due to the complexity and cost of vaccine development and production. There are also barriers to exit due to the complexity and cost of vaccine development and production. These barriers result in limited suppliers of innovative vaccines for a number of years, after which additional competitors may come to market with next-generation vaccines. There may sometimes even be barriers, or at least delays, to exit due to production timelines and potentially advance tenders. Market-shaping teams in global health organizations work to identify potential gaps in supply or affordability and provide incentives to suppliers to enter or remain in the market. The Healthy Markets Framework, developed jointly by Gavi, UNICEF, and the Bill & Melinda Gates Foundation (BMGF), is a tool that helps to support such teams in assessing the "health" of a given vaccine market and develop strategies to improve it (Gavi, 2020).

1.3.3.3 Market signals and their impact on product development

Given the significant scientific hurdles associated with vaccine R&D, vaccine developers face strong incentives to respond to the needs of high-income countries and governments with high abilities to pay or other lucrative markets (e.g., private travel vaccines). This means that private financing for R&D for vaccines that disproportionately affect poor populations tends to be insufficient—resulting in slower development or deprioritization of vaccines to target unmet health needs focused in low- and lower-middle-income countries. In addition, where vaccines do come to market, their characteristics do not always meet the specific needs of populations in lower-income countries, for example, in terms of serotype coverage (which influences efficacy).

Global donors and product development partnerships have played an important role in the vaccine supply landscape, providing incentives for vaccine companies to develop and sell products that meet health needs, where commercial incentives are insufficient to drive such R&D. These entities collaborate with vaccine companies to share the risk that their investments will not be recouped in the market (Cole & Iyer, 2016). One example is the Meningitis Vaccine Project, in which the WHO, PATH (formerly known as the Program for Appropriate Technology in Health), and Serum Institute of India, funded by the BMGF, worked with African public health officials to develop a low-cost meningitis A vaccine (MenAfriVac) designed specifically to meet the needs of populations along the African meningitis belt (PATH & WHO, 2017).

Furthermore, DCVMN members typically face different incentives than MNCs: the domestic markets they operate in provide incentives to develop products that meet the needs of local populations. In the case of Chinese and Indian DCVMN members, the combination of large domestic markets (in addition to demand from Gavi-eligible markets through pooled procurement) provides incentives for R&D to focus on meeting the needs of LMIC populations. DCVMN members' role in developing for and supplying to LMICs is expected to increase. For example, in 2019, the Serum Institute of India received Indian licensure and WHO prequalification for its PCV, which was designed to protect against ten serotypes of *Streptococcus pneumoniae* most likely to cause serious disease in Africa and Asia (Serum Institute of India & PATH, 2020). In addition to increasing fit to local disease burden in LMICs, this second-generation vaccine lowered the price of PCV immunization by one-third, compared to the lowest price offered by a competitor (Gavi, 2021c).

Suppliers benefit from country signals, which may indicate market appetite and stimulate vaccine development. These signals can include what products should be prioritized for development and under what conditions they would be preferred by countries. However, clear country signals on future demand for innovative vaccines are limited. Global think tanks, such as the Centre for Global Development, have proposed interventions to improve market signals and commitments to encourage product development. For example, the market-driven value-based advance commitment (Chalkidou, Garau, Silverman, & Towse, 2020), focuses on accelerating development of health products to minimize the burden of tuberculosis. The proposal is based on extending health technology assessments in-country to not only evaluate the value of potential products but also to commit to future procurement from interested countries provided products meet the required target product profile. Such demand signals and commitments may accelerate private sector development. In the absence of such signals, suppliers may be hesitant to invest the significant sums required to develop innovative vaccines.

1.3.4 Vaccine procurement

Vaccine procurement is the process whereby vaccines are purchased and delivered to governments or government agencies for public immunization programs, and to private purchasers for the private market. A range of procurement modalities exist—each with different eligibility criteria and implications for national immunization programs. This section first outlines the broad influence of procurement on vaccine economics, and then details the range of procurement modalities, followed by a discussion of trends and changes in the procurement landscape. It finishes with an exploration of innovative vaccine procurement mechanisms.

1.3.4.1 Impact of procurement levers on vaccine economics

The structure, eligibility, and processes used for different vaccine procurement modalities can influence the price, quality, availability, and supply security of different vaccine products. This is due to the influence that procurement modalities have on the relationship between supply and demand. The main levers are volume, visibility/predictability, country context, and extent of operational and regulatory requirements.

As explained above, suppliers typically wish to sell vaccines at scale and in an efficient manner. Procurement modalities that pool demand from a range of countries can be attractive to suppliers (ideally over multiple years), since they provide clear demand signals allowing allocation and potentially even expansion of production capacity to meet demand. This increased visibility and economic predictability of aggregated demand can enable suppliers to lower prices while ensuring economies of scale and "right sizing" of facilities. Typically, pooled and coordinated procurement modalities that procure larger volumes than individual countries can make lower prices accessible.

Suppliers also benefit from streamlined processes that simplify product presentation requirements (i.e., labelling, languages, doses per vial) since these lower the cost of consumables and labor required to prepare appropriate product presentations, shifting the cost curve. If aggregate volumes rise, but require diverse country-specific packaging, then suppliers will face increased costs to prepare different product presentations, which may counteract the benefits of scale. As a result, pooled/coordinated procurement mechanisms that agree on labelling harmonization may allow access to further lowered prices, provided cost savings from the supplier are passed onto purchasers.

Once clinical trials have been successfully completed, vaccines undergo quality and safety assurance steps through registration with a relevant regulatory authority for the production site. For in-country use, vaccines typically require local registration with the national regulatory authority and, potentially, further evidence of quality and safety—often in a different format and with different requirements to previous reviews. The existence of multiple different registration and licensure requirements across countries can limit access to vaccines in different geographies, due to the country-specific administrative requirements placed on suppliers. As a result, regulatory harmonization— such as acceptance of WHO prequalification in lieu of local regulatory assessment, and use of the WHO Collaborative Procedure for Accelerated Registration—can ease the market entry pathway in countries. This improves access to a wider range of vaccines as well as potentially increasing demand and lowering prices which reflect these greater efficiencies.

1.3.4.2 Procurement modalities

At the highest level, there are two main procurement modalities for vaccines: self-procurement and pooled procurement. In practice, many countries exploit a hybrid strategy with different products procured via different routes. Most high-income countries self-procure vaccines, and—due to the existence of and eligibility required for Gavi and the Pan American Health Organization (PAHO) (see section 1.3.4.2.2)—many LMICs procure through pooled procurement mechanisms.

1.3.4.2.1 Self-procurement
Self-procurement refers to the practice of procuring vaccines directly, either from internal domestic suppliers or bilaterally with international companies, and offers autonomy in terms of procurement schedule, tender frequency, product choice, and other, broader goals. Domestic suppliers are most

prevalent in high-income countries (e.g., the US, Europe, Japan, and South Korea) as well as some large middle-income countries (e.g., Brazil, China, India, Thailand, Indonesia, and Vietnam). Where countries have domestic vaccine companies, they often exhibit a preference for domestic supply—often due to the supply security offered and the ability to meet broader economic and domestic security goals. These domestic suppliers may also be subsidized by local governments, facilitating access to lower prices and enabling more control on domestic production (e.g., which vaccines are developed and what characteristics they have).

Access to affordable vaccines through self-procurement will typically depend on countries' requirements for vaccine registration and procurement, the volumes being secured, and negotiation power. If suppliers are required to conduct additional vaccine trials in the procuring country or navigate a complex registration process, this may decrease the number of interested suppliers. Bid prices may depend on population size (particularly if this is partnered with unique presentation requirements), meaning countries with small population sizes and complex registration requirements may encounter access or pricing challenges if they choose self-procurement.

Taking supplier preferences into account in tender and contract structures can lead to price reductions. Suppliers have communicated to countries and partners that they prefer longer duration tenders (e.g., 3 years) to shorter 1-year tenders. However, some countries may have cash flow or other financial restrictions, limiting the current tender and contract length and structure. Countries could investigate changes to the country-specific tender and contract processes, coordinated with any additional government procurement departments that may need to be involved in order to increase attractiveness to suppliers and potentially access lower prices.

In addition, countries can leverage publicly shared insights from comparable countries (i.e., in terms of income level or region) to understand market prices achieved via self-procurement and help negotiate a good price for the given country. Countries can refer to the WHO MI4A vaccine purchase database to review public procurement information (WHO: Immunization Vaccines and Biologicals, 2019), for example, reviewing vaccine prices categorized by product type, presentation, and volume.

1.3.4.2.2 Pooled procurement

Pooled procurement refers to the practice of central procurement agencies procuring on behalf of a group of countries, usually with defined conditions on eligibility. This section covers the two most prominent vaccine pooled procurement agencies: UNICEF Supply Division (SD) and the PAHO Revolving

Fund (RF). Both procurement bodies aggregate demand for a limited number of products for eligible countries. Other pooled procurement bodies have been proposed, for example, for the ASEAN region (Siripitayakunkit, 2018), and may emerge over time, as hurdles to achieve regulatory harmonization are overcome.

Most vaccines procured by UNICEF SD are accessible to all countries, provided they sign a memorandum of understanding with UNICEF SD—though prices depend on Gavi eligibility, and other income group criteria for PCV, HPV, and rotavirus vaccine prices in particular. Many countries procuring through UNICEF SD are Gavi eligible, based on country gross national income (GNI) per capita.

PAHO RF procurement is open to countries in the Americas—currently 34 economies in Latin America and the Caribbean have become PAHO members (Pan American Health Organization, 2020). Countries are required to pre-pay for orders placed through UNICEF SD or PAHO RF.

Pooled procurement bodies are typically responsible for some logistical, procedural, and regulatory steps in the procurement process such as shipping, tendering, and negotiations. It can be beneficial to countries to have these processes conducted by an independent body, since this decreases the in-country operational requirements and can leverage internationally accepted standards and processes that may not be available (or may be expensive to provide) in-country. This may come at a financial cost, for example, UNICEF SD's vaccines handling fee for Gavi countries is 1.4% (UNICEF, 2021). It may also be a requirement to accept specific tendering terms with regard to the timing or duration of tenders and deliveries in order to procure via the pooled procurement mechanism. This requires alignment in-country to forecast for the appropriate time period and organize the supply chain.

For countries participating in pooled procurement, the choice of vaccines will generally be limited to a predetermined menu—both in terms of products and product presentation (e.g., only multidose vials may be available). The consolidation of demand in a subset of products and product presentations facilitates lower prices and attracts suppliers that benefit from streamlined coordination of (stable) supply.

1.3.4.3 Trends in the procurement landscape

This section of the chapter describes some key trends in the procurement landscape that may shape the way vaccines are procured in the coming decade.

Table 1.3.1 Gavi classification and eligibility for support

Gavi classification	Eligibility conditions	Co-financing terms
Initial self-financing	GNI per capita below World Bank threshold for low-income countries	Countries pay flat rate of US $0.20/dose for each vaccine
Preparatory transition	GNI per capita above low-income country threshold, and below lower-middle-income country threshold	Country co-financing contributions increase 15% year-on-year
Accelerated transition	GNI per capita "Gavi eligibility threshold" (US $1,580 per capita in 2019)	Country co-financing requirements increase linearly year-on-year for 5 years to reach 100% at end
Fully self-financing	After 5 years of accelerated transition, provided GNI per capita remains above threshold	Countries pay the full procurement cost

1.3.4.3.1 Gavi transition

As a country's GNI per capita rises, it will transition out of Gavi support from full co-financing, to preparatory transition, to accelerated transition, to fully self-financing (see Chapter 5). Countries are classified based on where their average GNI per capita over the past 3 years falls compared to cut-off thresholds governing transition between phases (Gavi, 2018) (Table 1.3.1).

Growing independence from Gavi support has implications for procurement, particularly for the newly fully self-financing countries. Importantly, even when countries transition from Gavi support they are still eligible to continue to procure from UNICEF SD—offering continued logistical advantages. However, the prices they are eligible to access may evolve, depending on the status of post-transition pricing agreements. As it stands, post-transition pricing agreements exist for rotavirus and HPV vaccines as well as PCV (WHO, 2018). In the future, it is expected that middle-income countries that do not qualify for Gavi support may participate in pooled procurement for vaccines, given persistent barriers to accessing vaccines in these countries.

1.3.4.3.2 Switching procurement modalities

Driven by market intelligence and/or changes in country preferences, a country may wish to change how it procures a given vaccine, for example, from procuring via UNICEF SD to self-procuring or vice versa. Market intelligence on product options and variations in availability and price via different procurement mechanisms can be used to inform whether this is a beneficial decision and present an evidence base for the switch. It may be necessary to define new processes (e.g., in-country tendering procedures) or update agreements with the pooled procurement body to switch modality.

As vaccine markets evolve and the number of suppliers for each market increases, it will be important for policymakers and decision makers to leverage existing capacity, such as through National Immunization Technical Advisory Groups (2021) to switch products should new, alternative options better meet the country's needs.

1.3.4.4 Innovative procurement mechanisms

In recent years, innovative procurement mechanisms have been designed and implemented to encourage the development of vaccines essential for improving public health when market mechanisms are too slow, too expensive, or are simply ignoring diseases affecting citizens in lower-income countries. These innovative mechanisms are particularly important in augmenting demand signals and reassuring suppliers that development of potentially expensive, high-risk candidates could be profitable and sustainable for their businesses.

1.3.4.4.1 Advance market commitments

- *Pneumococcal Advance Market Commitment (Pneumococcal AMC).* Pneumonia is the leading vaccine-preventable cause of child mortality, and PCVs have complex development and production processes. To accelerate vaccine introduction and achieve affordable pricing for LMICs, the Pneumococcal AMC was set up in 2007. The AMC was a US $1.5 billion innovative financing "pull" fund put in place to incentivize development of PCVs to fit a target product profile to define suitability for use in low-income countries. As a "pull" mechanism, the AMC created financial incentives in the form of a "top-up" payment on top of the price paid (or co-financed by Gavi) for countries to encourage private sector engagement by creating viable market demand. During the 10-year window of the AMC (from 2010 to 2020), three PCV products were developed and received WHO prequalification, with 60/73 (83%) eligible Gavi countries rolling vaccines out nationwide (Gavi, 2021b).
- *The COVAX Facility.* The coronavirus disease 2019 (COVID-19) pandemic in 2020 required unprecedented acceleration of vaccine

development to control and respond to the novel coronavirus. Due to the speed of development required, the high risks of failure, and the need for an immense number of doses to respond to demand, global health partners worked to establish the COVAX Facility. The COVAX Facility is a global risk-sharing mechanism for pooled procurement and equitable distribution of COVID-19 vaccines to countries at all income levels (Gavi, 2021a). It uses both push and pull mechanisms, including an Advance Market Commitment for supply to lower-income countries, to incentivize manufacturers to develop COVID-19 vaccines according to a specific target product profile and to supply resulting products equitably at affordable prices and in adequate quantities to meet global need.

1.3.4.4.2 Volume guarantees

In volatile or uncertain markets, a lack of clear demand signals can disincentivize development or production of vaccines by suppliers. In these situations, volume guarantees—where a predetermined volume of vaccines is guaranteed to be procured or the delta in forecast revenues will be paid to the supplier at the end of a predetermined price window—can be used. An example of a volume guarantee comes from an agreement between the BMGF and a supplier of rotavirus vaccines, secured in 2010–2011. Through guaranteeing 132 million doses of sales to low- and lower-middle-income countries, the supplier was able to lower the cost of production per dose, and lower some of the risk premium that was initially factored into the pricing—thanks to increased predictability and amortizing costs over a larger volume. This allowed a 67% price reduction and a price of just $5 per immunized child (Gavi, 2012).

1.3.4.5 Other market-shaping levers

Alongside tools to shape procurement, other market-shaping levers that do not commit to procurement can be applied.

- *Push funding (or product development investments).* Suppliers may be able to receive investment (e.g., in the form of grants or attractive loan terms) to conduct clinical trials or expand manufacturing capacity for high-priority vaccines (e.g., from the BMGF, International Vaccine Institute, or other large donors). By subsidizing the cost of development, donors may put in place global access terms that set a ceiling price and/or a minimum production commitment to serve LMICs if successful. This form of market shaping is the most common.

- *Product development partnerships (PDPs).* In addition to the Meningitis Vaccine Project, the oral cholera vaccine was developed via a PDP. Partnerships between the International Vaccine Institute, suppliers across Sweden, Vietnam, India, and South Korea, alongside public and private funding accelerated the development of the oral cholera vaccine for the public sector (Odevall et al., 2018). PDPs are becoming less common, with a trend towards push funding.

1.3.5 Conclusion

For public health systems to ensure access to affordable vaccines, it is important that policymakers and decision makers understand what factors drive vaccine pricing, and supply sustainability. This chapter has demonstrated how firms' costs contribute to vaccine prices, and how market conditions also affect vaccine prices. Vaccine markets do not conform to the criteria for competitive markets due to a high degree of consolidation on both the supply and demand sides, high barriers to entry and exit, and imperfect information. This chapter has also provided an overview of the vaccine supply landscape, to provide an understanding of the range of vaccine companies and products that operate within vaccine markets. Suppliers often have power as price setters rather than price takers in vaccine markets. However, the development of pooled procurement systems—particularly focusing on lower-income countries—has enabled demand-side levers to lower prices and increase access to affordable vaccines globally.

References

Access to Medicine Foundation. (2017). *Access to Vaccines Index.* https://accesstomedicinefoundation.org/access-to-vaccines-index

André, F. E. (2002). How the research-based industry approaches vaccine development and establishes priorities. *Developments in Biologicals,* 25–29.

Batson, A. (2016, March 15). *Global vaccine market.* Paper presented at the Global Vaccine and Immunization Research Forum, Johannesburg (South Africa).

Bill & Melinda Gates Foundation. (2016). *Production economics for vaccines.* Seattle, WA: Bill & Melinda Gates Foundation.

Chalkidou, K., Garau, M., Silverman, R., & Towse, A. (2020). *Blueprint for a market-driven value-based advance commitment for tuberculosis.* Center for Global Development.

https://www.cgdev.org/publication/blueprint-market-driven-value-based-advance-com
mitment-tuberculosis

Cole, C. B., & Iyer, J. K. (2016). *Ensuring sustained incentives for pharma to develop medicine for the poor*. Access to Medicine Foundation. https://accesstomedicinefoundation.org/media/uploads/downloads/5bc5edfd5372e_2016-Ensuring-sustained-incentives-for-pharma-to-develop-medicine-for-the-poor.pdf

Gavi. (2012). *GAVI Alliance secures lower price for rotavirus vaccine* [Press release]. https://www.gavi.org/gavi-secures-lower-price-rotavirus-vaccine

Gavi. (2018). *Eligibility and transition policy*. https://www.gavi.org/programmes-impact/progr ammatic-policies/eligibility-and-transitioning-policy

Gavi. (2020). *Market shaping*. https://www.gavi.org/our-alliance/market-shaping

Gavi. (2021a). *COVAX*. https://www.gavi.org/covax-facility

Gavi. (2021b). *Pneumococcal vaccine support*. https://www.gavi.org/types-support/vaccine-support/pneumococcal

Gavi. (2021c). *Supply agreements*. https://www.gavi.org/investing-gavi/innovative-financing/pneumococcal-amc/manufacturers/supply-agreements

GlaxoSmithKline. (2019). *Tiered pricing and vaccines*. https://www.gsk.com/media/5683/tie red-pricing-and-vaccines-aug19.pdf

Heaton, P. M. (2020). Challenges of developing novel vaccines with particular global health importance. *Frontiers in Immunology, 11*, 517290. doi:10.3389/fimmu.2020.517290

Médecins Sans Frontières. (2010). *Giving developing countries the best shot: An overview of vaccine access and R&D*. https://msfaccess.org/giving-developing-countries-best-shot-overv iew-vaccine-access-and-rd

National Immunization Technical Advisory Groups. (2021). *The unique database on National Immunization Technical Advisory Groups*. https://www.nitag-resource.org/

Odevall, L., Hong, D., Digilio, L., Sahastrabuddhe, S., Mogasale, V., Baik, Y., . . . Lynch, J. (2018). The Euvichol story—development and licensure of a safe, effective and affordable oral cholera vaccine through global public private partnerships. *Vaccine, 36*(45), 6606–6614. doi:10.1016/j.vaccine.2018.09.026

Pan American Health Organization. (2020). *PAHO strategic fund*. https://www.paho.org/en/paho-strategic-fund

PATH, & World Health Organization. (2017). *Meningitis vaccine project*. https://www.mening vax.org/

Pronker, E. S., Weenen, T. C., Commandeur, H., Claassen, E. H. J. H. M., & Osterhaus, A. D. M. E. (2013). Risk in vaccine research and development quantified. *PloS One, 8*(3), e57755. doi:10.1371/journal.pone.0057755

Serum Institute of India, & PATH. (2020). *Fact sheet: Pneumococcal disease, pneumococcal conjugate vaccines, and Pneumosil*. https://pneumosil.com/wp-content/uploads/2020/07/path-fact-sheet.pdf

Siripitayakunkit, U. (2018). *Procurement policies—an example for ensuring vaccine security: The ASEAN vaccine security and self-reliance initiative*. https://dokumen.tips/download/link/procurement-policies-a-an-example-for-ensuring-vaccine-unchalee-siripitayakunkit. Accessed June 26, 2022.

UNICEF. (2021). *Handling fees*. https://www.unicef.org/supply/handling-fees

Vidor, E., & Soubeyrand, B. (2016). Manufacturing DTaP-based combination vaccines: Industrial challenges around essential public health tools. *Expert Review of Vaccines, 15*(12), 1575–1582. doi:10.1080/14760584.2016.1205492

Wolf, J., Bruno, S., Eichberg, M., Jannat, R., Rudo, S., VanRheenen, S., & Coller, B.-A. (2020). Applying lessons from the Ebola vaccine experience for SARS-CoV-2 and other epidemic pathogens. *NPJ Vaccines, 5*(1), 51. doi:10.1038/s41541-020-0204-7

World Health Organization. (2018). *Vaccine pricing: Gavi fully self-financing & accelerated transition countries.* https://cdn.who.int/media/docs/default-source/immunization/mi4a/factsheet_vacc_pricing_gavi_transitioning.pdf?sfvrsn=cc0e5566_6&download=true

World Health Organization: Immunization Vaccines and Biologicals. (2019). *MI4A: Market information for access to vaccines.* https://cdn.who.int/media/docs/default-source/immunization/mi4a/factsheet_vacc_pricing_gavi_transitioning.pdf?sfvrsn=cc0e5566_6&download=true

1.4

Vaccination as investment in human capital

J. P. Sevilla, David Bloom, Dan Salmon, and David Bishai

We present the economic view of vaccinations as investments in human capital. That is, they involve expenditures at a point in an individual's life that produce a stream of future benefits in terms of time spent alive with a high quality of life. These benefits have both intrinsic and instrumental value. The intrinsic value is the direct benefit of being healthy. The instrumental value includes the broad socioeconomic value of health as an input to achieve other goals. We discuss how conceptions of the value of vaccination have broadened in recent years from an initial narrow focus on health impacts on vaccinated individuals related to the averted treatment costs to the full public health and socioeconomic value of vaccination. We discuss how the broadened benefits from vaccine investments may not be captured by individual rational decision-making and how this leads to market failures. The decision-making challenges include the costs of rational decision-making encompassing misinformation, dynamic inconsistency, the use of heuristics, motivated cognition, and vaccine hesitancy. The market failures involve externalities, public goods, and merit goods. Important externalities include herd immunity and macroeconomic effects. These interactions imply that socially optimal vaccination requires both strong public sector involvement and pro-vaccination social norms. Public sector involvement includes public financing, subsidies and incentives, guidance, and mandates. The social norms involve altruism, personal and collective responsibility, and commitments not to free ride. Cultivating such norms requires non-economic policy instruments.

We discuss how existing vaccine valuation frameworks often adopt the health payer's perspective and cost–utility analysis (CUA), which can yield to undervaluation of, and underinvestment in, vaccination. This can be

J. P. Sevilla, David Bloom, Dan Salmon, and David Bishai, *Vaccination as investment in human capital* In: *Handbook of Applied Health Economics in Vaccines*. Edited by: David Bishai, Logan Brenzel and William V. Padula, Oxford University Press.

remedied by wider use of societal perspective cost–benefit analysis (CBA) and of social welfare functions to address equity issues. Finally, we discuss optimal investment in research and development (R&D), and how this raises the challenge of incentivizing innovation, promoting access and equity, and reducing deadweight losses and rents, all at the same time.

1.4.1 Health as human capital, and vaccinations as investments in human capital

Economists view health as a form of human capital (Becker, 2007), a stock or asset embodied in the states of our bodies and minds that yields a future stream of benefits in terms of time spent alive and free from morbidity or disability. It is a stock whose monetary value equals the expected present discounted monetary value of each moment within that stream. Health is a central element of human capital, along with education and work skills. Like any asset, health can depreciate through neglect, disease, poor living conditions or habits, aging, or other factors, thereby reducing the flow of benefits. But it can also be maintained and augmented through investments in the form of the provision of various sorts of security (e.g., physical and socioeconomic); good diet, exercise, and health habits; healthy environments (e.g., access to clean water and air); and the appropriate use of healthcare and health technologies, including vaccination. Many investments, such as vaccinations, are costly, and so appropriate levels of investment require quantifying and comparing such costs and benefits and undertaking those investments for which benefits exceed costs. These costs and benefits can be computed at the level of an individual, in which case any investment whose individual benefits exceed its individual costs can be called individually optimal. But these can also be computed at the level of society as a whole, in which case any investment whose societal benefits exceed its societal costs is socially optimal.

The word "investment" might suggest that vaccinations be valued for their impact on market-related outcomes such as wages, earnings, or gross domestic product. As we discuss below, such impacts are indeed part of vaccinations' value and often ignored in vaccine evaluation. Therefore, these are an important part of the economic view. However, it is equally important that economic theory, and rational choice theory more generally, defines value expansively: in terms of the satisfaction of individuals' preferences. Any situation an individual would want to occur—for example, having a long life; being able to spend time with friends and family; pursuing meaningful work or life projects whether paid or not; being happy, enjoying pleasurable activities and experiences, and minimizing pain; being active, free, independent, and self-determining; or anything else whether market-related or not—is a relevant aspect of value. Thus, the value of an investment in health is not limited to an investment's impact on market-related outcomes but extends to any impact individuals or societies care about.

The benefits of investment in health capital reflect health's intrinsic value (i.e., the extent to which health is valuable in and of itself to the individual whose health is at issue) and instrumental value (i.e., the extent to which improved health produces valuable socioeconomic and other non-health outcomes, whether for the individual or for society as a whole). The best way within economic theory to represent and distinguish these values is through a health-augmented lifecycle model. Let us think of a person's lifetime utility (we treat utility and well-being as synonyms, which is not uncontroversial), U, as depending on lifetime trajectories in longevity prospects, s (where "s" stands for survivorship), health-related quality of life, q, consumption of goods and services, c, and non-market time, l. We can represent this by a function:

Equation 1.4.1. A person's lifetime utility:

$$U(s,q,c,l)$$

Non-market time in turn consists of time spent on unpaid work and on leisure, where unpaid work includes such activities as housework, caregiving, and volunteering. The arguments of U are trajectories over a lifetime as opposed to levels at any point in that lifetime. U is a positive function of these trajectories: the higher these trajectories, the better. U is typically assumed to be concave in consumption and non-market time: stable and certain trajectories are superior to cyclical or risky ones. These four arguments are typically assumed to be natural complements or mutual enhancers of each other: the higher the level of any one quantity, the greater the value of improvements in any of the others (the way the value of having a left glove is enhanced by also having a right glove).

Healthier people can have higher levels of both consumption and non-market time. For example, higher health-related quality of life allows a person to be more productive during a workday and earn and consume more over a lifetime. A longer life allows more leisure time, for example, to build relationships with one's grandchildren. Health can also contribute to stabilizing consumption and non-market time such as reducing exposure to the often significant and sometimes catastrophic out-of-pocket costs of illness or risks of enforced inactivity when disabled. In recognition of these mechanisms for health's impact on consumption and non-market time, we can rewrite Equation 1.4.1 thus:

Equation 1.4.2. A person's lifetime utility (detailed):

$$U\big(s,q,c(s,q),l(s,q)\big)$$

In this fuller statement, health matters intrinsically: s and q are direct arguments in the utility function. But it also matters instrumentally: s and q determine the level, stability, and certainty of lifetime consumption and non-market time. Thus, properly valuing health requires measuring its intrinsic value (how much individuals value health in and of itself) and its instrumental value (how it affects levels and variability over a lifetime of consumption and non-market time). Health's impact on market-related outcomes such as earnings (the sick are less able to work, and often earn less from work) are therefore part of the value of health because earnings facilitate consumption. However, market-related outcomes do not tell the whole story. Health's intrinsic value, its impact on unpaid work and leisure, and the natural complementarities among health, consumption, and non-market time also matter.

The lifecycle aspect of this picture requires emphasis: vaccinations yield their benefits not only during the period immediately following their occurrence but potentially for the entire lifespan. A vaccine's effectiveness often exists for only a few years (e.g., a decade). Nevertheless, if it prevents death or severe disability during those years, this potentially raises survival probabilities, health-related quality of life, and economic productivity for significant and much longer chunks of the vaccinated person's lifetime.

The above theoretical picture can and should be extended beyond the individual being vaccinated to other individuals in society. For example, vaccination of an individual confers herd protection on the unvaccinated by reducing the number of people from whom the latter might catch a particular infection. The reduced mortality and morbidity risks enjoyed by the unvaccinated from herd protections have the same intrinsic and instrumental values as those of the vaccinated. Such protection is particularly valuable to those unable to be vaccinated because they are too old or young, immunocompromised, or lack access.

Finally, vaccinations can confer wholly instrumental benefits to communities and societies. Perhaps the most important and salient contemporary example of this is the coronavirus disease 2019 (COVID-19) pandemic, which the world is living (and dying) through as this chapter is being written.

Addressing infectious disease outbreaks like the global COVID-19 pandemic often requires shutting down broad swathes of socioeconomic activity, causing severe declines in economic activity, income, and employment, and dramatic increases in poverty and economic vulnerability. Vaccination reduces the need for such shutdowns, thus protecting people's livelihoods (and therefore their consumption) over and above any health benefits such vaccinations produce.

1.4.2 From narrow to broad conceptions of the value of vaccination

Historically, the field of vaccine valuation has had an excessively narrow focus. To the extent that health was seen as an important value element, vaccine evaluations adopted a "therapeutic paradigm," focusing only on the health impacts on the vaccinated individual, and impacts related to the vaccine's target pathogen (e.g., measles-related outcomes in measles vaccine recipients) (Gessner et al., 2017). From an economic perspective, the main element of value was seen to be the averted costs to the health system of treating disease. From the economic perspective, health expenditures were not explicitly seen as producing streams of economic benefits extending into the future, but implicitly seen as consumption expenditures rather than investments (Bloom & Canning, 2000).

The value focus has gratifyingly expanded in recent times. With respect to health benefits, there is a growing appreciation of the full public health value of vaccination (Gessner et al., 2017). A core element of this full value are the herd protections mentioned above. Since infections often result in hospitalization, vaccination also reduces difficult- and expensive-to-treat nosocomial (i.e., hospital-based) infections such as *Clostridium difficile*, *Staphylococcus aureus*, *Klebsiella*, and *Escherichia coli*. Some vaccines have nonspecific (sometimes also called heterologous or off-target) effects (Saadatian-Elahi et al., 2016). For example, measles-containing vaccine appears to promote general immune function and reduce all-cause mortality (Mina et al., 2019; Mina, Metcalf, de Swart, Osterhaus, & Grenfell, 2015). Childhood bacillus Calmette–Guérin vaccination is associated with diminished rates of lung cancer at older ages (Usher et al., 2019). Vaccination can reduce or slow down the progress of antimicrobial resistance in both targeted and bystander pathogens, either directly by preventing resistant infections or indirectly by reducing antibiotic treatments (Sevilla, Bloom, Cadarette, Jit, &

Lipsitch, 2018). Reduced use of antibiotics can also protect human health by preserving the gut microbiome (Cully, 2019). Severe disease case definitions often do not exist—for example, severe pneumonia is typically defined in terms of requiring hospitalization—so appreciating vaccinations' full health benefits requires appreciating the averted health burdens of severe disease (Wilder-Smith et al., 2017). Other elements of full public health value are disease control, including their elimination and eradication (which eliminates all downstream burdens of disease and vaccination costs; Xue & Ouellette, 2020); health system strengthening; and health equity (i.e., reductions in differences across socioeconomic/demographic groups in health outcomes and access and use of health services).

There is also a growing appreciation of the full socioeconomic value of vaccination. Vaccination can reduce various socioeconomic burdens of the acute stage of the disease, from the potentially catastrophic out-of-pocket costs paid by patients and their families and friends and caregivers to the economic costs (in terms of lost earnings and foregone uses of non-market time) of time lost seeking care, providing care, or recuperating. Over longer time horizons, vaccination is an enabler and driver of human capital accumulation, productivity, labor supply, income generation, and poverty alleviation. Vaccinated children tend to have better records of school attendance, higher levels of educational attainment, and better cognitive function—as evidenced, for example, in studies focused on a variety of vaccines (e.g., for measles, tetanus, *Haemophilus influenzae* type b, rotavirus, and pneumococcal disease) and different country contexts, including Bangladesh, China, Ethiopia, India, the Philippines, South Africa, and Vietnam (Anekwe, Newell, Tanser, Pillay, & Bärnighausen, 2015; Bloom, Canning, & Shenoy, 2011; Canning et al., 2011; Megiddo, Klein, & Laxminarayan, 2018; Nandi, Deolalikar, Bloom, & Laxminarayan, 2019; Nandi, Shet, et al., 2019; Oskorouchi, Sousa-Poza, & Bloom, 2020). Studies have also found that vaccinated individuals have higher trajectories of productive market and productive non-market activities (Bloom, Khoury, Algur, & Sevilla, 2020) than their (otherwise comparable but less healthy) unvaccinated counterparts (Sevilla et al., 2020; Sevilla et al., 2019).

Vaccination thereby translates into higher levels of consumption and savings at the micro level and more rapid economic growth at the macro level (Masia, Smerling, Kapfidze, Manning, & Showalter, 2018). The parents of vaccinated children also tend to have better records of work attendance and productivity, as well as greater peace of mind associated with reduced health and related financial risks associated with infectious disease.

The social benefits of vaccination include improvements in health and social equity and the distribution of economic well-being. Such benefits can
arise insofar as vaccination prevents diseases that disproportionately afflict
the poor and disadvantaged racial and ethnic minorities. Vaccination can also
confer intergenerational benefits. For example, to the extent that vaccination
of adolescents against human papillomavirus affords protection against subsequent development of cervical cancer, maternal survival will be improved
with concomitant benefits for the nurturing and development of children and
disruptions to intergenerational impulses regarding the transmission of poverty (Bärnighausen, Bloom, Cafiero, & O'Brien, 2012; Riumallo-Herl et al.,
2018; Verguet et al., 2015).

1.4.3 Individual decision-making

Whether a particular vaccination is individually optimal depends on the relative size of the vaccine's individual benefits (in terms of its individual intrinsic
and instrumental values) and individual costs. When a vaccine is part of the
national immunization program (NIP) such as an infant measles, mumps, and
rubella vaccine, individuals don't need to pay for vaccines out of pocket when
they get vaccinated. Instead, such vaccines are financed by a NIP that is in turn
financed by taxes or social health insurance premiums. For such vaccines, the
individual costs are largely the costs in terms of time, effort, and funds required to make an appointment, travel to a clinic, or take time off work; risk
of adverse reactions to the vaccine; and discomfort and distress resulting from
muscle aches, nausea, and a fear of needles. Of course, when vaccines are not
in the NIP, such as influenza vaccines for working age adults without risk factors, the individual costs will include the out-of-pocket costs for the vaccine
doses and administration. Later, we will see how cognitive dissonance, and
certain moral preferences and attitudes can also make vaccination costly to
the individual. The magnitude of the expected benefits to the individual are a
function of many of the various intrinsic and instrumental values described
above that accrue to vaccinated individuals. They are also a function of the
magnitude of the risk of infection, which in turn is a function of the incidence
or prevalence of the disease and the effectiveness of the vaccine. If individual
costs are sufficiently high (e.g., because vaccination clinics are not conveniently located and so are costly in terms of time, effort, and funds to access)
and benefits sufficiently low (e.g., because incidence or vaccine effectiveness

or severity of infection are low), then it would be individually rational not to get vaccinated.

Recall that vaccination is socially optimal if its social benefits (i.e., individual benefits summed across all individuals in society) exceed its social costs. Not all vaccinations are socially optimal: if infection risk, vaccine efficacy, and mortality and morbidity risks of infection are low or the vaccine is costly, then vaccination may not be individually or socially optimal.

From society's point of view, it would be ideal if individually optimal vaccination decisions coincided with socially optimal ones, in which case society could take a hands-off approach and simply leave vaccination choices to individuals. But there are multiple reasons why individual decisions may diverge from socially optimal ones.

First, even if we were to make the extreme assumption that individuals are perfectly (in the sense of being relatively well informed and capable of bearing the cognitive burden of thinking through complex decisions) and self-interestedly rational, externalities would often result in vaccination incentives faced by individuals falling short of what is socially optimal. Externalities are various consequences of a decision maker's choices that are borne by others in society and that for self-interested reasons decision makers do not factor into their decisions. Central externalities related to vaccination are herd protections, reductions in collectively financed treatment costs, benefits to the rest of the world and to future generations of disease eradication, and indeed most elements of the full public health and socioeconomic value of vaccination that are realized at a macro level (e.g., at the level of a community, society, or population).

Second, perfectly rational decision makers may, again for self-interested reasons, prefer to free ride. Herd protections are an example of what economists refer to as a pure public good. A pure public good is one that is both nonexclusive and non-rival. A nonexcludable good is a good for which there cannot be selective access. A non-rival good is one such that one person's use of the good does not deplete the stock available for others to use. Herd immunity is both non-excludable and non-rival. If herd protections are achieved, it is impossible to exclude anybody from enjoying them. And once the threshold for achieving any community immunity has been achieved, the marginal cost of letting one more person enjoy community immunity is zero.

The non-excludability of a public good gives people an incentive to free ride. According to economic theory, producing an efficient amount of a public good requires each person to contribute to financing the production of that good by an amount equal to their willingness to pay for it. However, non-excludability implies that people will not have an incentive to make those contributions. From a selfish perspective, it is better to let others contribute since once the public good has been produced, since it will be available to non-contributors as much as to contributors. Thus, it may be rational for individuals to forego vaccination, thereby avoiding the inconveniences and time and effort required, and hope that enough other people get vaccinated to provide everyone with protection. If there are sufficiently many free riders, vaccination uptake may fail to reach the threshold required to produce the herd effects, jeopardizing the production of the public good.

Third, rational decision-making about health is informationally and cognitively demanding. An individual must know or research probabilities of infections and of death and various kinds of disabilities that result from infection, the impact on quality of life and economic well-being of various disabilities, what actions they can take to prevent or treat disease, and the costs and effectiveness of those actions. It takes a lot of time, effort, funds, and thought to make informed rational choices. Facing those demands, we may end up being paralyzed into inaction.

Fourth, individuals fall prey to systematic departures from rationality in three areas: biases in the perception or understanding of information, the use of heuristics (or rules of thumb or cognitive shortcuts), and self-control problems (Sassi et al., 2015). Self-control problems (also referred to as time inconsistency and present bias) can lead individuals to overweight today's costs and benefits (such as the inconvenience of getting vaccinated today) over tomorrow's (such as reduced infection risk) (O'Donoghue & Rabin, 2015). (Such bias is distinct from discounting since one may prefer to get vaccinated tomorrow rather than face a higher infection risk 2 days from now.) Omission biases lead individuals to prefer potentially harmful inactions (such as a vaccine-preventable infection) to potentially harmful actions (such as vaccine-induced adverse effects) (Ritov & Baron, 1990). Ambiguity aversion or dread leads us to prefer known risks (risk of infection) to unknown risks (risks of adverse events) (Han, Reeve, Moser, & Klein, 2009). Affect heuristics make individuals' risk judgments depend more on positive or negative feelings toward some aspect of the risk than objective statistical information about disease risks and vaccine benefits (Betsch, Ulshöfer, Renkewitz, & Betsch, 2011). The availability heuristic makes individuals mistakenly judge outcomes of which they are aware (e.g., from acquaintances' experience or media reports) as more probable (Blumenthal-Barby & Krieger, 2015). Optimism bias leads people to overestimate the probability of good outcomes (such as not getting infected) and underestimate the probability of bad ones (such as getting infected) (Sharot, 2011). A naturalness bias leads individuals to prefer actions and outcomes perceived to be more natural (e.g., natural immunity) than those seen to be artificial, synthetic, or processed (e.g., vaccine-induced immunity) (daCosta DiBonaventura & Chapman, 2008).

Confirmation biases lead people to underweight information that conflicts with what they *already* believe, and motivated cognition leads individuals to underweight information that conflicts with what they *want* to believe (Stone & Wood, 2018). Both are forms of cognitive dissonance and can lead individuals to be overly sensitive to information about adverse events and resistant to information about vaccine benefits. The Dunning–Kruger effect can lead individuals to overestimate their own expertise (e.g., on the causes of autism) and underestimate those of others (like professional experts) (Motta, Callaghan, & Sylvester, 2018). Moral foundations theory suggests that moral preferences (e.g., commitments to individual liberty) can shape empirical judgments (Rossen, Hurlstone, Dunlop, & Lawrence, 2019). The "attitude roots" literature emphasizes how receptivity to scientific evidence can be shaped by underlying attitudes such as world views (especially individualistic and libertarian ones), conspiratorial ideation, vested interests, personal identity expression, social identity needs, fears and phobias (e.g., of needles), and disgust sensitivity (Hornsey & Fielding, 2017; Hornsey, Harris, & Fielding, 2018).

The above four decision-making obstacles contribute to vaccine hesitancy, which according to the World Health Organization is a top ten threat to global health (World Health Organization, 2019a) and "as contagious and dangerous as the diseases it helps to spread" (World Health Organization, 2019b). The World Health Organization defines the vaccine hesitant as "those who refuse some or all vaccines, delay some vaccine perhaps according to an 'alternative schedule', or accept all vaccines but remain concerned" (World Health Organization, 2014). Vaccine hesitancy should not be considered a single state but rather a spectrum of combinations of behaviors and attitudes (Dubé, Ward, Verger, & MacDonald, 2021). At one extreme are individuals who (behaviorally) reject all vaccines and (attitudinally) are very sure of their views, and at the other extreme are those who (behaviorally) accept all relevant vaccines and are equally (attitudinally) very sure of their views. In between these extremes are many intermediate behavioral and attitudinal combinations. Behaviorally, individuals may accept or reject some but not all vaccines, or they may delay or be genuinely undecided regarding certain vaccines. Attitudinally, people may vary in the certainty of their acceptance or rejection. Only those who reject all vaccines and are highly certain in such rejection can be thought of as hardcore anti-vaxxers. Anyone who accepts at least one vaccine, who entertains some uncertainty about any refusal, or who merely delays or is genuinely undecided, is potentially susceptible to pro-vaccine messaging. Attitudes can reflect concerns about vaccines, and even those who get vaccinated can be concerned about such vaccinations.

A fifth set of reasons individual vaccination choices may fall short of socially optimal ones relate to equity or distributional issues. Infectious disease-related risks and burdens are distributed unequally in society, often reflecting and interacting with socioeconomic/demographic inequalities, so that the poor and vulnerable often face higher risks and burdens. Many societies have strong commitments to reducing so-called socioeconomic gradients in health, that is, disparities in health outcomes and in access to and use of health services across socioeconomic/demographic groups. Vaccines, like many other health technologies, are also held by many to be merit goods for which access ought not to depend on ability to pay. Individuals' health-related decisions are influenced largely by self-interest, and the most important redistributive mechanisms are those within the capacity of governments, so we expect government as opposed to individual action to be the primary mechanisms for achieving equity-related goals. Merit goods also inherently require redistributive funding mechanism like taxes or subsidies (from those with ability to pay to those who do not) and cannot rely for financing exclusively or even primarily on out-of-pocket expenditures since these are, of course, constrained by ability to pay.

1.4.4 Optimal investment in vaccination cannot be left to markets but requires a strong government role

For reasons given above, we cannot expect individuals to invest socially optimal amounts in vaccination. We therefore cannot leave vaccination decisions to individuals and the market. Getting vaccinated is very different from, say, buying a pizza. Pizza purchases and consumption are typically left to decentralized market decisions with only two parties: buyers and sellers dealing directly with each other. Each person decides if they want pizza, what kind, and at what price, and is assumed perfectly capable of making these judgments for themselves and their children. Transactions between buyer and seller are voluntary, and so mutually beneficial. Consumers finance pizza production directly out of pocket. Prices are market determined, reflecting countless decentralized decisions. Governments don't regulate pizza prices to protect consumers since competition among pizza makers tends to keep prices low.

When markets determine aggregate outcomes—who gets pizza and who doesn't, who produces it, the reigning prices, and the quantities sold—we seldom worry that these outcomes fall short of some social goals. Innovation in pizza-making technology is not a matter of profound social concern, and we are quite happy to let market forces dictate its pace.

Vaccination is very different. Markets play much smaller roles and governments much bigger roles as intermediaries. Few countries leave vaccine choices entirely to people, instead relying on expert judgment as reflected in vaccination guidelines, mandates, and advice of healthcare professionals. Vaccine mandates compel people to act against their own preferences regarding their own health and that of their children, in part to solve the free-rider problem. This raises issues involving the balance of public health imperatives and the greater good on the one hand and freedom and self-determination on the other. Vaccine financing involves government setting and collecting taxes or social insurance premiums. Prices paid to suppliers often reflect bilateral negotiations between manufacturers and large regional or national vaccine purchasers. Who is eligible for vaccinations and with what copay are determined by public health officials and government and payer reimbursement decisions. Aggregate outcomes are scrutinized for efficiency (e.g., are enough people being vaccinated?) and equity (do the worse off have meaningful access?). Promoting vaccines innovation is often a significant global priority, forcing trade-offs between strengthening patent rights to promote innovation and weakening them to promote access.

Government policies attempt to shift individual perceptions of the net benefits of vaccination by lowering the cost to obtain vaccines and supplying information to raise demand. Costs of vaccine are lowered not only by providing them for zero out-of-pocket monetary costs, but also by offering convenient venues and low waiting time. Sometimes there are conditional cash transfers to compensate people for the effort and time taken to get vaccinated. Vaccine information campaigns use multiple channels including media, medical professionals, schools, social media, and faith-based initiatives to communicate facts about the safety and benefits of vaccines. Policy incentives to address heuristics surrounding benefit and risk perception are still an evolving area of communications research. Setting up narratives and stories to counter concerns that vaccines have dreaded and unknown properties needs to be done with care. Widely disseminating messages to the public in an impactful manner is challenging in many ways, including the need to individually tailor such messages. As described by the World Health Organization, "messages need to be tailored for the specific target group, because messaging

that too strongly advocates vaccination may be counterproductive, reinfor-
cing the hesitancy of those already hesitant" (Dubé et al., 2021).

1.4.5 Do governments invest enough in vaccination?

For reasons given above, we cannot expect individuals to invest socially optimal amounts in vaccination. Thus, governments must play a central role in
such investments. But there are challenges to socially optimal government investment as well.

Consider three different layers of governmental decision-making. First,
in many countries, a Department of Health (DOH) is often allocated a fixed
budget by the Department of Finance (DOF), and the DOH must in turn allocate that health budget across the different health sector activities, including
vaccination. The fixed budget implies that spending more on vaccines requires
spending less on other activities. The second layer involves the DOF, which
often operates with a fixed public sector budget set by the tax-and-transfer
policies set by legislatures. The DOF can expand the DOH budget, allowing
the DOH to, say, spend more on vaccines without having to sacrifice other
health expenditures. However, the fixed public sector budget implies that such
expansion requires the DOF to allocate less to other non-health departments
such as education, infrastructure, or social assistance. The third layer involves
the legislature, which has the power to set taxes and therefore determine what
share of national income gets reallocated to the DOF and what stays in private
hands. It can raise taxes, thereby facilitating higher public spending, but at the
expense of reducing households' after-tax income.

These three decision makers directly and indirectly affect levels of investment in vaccination. The DOH can spend more on vaccination but less on
other health technologies. The DOF can expand the DOH budget, allowing
vaccination spending to rise while protecting other health spending, but at the
cost of foregoing non-health sector public spending. And legislatures can expand the DOF budget, relaxing health versus non-health trade-offs in public
spending, but reducing household disposable income.

To achieve socially optimal decisions, each of these three decision makers
should compute the full social costs and benefits of each of its options and
then prioritize those options according to which yields the largest net social
benefit per dollar spent from the relevant budget. Thus, to achieve optimal
public spending on vaccination, we should measure the net social benefit
of vaccination per dollar spent out of the DOH budget (or equivalently, the

social rate of return to vaccination). The DOH should compare this social rate of return to that of other health spending, the DOF should compare it to that of non-health sector public spending, and the legislature should compare it to the social rate of return of extra household post-tax income.

Optimal public spending at all levels thus requires quantitative estimates of the full social benefits and costs per DOH dollar spent on vaccination. Such estimates must include all the elements of the intrinsic and instrumental values described earlier, including the full public health and socioeconomic values of vaccination. It also requires the three governmental decision makers to allow such social value estimates to drive their decisions. These are easier said than done.

Many DOHs, when deciding whether to include a vaccine in a NIP, will conduct an economic evaluation of that vaccine. Performing such evaluation requires making two specification choices. The first is the choice of perspective, the most important options being the health payer and societal perspective. The second is the choice of analysis, the most important options being CUA and CBA.

The health payer's perspective narrowly focuses only on two aspects of the value of vaccines: their health impacts (typically measured in quality-adjusted life years (QALYs) or disability-adjusted life years (DALYs)) and consequences for the DOH's budget (often the costs of the vaccination program offset by averted costs of treating infections and controlling outbreaks). The goal underlying the health payer perspective is to allocate the DOH budget to maximize the health. It therefore reimburses a vaccine only if its incremental cost-effectiveness ratio (the ratio of incremental DOH costs to the incremental QALYs/DALYs) falls below the incremental cost-effectiveness ratio of the marginal health technology (the technology likely to be displaced to accommodate the vaccine given the fixed DOH budget, which should be the currently reimbursed technology with the highest incremental cost-effectiveness ratio). This perspective assumes—or at least does not question—the optimality of the size of the DOH budget and does not attempt to inform the decisions of the DOF and of legislatures. The societal perspective, in contrast, considers the full public health and socioeconomic value of vaccines, and indeed of any policy whether health related or not, being considered for public funding out of the DOH or DOF budget.

CUA and CBA differ from each other in what each takes as the unit of value. CUA assumes that every QALY or DALY has equal value, which is sometimes called the "QALY is a QALY is a QALY" assumption. CBA assumes that every dollar has equal value, which we might call the "dollar is a dollar is a dollar" assumption. These views empirically diverge when the same size health gains can have differential socioeconomic implications. One critical example of such divergence comes from lifecycle variations in economic activity: since prime-aged adults are more likely to be working and less likely to be dependent on social pensions and assistance than the elderly, raising the health of prime-aged adults by 1 QALY may have more instrumental economic value for society as a whole than raising the health of the elderly by 1 QALY. Another example of such divergence might be between diseases with and without outbreak potential. As discussed earlier, addressing the COVID-19 pandemic in the absence of vaccines requires shutting down economic activity, which has negative macroeconomic effects. This implies that COVID-19 vaccines do not just raise population health but also facilitate a return to normal pre-pandemic levels of macroeconomic activity. Other vaccine-preventable infectious diseases (e.g., pneumococcal disease) may be less macroeconomically costly to control, so vaccines that address such diseases may have less macroeconomic value to them. CBA is better able than CUA to reflect heterogeneity in socioeconomic effects—whether driven by lifecycle or macroeconomic factors—of improved health.

CBA's equal value per dollar assumption, however, makes it give inappropriate priority to the health needs of the wealthy, who have greater ability to pay. Such problematic priority leads many to prefer the health payer perspective and CUA, which for all its shortcomings values the QALY gains of the poor as much as those of the rich. To eliminate such problematic priority, distribution-sensitive versions of CBA should be developed. The most promising such version involves using social welfare functions, which effectively scale individuals' willingness to pay by their marginal utility of income (to neutralize differences in ability to pay) and by distributional weights which are larger for the worse off (Adler, 2019). Combining CBA and social welfare functions allows economic evaluation of vaccines to robustly incorporate equity considerations.

Many DOHs worldwide adopt a health payer perspective CUA as the baseline specification for vaccine evaluation. Such adoption risks underinvestment in vaccines. The health payer's perspective, by focusing only on health gains and health payer budget impacts, ignores important socioeconomic instrumental value elements of vaccines. Vaccines may have disproportionate socioeconomic value relative to other health technologies because, for example, they prevent outbreaks (like the COVID-19 pandemic) that are accompanied by macroeconomic burdens. Because of such omission, there is a risk of suboptimally low vaccine spending out of the health payer's budget.

Another suboptimal aspect of the health payer's perspective is its unquestioning acceptance of the size of the health payer's budget. The fact that this perspective ignores socioeconomic values yet assumes the health payer's budget to be optimal implies that this perspective faces the risk of spending too little on health in general (and therefore vaccines in particular). From a societal perspective, public spending on health technologies should reflect both its intrinsic and instrumental value. The fact that the health payer perspective ignores socioeconomic value makes it likely that from a societal perspective, public spending on health is suboptimally low. The solution to such a problem is to raise the health payer's budget in recognition of the instrumental value of its expenditures, but the health payer perspective assumes that the existing budget is already optimal, thereby prohibiting the expansion of health expenditures merited by their instrumental value. This suggests that simply taking the health payer's budget as given and optimal risks underinvestment in health and vaccination relative to their socially optimal levels.

To facilitate setting the health payer's budget at a socially optimal level, and thereby facilitate optimal vaccination investment out of that budget, a shift from a health payer perspective to a societal one is critical. More generally, optimal spending and decision-making by DOHs, DOFs, and legislatures will require shifting from health payer perspective CUAs toward societal perspective CBAs. Such a shift of perspective would fully incorporate the full social benefits and costs of vaccination into economic evaluation, helping identify optimal levels of vaccine spending. A shift from CUA to CBA would allow more accurate estimation of the socioeconomic value of vaccination, unconstrained by simplifying assumptions such as equal values per QALY.

1.4.6 Research and development, or investment in future vaccines

We have so far discussed optimal investment in existing vaccines, but also important is optimal investment in R&D into future vaccines. R&D financing comes from three main sources: governments which often fund basic research, for-profit pharmaceutical companies, and non-government nonprofits like the Bill & Melinda Gates Foundation.

For-profits will invest in vaccine R&D only if they expect sufficient risk-adjusted return on such investment. The probable underspending on vaccination by national governments that we previously discussed therefore creates risks of sending adverse market signals to for-profits and risks of suboptimally low investment in vaccine R&D, which could harm future generations. Greater recognition of the full public health and socioeconomic value of vaccination, and superior quantification of such value using societal perspective

CBA and social welfare functions may therefore facilitate not just optimal investment by governments in existing vaccines but also optimal investment by for-profits in future vaccines. Such broader vaccine evaluation can also stimulate R&D funding by governments and nongovernmental nonprofits by providing more comprehensive estimates of the social value of future vaccines.

There is a tension, however, between trying to incentivize innovation on the one hand and trying to achieve widespread access and equity on the other. Pharmaceutical company R&D is responsive to expected profits, which in turn is facilitated by vaccine prices reflecting healthy markups above marginal production costs. But such markups, in turn, can make vaccines unaffordable, reduce access, and cause deadweight loss and inequity. There is, therefore, a potential trade-off between present and future generations, the former benefitting from low markups and the latter from the innovation enabled by higher markups. Of course, there may also be markups that are so high that they yield expected profits in excess of what is necessary to incentivize R&D. Any profits extracted from such markups are called rents. They are purely redistributive, causing deadweight loss, inequity, and lack of access without facilitating any innovation. If equity is a central policy goal, then all else being equal, such rents should be minimized. Reconciling innovation with access and equity, and minimizing rent, all at the same time, is a challenging policy balancing act. This has provoked research on possible responses like value-based pricing (Danzon, Towse, & Mestre-Ferrandiz, 2015), fair pricing (Moon, Mariat, Kamae, & Pedersen, 2020), innovative financing mechanisms like advanced market commitments (Kremer et al., 2020), and more radical proposals like eliminating patents (Boldrin & Levine, 2013).

Ultimately, the pathway to achieving investments in vaccines that get us closer to embracing their full value will require both private and public sector investors who are motivated by accounts that trace that value across the multiple ways that vaccines benefit society. The work of vaccine economics and the methods that account for the full value of vaccines are the subjects of the remainder of this book.

References

Adler, M. (2019). *Measuring social welfare: An introduction.* New York, NY: Oxford University Press.

Anekwe, T. D., Newell, M.-L., Tanser, F., Pillay, D., & Bärnighausen, T. (2015). The causal effect of childhood measles vaccination on educational attainment: A mother fixed-effects study in rural South Africa. *Vaccine, 33*(38), 5020–5026. doi:10.1016/j.vaccine.2015.04.072

Bärnighausen, T., Bloom, D. E., Cafiero, E. T., & O'Brien, J. C. (2012). Economic evaluation of vaccination: Capturing the full benefits, with an application to human papillomavirus. *Clinical Microbiology and Infection, 18*(s5), 70–76. doi.org/10.1111/j.1469-0691.2012.03977.x

Becker, G. (2007). Health as human capital: Synthesis and extensions. *Oxford Economic Papers, 59*(3), 379–410. doi.org/10.1093/oep/gpm020

Betsch, C., Ulshöfer, C., Renkewitz, F., & Betsch, T. (2011). The influence of narrative v. statistical information on perceiving vaccination risks. *Medical Decision Making, 31*(5), 742–753. doi:10.1177/0272989x11400419

Bloom, D. E., & Canning, D. (2000). Policy forum: public health. The health and wealth of nations. *Science, 287*(5456), 1207, 1209. doi:10.1126/science.287.5456.1207

Bloom, D. E., Canning, D., & Shenoy, E. S. (2011). The effect of vaccination on children's physical and cognitive development in the Philippines. *Applied Economics, 44*(21), 2777–2783. doi:10.1080/00036846.2011.566203

Bloom, D. E., Khoury, A., Algur, E., & Sevilla, J. P. (2020). Valuing productive non-market activities of older adults in Europe and the US. *De Economist, 168*(2), 153–181. doi:10.1007/s10645-020-09362-1

Blumenthal-Barby, J. S., & Krieger, H. (2015). Cognitive biases and heuristics in medical decision making: A critical review using a systematic search strategy. *Medical Decision Making, 35*(4), 539–557. doi:10.1177/0272989x14547740

Boldrin, M., & Levine, D. K. (2013). The case against patents. *Journal of Economic Perspectives, 27*(1), 3–22. doi:10.1257/jep.27.1.3

Canning, D., Razzaque, A., Driessen, J., Walker, D. G., Streatfield, P. K., & Yunus, M. (2011). The effect of maternal tetanus immunization on children's schooling attainment in Matlab, Bangladesh: Follow-up of a randomized trial. *Social Science & Medicine, 72*(9), 1429–1436. doi:10.1016/j.socscimed.2011.02.043

Cully, M. (2019, June 17). *Antibiotics alter the gut microbiome and host health.* Nature Research. https://www.nature.com/articles/d42859-019-00019-x

daCosta DiBonaventura, M., & Chapman, G. (2008). Do decision biases predict bad decisions? Omission bias, naturalness bias, and influenza vaccination. *Medical Decision Making, 28*(4), 532–539. doi:10.1177/0272989X07312723

Danzon, P. M., Towse, A., & Mestre-Ferrandiz, J. (2015). Value-based differential pricing: Efficient prices for drugs in a global context. *Health Economics, 24*(3), 294–301. doi:10.1002/hec.3021

Dubé, È., Ward, J. K., Verger, P., & MacDonald, N. E. (2021). Vaccine hesitancy, acceptance, and anti-vaccination: Trends and future prospects for public health. *Annual Review of Public Health, 42*(1), 175–191. doi:10.1146/annurev-publhealth-090419-102240

Gessner, B. D., Kaslow, D., Louis, J., Neuzil, K., O'Brien, K. L., Picot, V., . . . Nelson, C. B. (2017). Estimating the full public health value of vaccination. *Vaccine, 35*(46), 6255–6263. doi:10.1016/j.vaccine.2017.09.048

Han, P. K. J., Reeve, B. B., Moser, R. P., & Klein, W. M. P. (2009). Aversion to ambiguity regarding medical tests and treatments: Measurement, prevalence, and relationship to sociodemographic factors. *Journal of Health Communication, 14*(6), 556–572. doi:10.1080/10810730903089630

Hornsey, M. J., & Fielding, K. S. (2017). Attitude roots and Jiu Jitsu persuasion: Understanding and overcoming the motivated rejection of science. *American Psychologist, 72*(5), 459–473. doi:10.1037/a0040437

Hornsey, M. J., Harris, E. A., & Fielding, K. S. (2018). The psychological roots of anti-vaccination attitudes: A 24-nation investigation. *Health Psychology, 37*(4), 307–315. doi:10.1037/hea0000586

Kremer, M., Levin, J., & Snyder, C. M. (2020). Advance market commitments: Insights from theory and experience. *AEA Papers and Proceedings, 110*, 269–273. doi.org/10.1257/pandp.20201017

Masia, N. A., Smerling, J., Kapfidze, T., Manning, R., & Showalter, M. (2018). Vaccination and GDP growth rates: Exploring the links in a conditional convergence framework. *World Development, 103*(C), 88–99. doi:10.1016/j.worlddev.2017.1

Megiddo, I., Klein, E., & Laxminarayan, R. (2018). Potential impact of introducing the pneumococcal conjugate vaccine into national immunisation programmes: An economic-epidemiological analysis using data from India. *BMJ Global Health, 3*(3), e000636. doi:10.1136/bmjgh-2017-000636

Mina, M. J., Kula, T., Leng, Y., Li, M., de Vries, R. D., Knip, M., . . . Elledge, S. J. (2019). Measles virus infection diminishes preexisting antibodies that offer protection from other pathogens. *Science, 366*(6465), 599–606. doi:10.1126/science.aay6485

Mina, M. J., Metcalf, C. J., de Swart, R. L., Osterhaus, A. D., & Grenfell, B. T. (2015). Long-term measles-induced immunomodulation increases overall childhood infectious disease mortality. *Science, 348*(6235), 694–699. doi:10.1126/science.aaa3662

Moon, S., Mariat, S., Kamae, I., & Pedersen, H. B. (2020). Defining the concept of fair pricing for medicines. *BMJ, 368,* l4726. doi:10.1136/bmj.l4726

Motta, M., Callaghan, T., & Sylvester, S. (2018). Knowing less but presuming more: Dunning–Kruger effects and the endorsement of anti-vaccine policy attitudes. *Social Science & Medicine, 211,* 274–281. doi:10.1016/j.socscimed.2018.06.032

Nandi, A., Deolalikar, A. B., Bloom, D. E., & Laxminarayan, R. (2019). Haemophilus influenzae type b vaccination and anthropometric, cognitive, and schooling outcomes among Indian children. *Annals of the New York Academy of Sciences, 1449*(1), 70–82. doi:10.1111/nyas.14127

Nandi, A., Shet, A., Behrman, J. R., Black, M. M., Bloom, D. E., & Laxminarayan, R. (2019). Anthropometric, cognitive, and schooling benefits of measles vaccination: Longitudinal cohort analysis in Ethiopia, India, and Vietnam. *Vaccine, 37*(31), 4336–4343. doi:10.1016/j.vaccine.2019.06.025

O'Donoghue, T., & Rabin, M. (2015). Present bias: Lessons learned and to be learned. *American Economic Review, 105*(5), 273–279. doi:10.1257/aer.p20151085

Oskorouchi, H. R., Sousa-Poza, A., & Bloom, D. E. (2020). *The long-term cognitive and schooling effects of childhood vaccinations in China.* National Bureau of Economic Research, Inc. https://ideas.repec.org/p/nbr/nberwo/27217.html

Ritov, I., & Baron, J. (1990). Reluctance to vaccinate: Omission bias and ambiguity. *Journal of Behavioral Decision Making, 3*(4), 263–277. doi.org/10.1002/bdm.3960030404

Riumallo-Herl, C., Chang, A. Y., Clark, S., Constenla, D., Clark, A., Brenzel, L., & Verguet, S. (2018). Poverty reduction and equity benefits of introducing or scaling up measles, rotavirus and pneumococcal vaccines in low-income and middle-income countries: a modelling study. *BMJ Global Health, 3*(2), e000613. doi:10.1136/bmjgh-2017-000613

Rossen, I., Hurlstone, M. J., Dunlop, P. D., & Lawrence, C. (2019). Accepters, fence sitters, or rejecters: Moral profiles of vaccination attitudes. *Social Science & Medicine, 224,* 23–27. doi:10.1016/j.socscimed.2019.01.038

Sassi, F. et al. (2015) Introduction. In McDaid, David, Franco Sassi, and Sherry Merkur. *Promoting health, preventing disease: the economic case.* Open University Press, Maidenhead, UK. ISBN 9780335262267.

Saadatian-Elahi, M., Aaby, P., Shann, F., Netea, M. G., Levy, O., Louis, J., . . . Warren, W. (2016). Heterologous vaccine effects. *Vaccine, 34*(34), 3923–3930. doi:10.1016/j.vaccine.2016.06.020

Sevilla, J. P., Bloom, D. E., Cadarette, D., Jit, M., & Lipsitch, M. (2018). Toward economic evaluation of the value of vaccines and other health technologies in addressing AMR. *Proceedings of the National Academy of Sciences of the United States of America, 115*(51), 12911–12919. doi:10.1073/pnas.1717161115

Sevilla, J. P., Stawasz, A., Burnes, D., Agarwal, A., Hacibedel, B., Helvacioglu, K., . . . Bloom, D. E. (2020). Indirect costs of adult pneumococcal disease and the productivity-based rate of return to the 13-valent pneumococcal conjugate vaccine for adults in Turkey. *Human Vaccines & Immunotherapeutics, 16*(8), 1923–1936. doi:10.1080/21645515.2019.1708668

Sevilla, J. P., Stawasz, A., Burnes, D., Poulsen, P. B., Sato, R., & Bloom, D. E. (2019). Indirect costs of adult pneumococcal disease and productivity-based rate of return to PCV13 vaccination for older adults and elderly diabetics in Denmark. *Journal of the Economics of Ageing, 14*, 100203. doi.org/10.1016/j.jeoa.2019.100203

Sharot, T. (2011). The optimism bias. *Current Biology, 21*(23), R941–R945. doi:10.1016/j.cub.2011.10.030

Stone, D., & Wood, D. (2018). Cognitive dissonance, motivated reasoning, and confirmation bias: Applications in industrial organization. In V. J. Tremblay, E. Shroeder, & C. Horton Tremblay (Eds.), *Handbook of behavioral industrial organization* (pp. 114–137). Northampton, MA: Edward Elgar Publishing.

Usher, N. T., Chang, S., Howard, R. S., Martinez, A., Harrison, L. H., Santosham, M., & Aronson, N. E. (2019). Association of BCG vaccination in childhood with subsequent cancer diagnoses: A 60-year follow-up of a clinical trial. *JAMA Network Open, 2*(9), e1912014. doi:10.1001/jamanetworkopen.2019.12014

Verguet, S., Olson, Z. D., Babigumira, J. B., Desalegn, D., Johansson, K. A., Kruk, M. E., . . . Jamison, D. T. (2015). Health gains and financial risk protection afforded by public financing of selected interventions in Ethiopia: An extended cost-effectiveness analysis. *Lancet Global Health, 3*(5), e288–e296. doi:10.1016/s2214-109x(14)70346-8

Wilder-Smith, A., Longini, I., Zuber, P. L., Bärnighausen, T., Edmunds, W. J., Dean, N., . . . Gessner, B. D. (2017). The public health value of vaccines beyond efficacy: Methods, measures and outcomes. *BMC Medicine, 15*(1), 138. doi:10.1186/s12916-017-0911-8

World Health Organization. (2014). *Report of the Sage Working Group on Vaccine Hesitancy.* Retrieved from Geneva: https://www.asset-scienceinsociety.eu/sites/default/files/sage_working_group_revised_report_vaccine_hesitancy.pdf

World Health Organization. (2019a). *Ten threats to global health.* https://www.who.int/news-room/spotlight/ten-threats-to-global-health-in-2019

World Health Organization. (2019b). *WHO Director General statement on the role of social media platforms in health information* [Press release]. https://www.who.int/news-room/spotlight/ten-threats-to-global-health-in-2019

Xue, Q. C., & Ouellette, L. L. (2020). Innovation policy and the market for vaccines. *Journal of Law and the Biosciences, 7*(1), lsaa026. doi:10.1093/jlb/lsaa026

1.5

Economics of vaccine delivery

George Pariyo and Onaopemipo Abiodun

1.5.1 Introduction

Since the global recognition of immunization as one of the most effective and cost-effective ways to promote public health, countries have adopted different approaches to deliver vaccines. High-income countries often rely on private providers to deliver vaccines with financing through public and private health insurance (Cherian & Mantel, 2020; World Health Organization, 2018). On the other hand, most low- and middle-income countries (LMICs) deliver vaccinations mainly through government-funded national immunization programs (NIPs) (Cherian & Mantel, 2020). NIPs tend to deliver vaccines at dedicated clinics or through outreach and mobile services (Cherian & Mantel, 2020). However, in many LMICs which have a mixed public–private health delivery system, and especially in fragile states where government institutions are too weak to meet basic needs, private not-for-profit (PNFP) facilities are often contracted by governments to provide vaccinations (Levin & Kaddar, 2011). Private providers are also playing an increasingly important role in non-fragile LMICs. The level at which their services are integrated with those of public providers and regulated by the government varies widely. Effective coordination between the public and private sectors is essential, but there is no single way to achieve this since different contexts have different needs. For LMICs to enjoy the full benefits of immunization, they must be able to commit to long-term financing requirements (Results for Development, 2017). The aim of this chapter is to assess the advantages and disadvantages of various immunization delivery systems—public, private not-for-profit, private for-profit (PFP), and mixed delivery—across five domains: efficiency, which refers to immunization delivery at the lowest possible cost per dose; financial sustainability, which refers to the ability to finance immunization delivery in the long term; and equity, which means that every eligible individual can be immunized with all

George Pariyo and Onaopemipo Abiodun, *Economics of vaccine delivery* In: *Handbook of Applied Health Economics in Vaccines.* Edited by: David Bishai, Logan Brenzel and William V. Padula, Oxford University Press. © Oxford University Press 2023. DOI: 10.1093/oso/9780192896087.003.0006 appropriate vaccines (World Health Organization, 2013). We will also look at delivery strategies from the perspective of quality, which is delivering a service according to standards, as well as coverage, which refers to the proportion of those who would benefit from a service who receive it. While we are aware that it is impossible to strike a perfect balance among these five domains, the goal of this chapter is to support the critical assessment of immunization delivery systems. This is necessary to ensure the systems adequately serve those who rely on them. First, we consider these domains and their implications.

1.5.2 Efficiency

Efficiency refers to the ratio of input costs to desired outputs. In the context of immunization programs, we may measure efficiency as cost per dose of vaccine administered or cost per fully immunized child. In this chapter, we refer to efficiency in terms of cost per dose of vaccine administered, varying widely within and between countries with mixed delivery systems. A multi-country study conducted in Benin, Ghana, Honduras, Moldova, Uganda, and Zambia found that the average unit cost of routine immunization provided through public and nongovernmental organization facilities ranged from $2 in Benin to $18 in Moldova (Brenzel, Young, & Walker, 2015). While these differences may represent potential opportunities for efficiency gains, they may also be due to operational differences that cannot be readily altered, such as wages, site location, and health systems structure (Menzies, Suharlim, Resch, & Brenzel, 2020). In each country, high service volume was strongly associated with lower average cost per dose. On the other hand, higher per capita gross domestic product and outreach services were correlated with higher average cost per dose, hinting at the effect of country-level differences on efficiency measures as well as likely trade-offs between efficiency and efforts to extend access to hard-to-reach population. Nongovernmental organization facilities were also associated with a higher average cost per dose than public facilities (Menzies et al., 2017). This hints at a trade-off between efficiency and equity in public health policy. For instance, a country may choose to prioritize vaccinating all the citizens regardless of the fact that some harder-to-reach communities may significantly increase the unit costs of the program.

1.5.3 Financial sustainability

Sustainability has a wide interpretation in global health and may refer to financial, logistical, personnel, or political aspects of a program's ability to continue long term. In the context of this chapter, we are mainly referring to financial sustainability, the ability of a program to obtain ongoing funding from secure or predictable sources (World Health Organization, 2013). The financial sustainability of immunization delivery is under threat in many settings with a mixed mode of delivery. Oftentimes, this stems from a low prioritization of immunization by governments. In some LMICs, some policymakers may not allocate sufficient national budgetary funds to immunization with the expectation that international donors will step in to bridge the gap (Songane, 2018). In the US, private practice pediatricians and family physicians who function as small independent businesses are the main providers of early childhood vaccines (Berman, 2008). However, these physicians are at a disadvantage when negotiating vaccine prices as studies have found that vaccine prices are related to the amount ordered. As such, larger private practices usually receive lower prices than smaller practices. These small practices, instead, rely on insurance reimbursements, which they negotiate with health plans to cover the vaccine costs that they incur (O'Leary et al., 2014). Despite evidence showing the effectiveness of vaccines, insurance companies use their larger negotiating power, owing to their larger size, to negotiate reimbursements below costs (Berman, 2008; O'Leary et al., 2014). Due to the risk of uncompensated costs, some physicians have delayed offering vaccines or even outsourced immunizations (Beaulieu-Volk, 2014). In Ghana, the National Health Insurance Scheme (NHIS) only reimburses curative care (Results for Development, 2017). Indonesia operates a decentralized health system, where local governments are responsible for covering immunization service delivery costs using funds disbursed from the national level (Results for Development, 2017). Wide variation in managerial capability and commitment to immunization at the subnational level has resulted in varying immunization coverage throughout the country (Maharani & Tampubolon, 2014; Results for Development, 2017). To maintain the financial sustainability of mixed immunization delivery systems, government intervention is necessary. This could take the form of legislation mandating that immunization be funded at a rate that encourages providers to deliver this essential service (Berman, 2008).

1.5.4 Equity

Equity implies the absence of avoidable and unnecessary disparities in access to or utilization of a service based on individual or community characteristics such as geography, race and ethnicity, religious affiliation, or socioeconomic status. In assessing the equitability of immunization in mixed delivery systems, it is important to acknowledge existing societal inequities, which can be difficult to surmount. For instance, all adults aged 65 years and older in the US have access to the 13-valent pneumococcal conjugate vaccine (PCV13), which is universally recommended for them by the Centers for Disease Control and Prevention with no out-of-pocket costs because of full coverage by Medicare Part B. Yet, racial and socioeconomic differences in PCV13 uptake among adults in this age group remain (McLaughlin et al., 2019). These disparities are likely due to other healthcare barriers that minorities and low-income individuals often face, such as poor access to reliable transportation and primary care (O'Malley & Forrest, 2006; Silver, Blustein, & Weitzman, 2012). On the other hand, contractual relationships between the public and private sector with explicit equity goals can reduce disparities in immunization. This was the case in Cambodia, where results of a large-scale quasi-experiment showed that children in the poorest 50% of households in the districts served by contractors were more likely to be fully immunized than their counterparts in districts using the typical government model for health service delivery (Schwartz & Bhushan, 2004).

1.5.5 Quality

Quality broadly refers to performance according to standards. Quality in health has several different dimensions including safety, effectiveness, client centeredness, timeliness, efficiency, and equity (Mosadeghrad, 2012). All these aspects of quality are important with respect to immunizations. People should be vaccinated with an efficacious vaccine in a safe procedure, with little to no adverse effects, at a place and time that is convenient to them, and by friendly service providers who are knowledgeable and able to communicate effectively to respond to their questions and reassure them that vaccination is not only highly effective in preventing serious diseases but also very safe. This requires not only the right vaccines on the schedule but also effective cold chain and logistics facilities as well as knowledgeable and motivated personnel. Regular assessments of effective vaccine management, delivery, and cold chain systems conducted by countries with support of the World Health Organization and UNICEF have often found some deficiencies especially in LMICs (Gavi, 2018). Surveillance, monitoring, and reporting of adverse events following immunization is an important component of an immunization program.

1.5.6 Coverage

Coverage refers to the percentage of a population who would benefit from a service who can obtain the service (World Health Organization, 2010). Tanahashi (1978) described different aspects of coverage including availability, accessibility, acceptability, contact, and effective coverage. Effective coverage refers to those who eventually get in contact and receive effective care. In the context of immunization, this implies the percentage of those who would benefit who receive a safe and effective vaccine at the correct time and for the correct indication. Coverage rates are regularly reported through routine administrative systems and occasionally validated through immunization coverage surveys. Cross-country comparisons of immunization coverage rely on the annually reported World Health Organization and UNICEF estimates of national immunization coverage reports (Burton et al., 2009).

1.5.7 Options for increased vaccine delivery

As countries work toward sustainably financing their immunization programs, which delivery system will best position them to achieve this goal? The answer, as the available evidence shows, may be context specific. Some countries, like Malaysia, have achieved impressive levels of immunization coverage with a largely government-run system, while others, like Ghana and Indonesia, have adopted a mixed financing system (Results for Development, 2017).

1.5.7.1 Public delivery

Some countries have been able, using general government revenue, to provide immunizations for free at government-run health facilities (Box 1.5.1). As of 2015, over 90% of Malaysian states achieved three-dose diphtheria, tetanus, and pertussis (DTP3) vaccine coverage above 90%, while 60% achieved over 99% of coverage (Coe, Gergen, Mallow, Moi, & Phily, 2017). However, budget constraints are a major barrier to the adoption of new vaccines that address some of the vaccine-preventable diseases, such as dengue (Coe et al., 2017).

Public delivery is dependent on assured funding secured through the national budget process. Having established budget lines to fund vaccine purchase and delivery of immunizations through routine health service delivery is a great way to institutionalize sustainability of funding for immunization.

Box 1.5.1 Case study—Malaysia

Malaysia has achieved impressive levels of immunization coverage with a largely government-run system. Using general government revenue, Malaysia provides immunizations for free at government-run health facilities (Coe et al., 2017). As of 2015, over 90% of its states achieved DTP3 vaccine coverage above 90%, while 60% achieved over 99% of coverage (Coe et al., 2017). Yet these high percentages may mask concerning inequities. For instance, Malay ethnic children, who belong to the majority ethnic group, were found to have a significantly lower likelihood of receiving all recommended primary vaccine doses by the age of 12 months, as compared to minority Indian and other Bumiputera children (Lim et al., 2017).

Additionally, although Malaysia has been able to achieve high immunization coverage using general government revenue, budget constraints are a major barrier to the adoption of new vaccines for major disease burdens, such as dengue (Coe et al., 2017). The inability of public facilities to provide new vaccines has driven many Malaysians to seek them from private facilities, where they are required to pay out of pocket. Variations in people's ability to pay raises equity concerns (Coe et al., 2017). Private facilities are playing an increasingly important role in the health system, as they provide an alternative to the public system, which is struggling to keep up with a growing population (World Health Organization: Regional Office for the Western Pacific, 2012). However, the government has not been able to integrate and regulate the fast-growing private health sector. As a case in point, private providers are not mandated to follow the government immunization schedule (Ahmad, Jahis, Kuay, Jamaluddin, & Aris, 2017). This puts many children at risk of missing necessary immunizations. A study found that 10.7% of surveyed children aged 12–23 months did not complete their primary immunization due to lack of vaccine stock at private facilities, while another 6.2% did not complete their primary immunization because private healthcare centers advised that they were not yet due to be immunized, as reported by their mothers (Ahmad et al., 2017).

Malaysia's NHIS is being designed to facilitate integration between the public and private sectors, and improve access to vaccines (Coe et al., 2017; World Health Organization: Regional Office for the Western Pacific, 2012). It is also important the government enforces a standard immunization schedule for all children at all facilities, public or private, so that timely vaccination is available at all points of service delivery (Ahmad et al., 2017).

This means it can be a guaranteed source of funding if there is political commitment and national consensus that prioritizes immunization. Global agencies that help LMICs through funding for new vaccines and cold chain and logistics costs cover a substantial portion of the cost of immunization (Songane, 2018). Having immunization funding institutionalized in national and district health budgets helps prepare for the time external funding agencies phase out, ensuring better chances for sustainability of immunization financing. On the downside, it increases government expenditure and may suffer when the political priority of immunization and other health programs changes with successive governments. In many LMICs, public facilities may be the only available source of immunization services, particularly in rural areas, where other providers may have less incentive to operate. Ministries of health, through their NIPs, can exercise stronger supervision of standards and have the power to take corrective action. This helps to ensure quality, for instance, promptly investigating any reports of adverse events following immunization, and taking corrective action. In areas where the overall quality of government-run health services is low, immunization services may also be avoided due to low credibility and a trust deficit between the communities and public facilities. Public sector salaries are often lower than equivalently qualified workers in the private sector. However, public facilities are often perceived to be wasteful compared to their counterparts in PNFP or PFP facilities. The main sources of inefficiency may be due to high fixed costs for personnel and facility maintenance and utilities, as well as high slack capacity, especially in a context of low utilization.

1.5.7.2 Private not-for-profit providers

PNFP facilities are common in many LMICs and may contribute up to 40% of health service outputs such as vaccinations (Levin & Kaddar, 2011). They are often located in rural or other hard-to-reach areas of a country and thus serve as a source of much-needed services where public facilities do not exist and where there may be no incentive for PFP clinics to operate. This promotes equity in immunization delivery. The fact that they often depend on unpredictable donations, either from local sources or from foreign donors, makes their sustainability rather uncertain. Nevertheless, these facilities often benefit from government subsidies when conducive policies exist. Given that many of these PNFPs may have a faith-based orientation, at least in their origins and often in their management, they may be perceived to be community oriented and motivated by a strong sense of service and community solidarity. However, some segments of the population may hesitate to access them if they do not feel welcome due to being of a different faith. There have also been concerns about PNFP facilities, for budgetary reasons, employing staff who have fewer professional qualifications than their public facility counterparts. General technical competence was found to be lower in private facilities than public in one review of the literature (Berendes, Heywood, Oliver, & Garner, 2011). Health workers' knowledge of immunization schedules, waste, and vaccine management practices were found lacking in private facilities in a study of Cambodia (Soeung, Grundy, Morn, & Samnang, 2008).

1.5.7.3 Private clinics and practitioners

Private sector vaccine delivery offered by PFP clinics may exacerbate health inequities. A study of private sector *Haemophilus influenzae* type b vaccine coverage in India found that coverage was mainly limited to richer and more urbanized states (Sharma, Kaplan, Chokshi, Hasan Farooqui, & Zodpey, 2015).

In the US, adult immunization is mainly performed by private providers (Hinman, Orenstein, & Rodewald, 2004). Private providers recover costs through public and private insurance reimbursements for vaccine purchase and administration (O'Leary et al., 2014). However, a national survey carried out among private pediatricians and family physicians found that many of them are dissatisfied with insurance payments for immunization (O'Leary et al., 2014). Vaccine costs, which made up a minor part of the overheads of a private pediatric practice in the 1980s, are now one of the top overhead expenses largely due to new vaccines. This increases the risk of uncompensated costs to private providers in the US (American Academy of Pediatrics, 2006). Many physicians reported delaying offering vaccines to patients if insurance coverage is not certain (Hurley et al., 2017; O'Leary et al., 2014). This is a concerning trend, since physician recommendation has been found to play a crucial role in a patient's vaccination (Hurley et al., 2017).

Although PFP providers deliver a limited proportion of immunization services in LMICs, their activities are garnering more attention. In addition to providing traditional World Health Organization Expanded Program on Immunization vaccines to those who can afford to pay, private providers also introduce new and underutilized vaccines (Levin & Kaddar, 2011). However, they are more susceptible to market pressures than public providers. As such, they are often targeted by pharmaceutical marketing campaigns to introduce new and costly vaccines, and sometimes deviate from national immunization schedules (Levin & Kaddar, 2011; World Health Organization, 2018). Deviating from the national immunization schedule can have deleterious effects, such as increasing the risk of vaccine-preventable diseases or confusing the population, thereby reducing trust in the health system (World Health Organization, 2018). Nevertheless, individuals may choose private providers over public providers for immunization for a variety of reasons, including convenience from being closer or operating at better hours; they are the only providers of a particular vaccine; or they are perceived to provide better quality services than public providers (Amarasinghe, Davison, & Diorditsa, 2018; Levin & Kaddar, 2011). Yet, studies from several countries have revealed a number of quality concerns that can limit the efficiency of PFP immunization services, such as substandard vaccine storage practices and lack of knowledge on waste and vaccine management practices (Levin & Kaddar, 2011; Soeung et al., 2008). While the financial sustainability of PFP immunization may not be of concern, since providers mainly cater to those who can afford it, this attribute raises equity concerns. Studies conducted in LMICs confirm these concerns as they show that individuals who seek immunization services from these providers tend to be of a higher socioeconomic status or have a higher income (Levin & Kaddar, 2011).

1.5.7.4 Mixed delivery

Each financing and delivery system has its advantages and disadvantages. Some countries have opted for a mixed approach, which includes public and private funding and delivery of immunization.

For instance, Ghana and Indonesia provide free immunizations to their populations through private and public providers using mostly government budgetary funds with some contributions from their NHISs (Results for Development, 2017). While still adopting a mixed-financing system, Thailand provides all health services, including immunization, through a social health insurance scheme that is funded through general taxation (Results for Development, 2017).

Since 2016, he Malaysian government has been establishing an NHIS to facilitate integration between the public and private sectors and improve access to vaccines (Coe et al., 2017). However, mixed financing systems pose certain challenges. While funds from their NHISs have helped to diversify Ghana's and Indonesia's immunization financing, there is the risk of curative services being prioritized over immunization and other preventive care for different reasons. In Ghana, salaries are taking up an increasing proportion of the Ministry of Health budget, which has made public facilities more dependent on NHIS claims for payments for immunization delivery. However, these payments are only received for curative care (Results for Development, 2017). In Indonesia, capitation payments made by the NHIS, known as JKN, to primary care providers for immunization are sometimes diverted to curative care due to confusion among providers and local governments, which are responsible for covering service delivery costs in Indonesia's decentralized health system (Results for Development, 2017).

As many LMICs move toward mixed financing and health insurance scheme models for immunization, they can learn from the experiences of high-income countries, like the US, with similar financing models. In the US, immunization is provided through a mix of public and private providers via government and private financing. In 1993, the US government passed the Vaccines for Children (VFC) Act, which sets aside funding to immunize children who are uninsured, on Medicaid, or who are American Indians/Alaska Natives free of charge (Hinman et al., 2004; Robinson, Sepe, & Lin, 1993). The VFC Act also provides free vaccines at federally qualified health centers for insured children without immunization coverage (Robinson et al., 1993). Through the VFC program, the federal government purchases a sizeable share of pediatric vaccines. However, approximately half of pediatric vaccines are purchased by private pediatricians and family physicians, who vaccinate most US children (Hill, Elam-Evans, Yankey, Singleton, & Kang, 2018; Tayloe, 2009).

While collaboration with the private sector has helped many governments to improve their NIPs, there have also been drawbacks. For instance, public financing is not always sufficient to meet the needs of private practices. In the US, many private providers participating in the VFC program have expressed dissatisfaction with reimbursements they receive from public insurers (O'Leary et al., 2014). As of 2016, it was reported that private practices lose approximately $5–$15 for each dose of VFC vaccine administered (Diasio, 2016).

1.5.8 Discussion

We have discussed the pros and cons of using public, PNFP, PFP, and mixed immunization delivery options from the perspectives of the five domains of efficiency, sustainability, equity, quality, and coverage (immunization financing is further discussed in Chapter 5). While there is no single best solution, some lessons emerge and can guide country immunization policymakers in choosing the approach which works best in their setting. For LMICs to enjoy the full benefits of immunization, they must be able to commit to long-term financing requirements (Results for Development, 2017). From 2000, Gavi, the Vaccine Alliance financed the provision of vaccines that contributed to saving the lives of millions of children in over 75 of the world's poorest countries (Gavi, 2019). With or without external donor support, countries need to find new ways to finance their national immunization portfolios in the context of increasing cost of new vaccines (Saxenian et al., 2015). One estimate suggested that African countries needed approximately US $17 billion to finance vaccine purchases and service delivery between 2016 and 2020 (Songane, 2018).

Unsurprisingly, there appears to be no universally successful approach to immunization financing and no one vaccine delivery approach works best in different contexts even in the same country. All countries, and especially LMICs, need to adopt flexible vaccine delivery and financing models that best suit their various contexts. However, country experiences show a few commonalities in terms of factors to consider in the design and adoption of vaccine delivery systems. These include the need for clearly defined responsibilities in the system, leveraging both public and private sector mechanisms, strong supervision of both public and private sector providers to ensure performance according to international and national standards, as well as approaches to reduce inequities and ensure that immunization is prioritized in the health system as a public good. Private providers of immunization need access to public resources such as technical support, skills building and training opportunities, and financial subsidies in recognition of their contribution to the public good.

In order to achieve equity of immunizations, countries need to deliver vaccines through providers who are more readily accessible to communities near to where they live regardless of whether these are public, PNFP, or PFP providers. Achieving efficiency does not have to come at the cost of equity if all the resources available in the community are leveraged. Involving the private sector to deliver immunizations in countries where the public facilities offer the bulk of immunizations will help alleviate the burden on these often-underfunded services, while leveraging the innovation and additional infrastructure and personnel resources of the private sector. However, private facilities will need additional support through skills-based training funded by the public sector, as well as access to guidelines and technical support available in the public sector to ensure adherence to national and international standards.

1.5.9 Conclusion

An integrated immunization delivery system which leverages the respective strengths of the public and private sectors, delivering the life-saving and cost-effective vaccines to whomever and wherever they are needed, will contribute to socioeconomic development and help reduce inequities in health status. For countries where immunization is traditionally largely delivered through expensive, inefficient public delivery systems, it is time to try a new approach which prioritizes immunization regardless of who is delivering it. Finding ways to leverage available private sector providers in a way that does not impose too much of a financial burden on them will yield better coverage rates and healthier people, while ensuring better prospects for achieving health goals sustainably.

References

Ahmad, N. A., Jahis, R., Kuay, L. K., Jamaluddin, R., & Aris, T. (2017). Primary immunization among children in Malaysia: Reasons for incomplete vaccination. *Journal of Vaccines & Vaccination, 8*(3), 358. doi:10.4172/2157-7560.1000358

Amarasinghe, A., Davison, L., & Diorditsa, S. (2018). Engagement of private providers in immunization in the Western Pacific region. *Vaccine, 36*(32, Part B), 4958–4962. doi:10.1016/j.vaccine.2018.01.008

American Academy of Pediatrics. (2006). *The business case for pricing vaccines and immunization administration*. Washington, DC: American Academy of Pediatrics.

Beaulieu-Volk, D. (2014). Immunizations: How to make this vital service financially viable. Experts offer best practices related to smart purchasing, inventory control, and reducing waste. *Medical Economics, 91*(3), 68–72. https://pubmed.ncbi.nlm.nih.gov/25211950/

Berendes, S., Heywood, P., Oliver, S., & Garner, P. (2011). Quality of private and public ambulatory health care in low and middle income countries: Systematic review of comparative studies. *PLoS Medicine, 8*(4), e1000433. doi:10.1371/journal.pmed.1000433

Berman, S. (2008). Is our vaccine system at risk for a future financial "meltdown?" *Pediatrics, 122*(6), 1372. doi:10.1542/peds.2008-2881

Brenzel, L., Young, D., & Walker, D. G. (2015). Costs and financing of routine immunization: Approach and selected findings of a multi-country study (EPIC). *Vaccine, 33*, A13–A20. doi:10.1016/j.vaccine.2014.12.066

Burton, A., Monasch, R., Lautenbach, B., Gacic-Dobo, M., Neill, M., Karimov, R., . . . Birmingham, M. (2009). WHO and UNICEF estimates of national infant immunization coverage: Methods and processes. *Bulletin of the World Health Organization, 87*(7), 535–541. doi:10.2471/blt.08.053819

Cherian, T., & Mantel, C. (2020). National immunization programmes. *Bundesgesundheitsblatt—Gesundheitsforschung—Gesundheitsschutz, 63*(1), 16–24. doi:10.1007/s00103-019-03062-1

Coe, M., Gergen, J., Mallow, M., Moi, F., & Phily, C. (2017). *Sustainable immunization financing in Asia Pacific.* Washington, DC: ThinkWell.

Diasio, C. (2016, February 9). Pediatric vaccination: Who bears the burden? *HealthAffairs.* https://www.healthaffairs.org/do/10.1377/hblog20160209.053058/full/

Gavi. (2018). *Annual program report.* https://www.gavi.org/sites/default/files/publications/progress-reports/Gavi-Progress-Report-2018.pdf

Gavi. (2019). *Annual program report.* https://www.gavi.org/sites/default/files/programmes-impact/our-impact/apr/Gavi-Progress-Report-2019_1.pdf

Hill, H. A., Elam-Evans, L. D., Yankey, D., Singleton, J. A., & Kang, Y. (2018). Coverage among children aged 19–35 months—United States, 2017. *Morbidity and Mortality Weekly Report, 67*, 1123–1128. doi:10.15585/mmwr.mm6740a4

Hinman, A. R., Orenstein, W. A., & Rodewald, L. (2004). Financing immunizations in the United States. *Clinical Infectious Diseases, 38*(10), 1440–1446. doi:10.1086/420748

Hurley, L. P., Lindley, M. C., Allison, M. A., Crane, L. A., Brtnikova, M., Beaty, B. L., . . . Kempe, A. (2017). Primary care physicians' perspective on financial issues and adult immunization in the Era of the Affordable Care Act. *Vaccine, 35*(4), 647–654. doi:10.1016/j.vaccine.2016.12.007

Levin, A., & Kaddar, M. (2011). Role of the private sector in the provision of immunization services in low- and middle-income countries. *Health Policy and Planning, 26*(Suppl 1), i4–i12. doi:10.1093/heapol/czr037

Lim, K. K., Chan, Y. Y., Noor Ani, A., Rohani, J., Siti Norfadhilah, Z. A., & Santhi, M. R. (2017). Complete immunization coverage and its determinants among children in Malaysia: Findings from the National Health and Morbidity Survey (NHMS) 2016. *Public Health, 153*, 52–57. doi:10.1016/j.puhe.2017.08.001

Maharani, A., & Tampubolon, G. (2014). Has decentralisation affected child immunisation status in Indonesia? *Global Health Action, 7*, 24913. doi:10.3402/gha.v7.24913

McLaughlin, J. M., Swerdlow, D. L., Khan, F., Will, O., Curry, A., Snow, V., . . . Jodar, L. (2019). Disparities in uptake of 13-valent pneumococcal conjugate vaccine among older adults in the United States. *Human Vaccines & Immunotherapeutics, 15*(4), 841–849. doi:10.1080/21645515.2018.1564434

Menzies, N. A., Suharlim, C., Geng, F., Ward, Z. J., Brenzel, L., & Resch, S. C. (2017). The cost determinants of routine infant immunization services: A meta-regression analysis of six country studies. *BMC Medicine, 15*(1), 178. doi:10.1186/s12916-017-0942-1

Menzies, N. A., Suharlim, C., Resch, S. C., & Brenzel, L. (2020). The efficiency of routine infant immunization services in six countries: A comparison of methods. *Health Economics Review, 10*(1), 1. doi:10.1186/s13561-019-0259-1

Mosadeghrad, A. M. (2012). A conceptual framework for quality of care. *Materia Socio-medica, 24*(4), 251–261. doi:10.5455/msm.2012.24.251-261

O'Leary, S. T., Allison, M. A., Lindley, M. C., Crane, L. A., Hurley, L. P., Brtnikova, M., . . . Kempe, A. (2014). Vaccine financing from the perspective of primary care physicians. *Pediatrics, 133*(3), 367–374. doi:10.1542/peds.2013-2637

O'Malley, A. S., & Forrest, C. B. (2006). Immunization disparities in older Americans: Determinants and future research needs. *American Journal of Preventive Medicine, 31*(2), 150–158. doi:10.1016/j.amepre.2006.03.021

Results for Development. (2017). *Immunization financing: a resource guide for advocates, policymakers, and program managers.* https://r4d.org/resources/immunization-financing-resource-guide-advocates-policymakers-program-managers/

Robinson, C. A., Sepe, S. J., & Lin, K. F. (1993). The president's child immunization initiative—a summary of the problem and the response. *Public Health Reports (Washington, D.C.: 1974)*, *108*(4), 419–425. https://www.ncbi.nlm.nih.gov/pmc/articles/PMC1403402/

Saxenian, H., Hecht, R., Kaddar, M., Schmitt, S., Ryckman, T., & Cornejo, S. (2015). Overcoming challenges to sustainable immunization financing: Early experiences from GAVI graduating countries. *Health Policy and Planning*, *30*(2), 197–205. doi:10.1093/heapol/czu003

Schwartz, J. B., & Bhushan, I. (2004). Improving immunization equity through a public-private partnership in Cambodia. *Bulletin of the World Health Organization*, *82*(9), 661–667. https://www.ncbi.nlm.nih.gov/pmc/articles/PMC2622985/

Sharma, A., Kaplan, W. A., Chokshi, M., Hasan Farooqui, H., & Zodpey, S. P. (2015). Implications of private sector Hib vaccine coverage for the introduction of public sector Hib-containing pentavalent vaccine in India: Evidence from retrospective time series data. *BMJ Open*, *5*(2), e007038. doi:10.1136/bmjopen-2014-007038

Silver, D., Blustein, J., & Weitzman, B. C. (2012). Transportation to clinic: Findings from a pilot clinic-based survey of low-income suburbanites. *Journal of Immigrant and Minority Health*, *14*(2), 350–355. doi:10.1007/s10903-010-9410-0

Soeung, S. C., Grundy, J., Morn, C., & Samnang, C. (2008). Evaluation of immunization knowledge, practices, and service-delivery in the private sector in Cambodia. *Journal of Health, Population and Nutrition*, *26*(1), 95–104. https://www.ncbi.nlm.nih.gov/pmc/articles/PMC2740687/

Songane, M. (2018). Challenges for nationwide vaccine delivery in African countries. *International Journal of Health Economics and Management*, *18*(2), 197–219. doi:10.1007/s10754-017-9229-5

Tanahashi, T. (1978). Health service coverage and its evaluation. *Bulletin of the World Health Organization*, *56*(2), 295–303. https://www.ncbi.nlm.nih.gov/pmc/articles/PMC2395571/

Tayloe, D. T. (2009). Immunization financing: Key area for American Academy of Pediatrics advocacy. *Pediatrics*, *124*(Suppl 5), S455. doi:10.1542/peds.2009-1542C

World Health Organization. (2010). *Monitoring the building blocks of health systems: A handbook of indicators and their measurement strategies.* https://apps.who.int/iris/bitstream/handle/10665/258734/9789241564052-eng.pdf

World Health Organization. (2013). *Global vaccine action plan 2011–2020.* https://www.who.int/publications/i/item/global-vaccine-action-plan-2011-2020

World Health Organization. (2018). *WHO guidance note: Engagement of private providers in immunization service delivery. Considerations for national immunization programmes.* https://www.who.int/publications/i/item/WHO-IVB-17.15

World Health Organization: Regional Office for the Western Pacific. (2012). *Malaysia health system review.* https://apps.who.int/iris/handle/10665/206911

2

ESTIMATING THE COST OF IMMUNIZATION SERVICES

Edited by Logan Brenzel

2.0
Section introduction: estimating the cost of immunization services

Logan Brenzel

Immunization costing is concerned with identifying, measuring, and valuing the resources used to deliver immunization services. Resources are defined as the inputs used to vaccinate, such as labor time, vaccines, and medical supplies. Immunization services pertain to vaccinations offered through the national immunization program, at a district level, as part of a campaign or other delivery strategy, or through a new vaccine introduction initiative.

It is useful to distinguish primary costing studies from cost modeling exercises. When resources have been (or are being) consumed to deliver an already-implemented immunization service, a primary costing study is carried out to estimate the quantities of resources consumed and their associated monetary value. The study will involve collecting and analyzing primary data on resource use, program output, and other program characteristics. Data sources typically include a mix of sources including financial and other administrative records, surveys, interviews, and—sometimes—direct observation.

In contrast, some costing modeling exercises aim to forecast the cost of implementing a new immunization service, scaling up existing services, or some other change to immunization policy, prior to these changes occurring, in order to set budgets, mobilize resources, or inform decisions about whether or not to move forward with a proposed policy change. These cost modeling exercises typically draw on information regarding the cost of immunization services that have already been implemented, and thus depend, in part, on information from primary costing studies.

This section of the handbook covers methods for primary costing studies of implemented vaccine programs as well as cost modeling exercises for projecting the resource requirement of (future) new vaccine introduction.

Logan Brenzel, *Section introduction: estimating the cost of immunization services* In: *Handbook of Applied Health Economics in Vaccines*. Edited by: David Bishai, Logan Brenzel and William V. Padula, Oxford University Press. © Oxford University Press 2023. DOI: 10.1093/oso/9780192896087.003.0007

Chapter 2.1 motivates the section with an overview of the many uses of cost estimates from primary studies, and helps readers navigate a large set of existing guides, tools, and other technical resources for immunization costing. Chapter 2.2 provides an overview of key concepts and definitions. Chapter 2.3 covers key elements of costing study design. Chapter 2.4 covers the methods for data analysis. Chapter 2.5 illustrates how to apply methods for evaluating new vaccine introduction. This section also links to two appendices that contain exercises related to costing a routine immunization program (Appendix 1, Costing Exercise) and introducing a new vaccine (Appendix 2, Costing New Vaccine Introduction). ⬛ Additional content on (Costing Exercise and Costing New Vaccine Introduction) is available online, 10.1093/oso/9780192896087.012.0001.

2.1

Why costing studies are needed

Ann Levin, Stephen Resch, and Logan Brenzel

2.1.1 Introduction

Information regarding the cost of immunization services can be useful for a range of policy and program management processes. Estimating the cost of immunization programs is important for several reasons, including: (1) strategic planning and program budgeting; (2) assessing variation in service delivery costs and analysis of program efficiency or quality; (3) developing cost benchmarks; and (4) conducting cost-effectiveness analysis (CEA), cost–benefit analysis (CBA), and return on investment analysis to inform resource allocation decisions. The intended purpose of the analysis will determine subsequent study design choices, including the methods and the type of data to be collected.

2.1.2 Immunization program strategic planning and budgeting

Program managers can use information on the cost of immunization services to plan for implementation of their program activities, prepare immunization program budgets, develop multi-year strategic plans, and inform policy decisions such as whether to introduce a new vaccine. Managers can understand the relative magnitude of resource requirements for different vaccination activities, including the inputs or activities that account for the largest shares of total cost (cost drivers). Costing studies can offer insights regarding the share of program cost attributable to categories of resources (vaccines, labor), program activities (supply chain, facility-based vaccine administration, outreach), or organizational level (health facility, district, national). Understanding what may be driving up costs of services can lead to

Ann Levin, Stephen Resch, and Logan Brenzel, *Why costing studies are needed* In: *Handbook of Applied Health Economics in Vaccines*. Edited by: David Bishai, Logan Brenzel and William V. Padula, Oxford University Press. © Oxford University Press 2023. DOI: 10.1093/oso/9780192896087.003.0008 better management choices in how resources can be utilized. Another output of costing studies useful for program planning is a set of activity-specific unit costs such as cost per dose delivered via campaigns, or cost per dose delivered via routine facility-based services.

Evidence generated by costing studies can subsequently be used in cost modeling exercises to project the resources required in the future under different policy scenarios. This type of cost modeling is a common part of strategic planning used to ensure program goals are aligned with the expected available resources and to support mobilization of additional resources when needed. Estimates of annual or multi-year resource requirements can be used to advocate for funding for the program or new interventions such as a new vaccine introduction. Cost projections can also factor into budget impact analysis of adding a new vaccine or delivering services in a different manner.

2.1.3 Assessing variation in the cost of immunization service delivery

The analyst can use information on unit costs to compare variation in the cost of vaccination among health facilities, districts, or other administrative levels, or for different types of service delivery.

Cost estimation is important for assessing the technical efficiency of vaccination, which is how effective the program is in turning a set of inputs into a performance output (vaccinated child or dose delivered). A recent analysis (Geng, Suharlim, Brenzel, Resch, & Menzies, 2017) compares total and unit costs of delivering a dose of vaccine for a sample of facilities and subnational administrative units in six countries to determine which locations provided the greatest level services for the least amount of cost. Sites that were the most efficient were those that had lower shares of labor costs, either because of less time allocated or different staff complements, or both. This information can then be used to identify ways to improve the efficiency of service delivery. Hence, cost information can be used to determine whether specific inputs, such as personnel time, are translating into productive outputs.

2.1.4 Developing benchmarks

Another reason to estimate immunization costs is to develop unit cost benchmarks such as cost per vaccine dose administered or cost per fully immunized child. If country-specific information is unavailable, cost benchmarks can be helpful in filling the gap in information. A recent dataset of immunization delivery costs was developed (Portnoy et al., 2020). The World Health Organization (WHO) Choosing Interventions that are Cost-Effective (CHOICE) program created benchmarks for a range of healthcare costs (Stenberg, Lauer, Gkountouras, Fitzpatrick, & Stanciole, 2018). Benchmarks can also be used to develop or evaluate grant applications or as inputs to cost modeling exercises projecting financial requirements of a policy change.

2.1.5 Economic evaluations

Economic evaluations such as CEA, CBA, and return on investment calculations can be used to make choices among vaccination delivery strategies, among new vaccines, and among new vaccination technologies to maximize the use of available resources to obtain health impacts. To conduct these analyses, it is necessary to have data on both costs and effectiveness or benefits.

CEA and CBA are useful for determining whether a health intervention provides good value for money (compared to some alternative) and are used to inform resource allocation decisions. A CEA reflects the change in costs associated with a new intervention such as new vaccine introduction, compared to a change in effectiveness of the program, such as number of deaths or disability adjusted life-years (DALYs) averted. For instance, a policymaker might be interested to know whether it is a good investment to introduce a measles–rubella vaccine into their program: a study comparing the incremental costs with the incremental benefits would provide the answer to that question. There is an extensive literature on the cost-effectiveness of vaccines and technologies for the immunization program (Edoka et al., 2021; Jit, Brisson, Portnoy, & Hutubessy, 2014; Le et al., 2015; Levin, Levin, Kristensen, & Matthias, 2007; Novaes et al., 2015; Ozawa et al., 2017). A systematic review found that the cost/DALY of new vaccines ranges from less than $100 to less than $1,000 per DALY averted (Ozawa, Mirelman, Stack, Walker, & Levine, 2012). Chapters 3 and 4 go into further detail on how to conduct these types of analyses.

CBAs are similar to CEAs except that the benefits of the interventions are monetized rather than expressed as units of health such as deaths, life-years, or DALYs. A CBA calculates the net monetary benefit of a program (compared to a next-best alternative). This allows for the immunization program to be compared to other health and non-health interventions, such as comparing with a nutrition program to determine the best allocation of resources.

Return on investment analyses are used to estimate the ratio between the monetary benefits of a vaccination program divided by the costs. For instance, a recent study showed that for every $1 invested in the vaccines supported by Gavi, countries would yield a return of $21 based on productivity losses due to illness (Sim et al., 2020). A key driver of vaccine value is often treatment costs that are averted. Some economic evaluations may also include health-care costs related to vaccination or vaccine-preventable disease, as well as productivity impacts.

2.1.6 Resources available on immunization costing

This part of the chapter describes the key resources for readers related to costing methodologies and application to field-based studies.

2.1.6.1 Resource guides

A number of resource guides are available on methods for immunization costing. Several resource guides have come out of a Community of Practice on immunization economics, including " How to cost immunization programs: A practical guide for primary data collection and analysis." This guide discusses methods involved for cross-sectional retrospective costing of routine immunization services, derived from a sample of health facilities and provides standardized terminology and costing units, approaches to data collection and data requirements, guidance on facility sampling, and recommendations for analysis, write-up, and presentation (Resch et al., 2020).

Another resource, "How to conduct an immunization campaign costing study: Methodological guidance," provides guidance on costing of a wide variety of immunization campaigns, such as a national planned campaign, an integrated campaign that provides multiple vaccines or vaccines and other health services, or outbreak response campaigns (ThinkWell, 2021).

The Global Health Cost Consortium's reference case was developed for improving the comparability and quality of cost estimates for health interventions and is also relevant to immunization programs. This guide focuses not only on definitions of costing terms but also on principles of "good" costing organized around a checklist (Vassall et al., 2017). For example, one principle is to define the study design: purpose of the analysis, the perspective, types of cost, time horizon, and the definition of units. Other principles are resource use measurement (such as scope of costing, measuring resource use, and sampling), pricing and valuation (sources of price data, valuing capital inputs, and discount, inflation, and conversion rates), and analyzing and presenting results (exploring cost functions and heterogeneity, uncertainty, and transparency).

The Second US Panel on Cost-Effectiveness in Health and Medicine also provides useful guidance (Neumann, Ganiats, Russell, Sanders, & Siegel, 2016). This update to the first US Panel on Cost-effectiveness in Health and Medicine (Gold, Siegel, Russell, & Weinstein, 1996) provides recommendations on methods for costing and CEA, such that reference case analyses should include societal as well as health sector perspectives. Regarding costs, it makes recommendations about the components that should be included in costing of health services, inclusion of future costs, and discounting.

The WHO also has developed some resource guides and tools for costing. The WHO "Guideline for estimating the costs of introducing new vaccines into the national immunization system" contains a useful framework for identifying which cost elements will be affected by new vaccine introduction and how to project incremental costs. For instance, new vaccines will require additional space in the national cold chain and the guide highlights methods for estimating additional needs and associated costs (WHO: Immunization Vaccines and Biologicals, 2002). The WHO "Guide for standardization of economic evaluations of immunization programs" focuses on methods associated with different types of economic evaluations, and includes approaches to modeling, discounting, and interpretation of results (WHO: Immunization Vaccines and Biologicals, 2019).

The Pan American Health Organization developed COSTVAC which provides a template for selecting a sample of facilities, and analyzing cost data (Pan American Health Organization, 2019).

The WHO also has developed costing tools for estimation of incremental costs of either introducing new vaccines or estimating retrospective costs of single-vaccine implementation. These costing tools focus specifically on introduction of a single antigen, such as the Cervical Cancer Prevention and Control Costing Tool (Hutubessy et al., 2012) for estimation of human papillomavirus vaccination cost and the Seasonal Influenza Immunization Costing Tool (Pallas et al., 2020) for estimation of annual costs of introducing seasonal influenza vaccination to populations at highest risk, such as pregnant women and health workers. Other tools developed jointly with the International Vaccine Institute include CholTool, which can be used to estimate projected or retrospective incremental costs of preventive and outbreak responses with oral cholera vaccine campaigns (Morgan, Levin, Hutubessy, & Mogasale, 2020), and the Typhoid Conjugate Vaccine Costing Tool (TCVCT). Finally, WHO and UNICEF developed a spreadsheet tool to estimate the resource requirements for implementing the national immunization programs (comprehensive Multi-Year Plan Costing Tool; WHO: Immunization Vaccines and Biologicals, 2014). This tool helps countries to plan and identify needed financing for the program in order to achieve programmatic objectives.

Table 2.1.1 compares and contrasts the recommended uses of the various resources and tools available. This handbook draws from much of the work that has proceeded, and readers are encouraged to utilize this core material.

Table 2.1.1 Comparison of guides and tools for costing immunization programs

Resource guides and costing tools	Main emphasis	Recommended use
How to cost immunization programs: A practical guide for primary data collection and analysis	Application of costing methods to retrospective primary cost data collection, analysis, and policy dialogue on costs of routine immunization programs	Methodological guidance, design, and implementation of field-based studies in lower-income settings
How to conduct an immunization campaign costing study: Methodological guidance	Application of costing methods to retrospective primary cost data collection, analysis, and policy dialogue on costs of immunization campaigns	Design and implementation of field-based studies in lower-income settings
Global Health Cost Consortium reference case	Definitions and methods	Reference and methodological guidance
Second Panel on Cost-Effectiveness in Health and Medicine	Methods for costing and CEA	Reference and methodological guidance
WHO guideline for estimating the costs of introducing new vaccines into the national immunization system	Application of costing methods to retrospective primary cost data collection, analysis, and policy dialogue on costs of introducing new vaccines	Methodological guidance, design, and implementation of field-based studies in lower-income settings
WHO guide for standardization of economic evaluations of immunization programs	Methods for different types of economic evaluations	Reference and methodological guidance
PAHO COSTVAC	Methodology and tool for analyzing health facility immunization costs	Methods, sampling, and practical cost estimation tool

Table 2.1.1 Continued

Resource guides and costing tools	Main emphasis	Recommended use
WHO Cervical Cancer Prevention and Control Costing Tool	Data collection and analysis, policy dialogue	Estimating the cost of human papillomavirus vaccination and other interventions to control cervical cancer
WHO vaccine-specific costing tools (Seasonal Influenza Immunization Costing Tool; CholTool; TCVCT)	Data collection and analysis, policy dialogue	Estimating the cost of influenza, cholera, and typhoid vaccination
Comprehensive Multi-Year Plan Costing Tool	Estimation of immunization-specific and shared costs for achieving national program objectives	3–5-year planning of the resource needs for the national immunization program
National Immunization Strategy Costing Tool	Estimation of costs and budgets for achieving national program objectives	Annual and up to 5-year planning and budgeting for the national immunization program
Consensus Statement	Review and recommendation for future costing work	Reference
Immunization Delivery Cost Compendium (IDCC)	Up-to-date compendium of published and unpublished immunization costing studies	Reference, country results, and comparisons
DataVerse	Datasets from country immunization costing studies	Data analysis
Teaching Vaccine Economics Everywhere (TVEE)	Teaching materials related to economic evaluation of immunization programs	Teaching

2.1.6.2 Other resources

The various resources on immunization and health costing have commonalities as well as differences in their methodologies. Most of these differences can be attributed to the distinct purposes and objectives of the guides. Four dimensions of immunization cost estimation have been identified: (1) retrospective routine immunization cross-sectional costs, (2) retrospective single-vaccine costs, (3) projection of new vaccine introduction costs, and (4) projection of national immunization program costs. Recently, the WHO led the development of a Consensus Statement in order to harmonize and better align the principles, terminologies, and approaches used for immunization costing studies (Levin et al., 2022). The Consensus Statement will serve as a reference point to promote continued improvement and innovation in methods and tools, as well as to inform the principles and definitions that will make costing results more easily interpretable and useful.

The Immunization Delivery Cost Catalogue contains a wealth of published and unpublished immunization costing studies (ThinkWell, 2020). This downloadable database provides estimates on cost per dose and cost per child, as well as the characteristics and details on the methods used in the individual studies. This resource contains 192 datapoints from 62 individual country studies from 2015.

Downloadable datasets from immunization costing studies from a variety of countries and covering a range of immunization strategies are available from DataVerse (https://dataverse.harvard.edu/dataverse/EPIC).

Finally, teaching materials, course outlines, case studies, and curricula related to economic evaluation of immunization programs can be accessed online (Teaching Vaccine Economics Everywhere, 2021).

2.1.7 Conclusion

Immunization costing studies generate essential strategic information that program managers and policymakers require for planning and budgeting, policy decision-making, assessing technical efficiency, developing benchmarks, and economic evaluation to inform resource allocation decisions. While primary costing studies measure resource use for immunization services that have been implemented or are ongoing, the resulting cost estimates can be used as an input to cost modeling exercises designed to inform decisions about future immunization activities.

References

Edoka, I., Kohli-Lynch, C. N., Fraser, H., Hofman, K., Tempia, S., McMorrow, M., . . . Cohen, C. (2021). A cost-effectiveness analysis of South Africa's seasonal influenza vaccination programme. *Vaccine*, *39*(2), 412–422. doi:10.1016/j.vaccine.2020.11.028

Geng, F., Suharlim, C., Brenzel, L., Resch, S. C., & Menzies, N. A. (2017). The cost structure of routine infant immunization services: A systematic analysis of six countries. *Health Policy and Planning*, *32*(8), 1174–1184. doi:10.1093/heapol/czx067

Gold, M. R., Siegel, J., Russell, L., & Weinstein, M. (1996). *Cost-effectiveness in health and medicine*. New York, NY: Oxford University Press.

Hutubessy, R., Levin, A., Wang, S., Morgan, W., Ally, M., John, T., & Broutet, N. (2012). A case study using the United Republic of Tanzania: Costing nationwide HPV vaccine delivery using the WHO cervical cancer prevention and control costing tool. *BMC Medicine*, *10*(1), 136. doi:10.1186/1741-7015-10-136

Jit, M., Brisson, M., Portnoy, A., & Hutubessy, R. (2014). Cost-effectiveness of female human papillomavirus vaccination in 179 countries: A PRIME modelling study. *Lancet Global Health*, 2(7), e406–414. doi:10.1016/s2214-109x(14)70237-2

Le, P., Griffiths, U. K., Anh, D. D., Franzini, L., Chan, W., & Swint, J. M. (2015). Cost-effectiveness of Haemophilus influenzae type b vaccine in Vietnam. *Vaccine*, 33(36), 4639–4646. doi:10.1016/j.vaccine.2015.05.050

Levin, A., Levin, C., Kristensen, D., & Matthias, D. (2007). An economic evaluation of thermostable vaccines in Cambodia, Ghana and Bangladesh. *Vaccine*, 25(39), 6945–6957. doi:10.1016/j.vaccine.2007.06.065

Levin, A., Boonstoppel, L., Brenzel, L., Griffiths, U., Hutubessy, R., Jit, M., . . . Yeung, K.H.T. (2022). WHO-led consensus statement on vaccine delivery costing: Process, methods and findings. *BMC Medicine*, 20(1), 88. doi:10.1186/s12916-022-02278-4

Morgan, W., Levin, A., Hutubessy, R. C., & Mogasale, V. (2020). Costing oral cholera vaccine delivery using a generic oral cholera vaccine delivery planning and costing tool (CholTool). *Human Vaccines & Immunotherapeutics*, 16(12), 3111–3118. doi:10.1080/21645515.2020.1747930

Neumann, P., Ganiats, T., Russell, L., Sanders, G., & Siegel, J. (2016). *Cost-effectiveness in health and medicine*. New York, NY: Oxford University Press.

Novaes, H. M., de Soárez, P. C., Silva, G. A., Ayres, A., Itria, A., Rama, C. H., . . . Resch, S. (2015). Cost-effectiveness analysis of introducing universal human papillomavirus vaccination of girls aged 11 years into the National Immunization Program in Brazil. *Vaccine*, 33(Suppl 1), A135–A142. doi:10.1016/j.vaccine.2014.12.031

Ozawa, S., Clark, S., Portnoy, A., Grewal, S., Stack, M. L., Sinha, A., . . . Walker, D. (2017). Estimated economic impact of vaccinations in 73 low- and middle-income countries, 2001–2020. *Bulletin of the World Health Organization*, 95(9), 629–638. doi:10.2471/blt.16.178475

Ozawa, S., Mirelman, A., Stack, M. L., Walker, D., & Levine, O. S. (2012). Cost-effectiveness and economic benefits of vaccines in low- and middle-income countries: A systematic review. *Vaccine*, 31(1), 96–108. doi:10.1016/j.vaccine.2012.10.103

Pallas, S. W., Ahmeti, A., Morgan, W., Preza, I., Nelaj, E., Ebama, M., . . . Bino, S. (2020). Program cost analysis of influenza vaccination of health care workers in Albania. *Vaccine*, 38(2), 220–227. doi:10.1016/j.vaccine.2019.10.027

Pan American Health Organization. (2019). *COSTVAC.* http://immunizationeconomics.org/recent-activity/2019/9/23/update-of-pahos-provac-e-toolkit

Portnoy, A., Vaughan, K., Clarke-Deelder, E., Suharlim, C., Resch, S. C., Brenzel, L., & Menzies, N. A. (2020). Producing standardized country-level immunization delivery unit cost estimates. *PharmacoEconomics*, 38(9), 995–1005. doi:10.1007/s40273-020-00930-6

Resch, S. C., Menzies, N. A., Portnoy, A., Clarke-Deelder, E., O'Keefe, L., Suharlim, C., & Brenzel, L. (2020). *How to cost immunization programs: A practical guide for primary data collection and analysis.* ImmunizationEconomics.org. http://www.immunizationeconomics.org/epic

Sim, S. Y., Watts, E., Constenla, D., Brenzel, L., & Patenaude, B. N. (2020). Return on investment from immunization against 10 pathogens in 94 low-and middle-income countries, 2011–30. *Health Affairs*, 39(8), 1343–1353. doi:10.1377/hlthaff.2020.00103

Stenberg, K., Lauer, J. A., Gkountouras, G., Fitzpatrick, C., & Stanciole, A. (2018). Econometric estimation of WHO-CHOICE country-specific costs for inpatient and outpatient health service delivery. *Cost Effectiveness and Resource Allocation*, 16(1), 11. doi:10.1186/s12962-018-0095-x

Teaching Vaccine Economics Everywhere. (2021). *Teaching vaccine economics everywhere.* http://www.immunizationeconomics.org/tvee

ThinkWell. (2020). *Immunization delivery cost catalogue.* http://www.immunizationeconomics.org/ican

ThinkWell. (2021). *How to conduct an immunization campaign costing study: Methodological guidance.* http://immunizationeconomics.org/ican-idcc-methodology

Vassall, A., Sweeney, S., Kahn, J., Gomez, G. B., Bollinger, L., Marseille, E., . . . Levin, C. (2017). *Reference case for estimating the costs of global health services and interventions.* LSHTM Research Online. https://researchonline.lshtm.ac.uk/id/eprint/4653001/1/vassall_etal_2018_reference_case_for_estimating_costs_global_health_services.pdf

World Health Organization: Immunization Vaccines and Biologicals. (2002). *Guidelines for estimating costs of introducing new vaccines into the national immunization system.* https://apps.who.int/iris/handle/10665/67342

World Health Organization: Immunization Vaccines and Biologicals. (2014). *Comprehensive multi-year plan costing tool.* https://apps.who.int/iris/bitstream/handle/10665/128051/WHO_IVB_14.06_eng.pdf

World Health Organization: Immunization Vaccines and Biologicals. (2019). *WHO guide for standardization of economic evaluations of immunization programmes.* https://apps.who.int/iris/bitstream/handle/10665/329389/WHO-IVB-19.10-eng.pdf

2.2

Defining immunization costs

Logan Brenzel

2.2.1 Defining costs

Chapters 1.4 and 1.5 provide an overview of why immunizations and vaccines might be undersupplied and under-consumed because of its dual public and private goods nature. In competitive markets, prices are equal to the marginal cost of the inputs that go into producing a product (McCaffrey, 2018). Total cost is a function of outputs, prices, and other factors. A cost function describes the relationship between exogenous prices and volume of outputs produced. Imperfect markets, like the one for vaccines, do not lead to a situation where marginal costs are equal to prices.

The assumption of cost minimization applies to competitive markets where there are many buyers and sellers all making a similar product, limited barriers to entry, and full information. However, this scenario does not necessarily apply to health service provision in the public sector given the heterogeneity and uncertainty of healthcare needs and services, the imbalance of information between the patient and the healthcare provider, as well as the possible absence of incentives. In some countries, public healthcare workers are paid the same wage whether they vaccinate 100 or 10 children per day, or whether they provide a high or low quality of care. The management and use of health sector inputs, such as medicines, vaccines, and equipment, may not be directed toward cost minimization in environments, due to supply constraints, poor information, and lack of data to be able to continually value and monitor costs.

Chapter 2.1 laid out different reasons for conducting an analysis of immunization programs and service delivery costs. Dedicated costing studies of vaccines and immunization programs in lower-income settings have been conducted since the 1980s, at a time when countries were focused on achieving universal childhood immunization (Brenzel & Claquin, 1994).

Logan Brenzel, *Defining immunization costs* In: *Handbook of Applied Health Economics in Vaccines*. Edited by: David Bishai, Logan Brenzel and William V. Padula, Oxford University Press. © Oxford University Press 2023. DOI: 10.1093/oso/9780192896087.003.0009

Because of weaknesses in financial and data systems in lower-income countries, costing is usually accomplished through an analysis of the inputs required to deliver services, assigning prices, and approximate usage for the program if inputs are shared. Presently, the population-weighted average economic delivery cost per dose (net of vaccine costs) is $1.87, with labor costs accounting for the greatest proportion of costs (Portnoy et al., 2020). The total cost of fully vaccinating a child against measles, pertussis, diphtheria, polio, rotavirus, human papilloma virus, and pneumococcal disease is approximately $54, though this will vary depending upon the delivery context (Sim, Watts, Constenla, Brenzel, & Patenaude, 2020).

Variation in the unit cost per dose across different geographical areas and between different types of providers has been documented in the literature (Brenzel, Young, & Walker, 2015; Chatterjee et al., 2018; Fox-Rushby, Kaddar, Levine, & Brenzel, 2004; Geng, Suharlim, Brenzel, Resch, & Menzies, 2017; Menzies et al., 2017; ThinkWell, 2020). Variation also exists between the costs of delivering immunization services through different strategies, such as routine services provided through fixed facilities or a campaign approach. A compendium of immunization delivery costs finds that most studies have been conducted in African countries. Immunization costs also appear to vary by socioeconomic level of the country, with a lower average cost per dose in lower-income countries (Sim et al., 2020).

2.2.2 Cost definitions and categorizations

Methods for evaluating the costs of immunization programs involve measuring economic, financial, or fiscal costs (Resch et al., 2020). An *economic cost* is the value of all inputs used to provide immunization services with respect to trade-offs of where else those same inputs could have been employed. Economic costs include the value of time spent by health workers, value of donated goods and items, and the proportional value of shared inputs, such as transport or equipment. For each one of these inputs, choices must be made on investments in health or other common alternatives uses. Thus, economic costs are resources foregone by society and are viewed from the perspective of society.

Economic costs can also be thought of as the opportunity cost of investing in one program relative to investing in another to achieve the same set of outcomes. If a country has a fixed level of resources to devote to saving children's lives, the policymaker can invest that money in a range of services and must decide about how to allocate those resources. If resources are invested in immunization programs, those resources are not available for other uses. However, the return on investment in immunization may far outweigh that for other services (Vaughan et al., 2019). Evaluating trade-offs between programs is the domain of cost-effectiveness analysis (see Chapter 4).

A *financial cost* focuses on the cash outlays incurred for the delivery of a program. In viewing costs in this way, donated goods would be free and therefore not included. Financial costs can be viewed from the perspective of the payer (see Chapter 2.3), and costs are resources foregone by the payor. Financial costs are often used in immunization costing evaluations as these can be linked to key policy considerations of affordability, sustainability, and budget impact.

A further refinement of financial cost is *fiscal cost*, which refers to actual expenditures made. For instance, the entire amount spent on cold chain equipment could be assigned to the time period in which the purchase occurred. For instance, a refrigerator purchased for $1,000 in September 2020 will represent $1,000 of fiscal expenditure in 2020. While in a financial cost analysis, the refrigerator is assumed to be used over a period of several years, and the corresponding cost is annualized for each year.

The language around costs can be confusing. Published costing studies may not have explicitly stated what type of costs are being evaluated (Brenzel, 2014). Readers of this handbook are encouraged to carefully classify, characterize, and report the type of costs in their analysis. Furthermore, the terms cost, budget, expenditures, and prices are often used interchangeably, but these represent different values. A budget is planned spending which has not yet occurred. In the absence of expenditure data, one might use budgeted amounts as a proxy for spending. But actual expenditure can vary substantially from budgets because of delays in disbursement and lower expenditure rates.

In order to reflect the societal perspective in costing studies, the analysis should take into consideration the costs incurred by households to seek immunization services. These costs can include transportation and waiting times, as well as lost productivity from missing work. Few immunization costing studies incorporate the full societal perspective and include household costs, primary because of the additional cost for data collection through household surveys or facility exit interviews. Nevertheless, when evaluating the costs of different strategies, households may incur varying levels of costs. Fixed facility services require families to visit facilities which are often far away, entailing missed work time and often long waiting times. Campaigns that are offered in central locations may be closer to the community and the household, though the density of the population may entail longer waiting times. Outreach services in which providers go to remote areas are likely to reduce the costs for households in seeking services.

2.2.3 Immunization program cost characterization

Table 2.2.1 illustrates the range of inputs that are evaluated in a typical immunization costing study. Labor costs entail the time spent by a range of health workers, such as medical doctors, nurses, nurse aides, and community health workers, to administer the vaccine dose, and also to undertake record keeping, travel to obtain vaccines and supplies, advocate within the community to come for vaccination, and to repair and maintain equipment. Because vaccines need to be maintained at lower temperatures (2–8°C for most vaccines), the use of vaccine carriers, cold boxes, refrigerators, and freezers is critical to successful vaccination delivery. These appliances need to be maintained and have associated running costs. Often, immunization services are provided in fixed facilities or through outreach and immunization campaigns. Travel to vaccination sites (urban or remote) entails use of resources (vehicles, fuel, per diem) that need to be included in costing studies. In economic cost studies, the economic value of use of building space is also valued. Strategies and approaches to data collection and analysis for costing studies are presented and discussed in Chapters 2.3–2.5.

Costing studies require information on the prices of inputs. Historical prices are known from records, but they are not reflective of the opportunity cost of future resources. As such, replacement prices are preferred to historical prices, particularly for capital inputs in cost analysis. Prices for various cadres of healthcare workers and administrative personnel include salaries and allowances and other benefits. Prices may not be available for volunteer labor and studies often use an average daily wage which can be obtained from government surveys or the International Labor Organization (2021).

Because prices may reflect the quality of inputs, it is important to control for differences in quality of care in the cost evaluation. Selecting a best practice standard for an input may help in this regard. The prices of some inputs such as fuel can vary within a country, and it may be useful to collect price information in the sample areas to account for this. The prices of vaccines or cold chain equipment should also reflect costs related to shipping, international freight, and insurance. The freight-on-board price reflects additional costs for loading and unloading, taxes and other fees to the point of delivery.

Table 2.2.1 Comparison of economic and financial cost inputs

Line item	Economic cost	Financial cost
Paid labor	Value of time allocated to immunization for existing or new staff	Expense made for hiring new staff for immunization-specific activities
Volunteer labor	Value of time allocated to immunization benchmarked against average daily wage	Not included
Per diem	Value of per diems given to health workers	Expenditures on per diems
Vaccines	Value of vaccines administered and wasted	Purchase expense for vaccines
Injection supplies	Value of syringes, wastage containers used and wasted	Purchase expense for syringes, wastage containers
Fuel and transportation	Value related to use of fuel for immunization-specific activities	Expense on fuel and transportation
Vehicle maintenance	Value of maintenance related to immunization-specific activities	Expense for maintenance
Cold chain energy costs	Estimated value of cold chain energy costs	Expense for butane or other energy to run the cold chain
Waste disposal	Value of waste boxes and incineration of used vaccination supplies (syringes, vaccine vials, gauze, etc.)	Purchase of waste boxes, and expense for incineration adjusted using straight line depreciation
Printing	Estimated value of printing based on unit price and volume	Expense for printing
Utilities	Estimated value of utilities and communications based on immunization share to total services	Expense for utilities
Other recurrent inputs	Estimated value of other recurrent inputs based on unit prices, allocation to immunization and quantity used	Expenses for other inputs related to immunization
Cold chain equipment	Annualized and discounted value of cold chain equipment used	Expense for cold chain adjusted using straight line depreciation
Vehicles	Annualized and discounted value of vehicles used	Expense for vehicles used for immunization adjusted using straight line depreciation
Other equipment	Annualized and discounted value of other equipment (computers) used	Expense for other equipment adjusted using straight line depreciation
Buildings	Annualized and discounted value of building space used based on useful life and discount rate	Expense for constructing buildings related to immunization services adjusted using straight line depreciation

The cost, insurance, and freight price covers insurance, customs duties, and rerouting costs associated with the shipment before loading.

Prices may also reflect market distortions. Countries may impose trade and exchange rate barriers or subsidize the cost of production. Prices reflect include taxes and government fees that are transfers. An input may be produced in noncompetitive markets, such as monopolies.

Total immunization costs can be evaluated and reported by input line item as in Table 2.2.1, or by the type of immunization activity defined in Table 2.2.2. Activities are comprised of a combination of line items. For instance, social mobilization and advocacy might entail the cost of television advertising, as well as travel to communities to bring greater awareness of the benefits of vaccination. Appendix 3 provides an example of a crosswalk between line items and activities for an immunization program.

Table 2.2.2 Immunization service cost activity definitions

Immunization activity	Definition
Routine facility-based immunization delivery	Labor time and other resources required to administer vaccines in a facility, including supplies, use of cold chain equipment, waste disposal, etc.
Outreach immunization delivery	Labor time and other resources required to administer vaccines outside of the facility, including supplies, transportation, use of vehicles, use of cold chain, per diem, waste disposal, etc.
Record keeping and data management	Labor time and resources required to record and manage immunization records
Social mobilization and advocacy	Labor time and resources required to motivate, sensitize, and mobilize the population for vaccination services, including radio and television broadcasting, developing and printing posters, supporting community events, etc.
Program management	Time and resources required to plan, budget, and manage the delivery of immunization services within a facility or to a population
Vaccine collection, distribution, and storage	Time and resources required to collect distribute and store vaccines (from port to delivery point), including transportation, per diem, use of vehicles, etc.
Cold chain maintenance	Time and resources required to maintain temperature control for vaccines
Supervision	Time and resources required to undertake supervisory activities
Training	Time and resources required (per diem and travel of participants, developing and printing of materials, renting venues, refreshments, etc.) to provide in-service training to vaccinators and administrators
Surveillance	Time and resources required to undertake case detection, follow up on adverse events or other surveillance activities, including travel, per diem, and other resources

If the focus of the study is to understand and evaluate the total costs of a national immunization program or the different strategies of that program, all inputs utilized in the program or strategy need to be included and measured. If the purpose of the analysis is to determine the cost of introducing a new vaccine, then an incremental cost analysis would be conducted. An incremental analysis would only focus on the additional labor time, or the additional use of vehicles and equipment for the new vaccine. Chapter 2.5 presents an approach to evaluating the introduction of new vaccines.

Other approaches to costing health services can be applied to costing immunization programs. For instance, a cost accounting approach called step-down cost accounting allocates costs to different departments in a facility in a sequential process, starting with support services (e.g. administration) (Conteh & Walker, 2004). Activity-based costing is another approach that measures the relationship between resources, activities, and performance or outputs (Baker, 1998). This approach can be widely applied in healthcare and may be useful for estimating the cost of achieving coverage targets.

2.2.4 Conclusion

This chapter has provided the basic structure and concepts for immunization program costing. For cost-effectiveness and other economic evaluations, economic costs should be estimated to reflect the full economic costs of services. Financial costs are more relevant if the policy question relates to the resources that need to be mobilized or the budget impact of the program. Household costs are rarely considered in immunization costing studies, although more work would be useful in this area, as service delivery modalities have varying impacts on household costs. More detailed methods and approaches are found in the following chapters.

References

Baker, J. J. (1998). *Activity-based costing and activity-based management for health care.* Gaithersburg, MD: Aspen Publishers.

Brenzel, L. (2014). Working Paper: Common approach for the costing and financing analyses of routine immunization and new vaccine introduction costs (EPIC). Mimeograph. Bill & Melinda Gates Foundation. www.immunizationeconomics.org/epic-info.

Brenzel, L., & Claquin, P. (1994). Immunization programs and their costs. *Social Science & Medicine, 39*(4), 527–536. doi:10.1016/0277-9536(94)90095-7

Brenzel, L., Young, D., & Walker, D. G. (2015). Costs and financing of routine immunization: Approach and selected findings of a multi-country study (EPIC). *Vaccine, 33*, A13–A20. doi:10.1016/j.vaccine.2014.12.066

Chatterjee, S., Das, P., Nigam, A., Nandi, A., Brenzel, L., Ray, A., . . . Laxminarayan, R. (2018). Variation in cost and performance of routine immunisation service delivery in India. *BMJ Global Health, 3*(3), e000794. doi:10.1136/bmjgh-2018-000794

Conteh, L., & Walker, D. (2004). Cost and unit cost calculations using step-down accounting. *Health Policy and Planning, 19*(2), 127–135. doi:10.1093/heapol/czh015

Fox-Rushby, J., Kaddar, M., Levine, R., & Brenzel, L. (2004). The economics of vaccination in low- and middle-income countries. *Bulletin of the World Health Organization, 82*, 640. doi:10.1590/S0042-96862004000900002

Geng, F., Suharlim, C., Brenzel, L., Resch, S. C., & Menzies, N. A. (2017). The cost structure of routine infant immunization services: A systematic analysis of six countries. *Health Policy and Planning, 32*(8), 1174–1184. doi:10.1093/heapol/czx067

International Labor Organization. (2021). *Global wage report 2020–21: Wages and minimum wages in the time of COVID-19.* https://www.ilo.org/wcmsp5/groups/public/---dgreports/---dcomm/---publ/documents/publication/wcms_762534.pdf

McCaffrey, M. (2018). *The economic theory of cost: Foundation and new directions.* London: Routledge.

Menzies, N. A., Suharlim, C., Geng, F., Ward, Z. J., Brenzel, L., & Resch, S. C. (2017). The cost determinants of routine infant immunization services: A meta-regression analysis of six country studies. *BMC Medicine, 15*(1), 178. doi:10.1186/s12916-017-0942-1

Portnoy, A., Vaughan, K., Clarke-Deelder, E., Suharlim, C., Resch, S. C., Brenzel, L., & Menzies, N. A. (2020). Producing standardized country-level immunization delivery unit cost estimates. *PharmacoEconomics, 38*(9), 995–1005. doi:10.1007/s40273-020-00930-6

Resch, S. C., Menzies, N. A., Portnoy, A., Clarke-Deelder, E., O'Keefe, L., Suharlim, C., & Brenzel, L. (2020). *How to cost immunization programs: A practical guide for primary data collection and analysis.* ImmunizationEconomics.org. http://www.immunizationeconomics.org/epic

Sim, S. Y., Watts, E., Constenla, D., Brenzel, L., & Patenaude, B. N. (2020). Return on investment from immunization against 10 pathogens in 94 low-and middle-income countries, 2011–30. *Health Affairs, 39*(8), 1343–1353. doi:10.1377/hlthaff.2020.00103

ThinkWell. (2020). *Immunization delivery cost catalogue.* http://www.immunizationeconomics.org/ican

Vaughan, K., Ozaltin, A., Mallow, M., Moi, F., Wilkason, C., Stone, J., & Brenzel, L. (2019). The costs of delivering vaccines in low- and middle-income countries: Findings from a systematic review. *Vaccine: X, 2*, 100034. doi:10.1016/j.jvacx.2019.100034

2.3

Designing a primary costing study or analysis

Ijeoma Edoka, Stephen Resch, and Logan Brenzel

This chapter presents and highlights critical elements related to the design, purpose, scope, and perspective of the study. In addition, approaches for data collection, and sampling are addressed.

2.3.1 Design considerations

When planning and designing an immunization costing study, the purpose and use of the results and by whom should be identified as a first step. This may entail elaborating the main question(s) the study will address. This is an important step as this will guide the subsequent design and approach for the costing study. In discussion with policymakers and other relevant stakeholders, it will be useful to specify the immunization service(s) to be costed, and to understand how the results of the study are going to be used by the government or funder. This will help to set the expectations for the exercise.

2.3.1.1 Scope

Defining the scope of the costing study is important for identifying the types of resources to be counted and included in the study which allows the analyst to set boundaries for the costing exercise. The scope of the study will depend on the purpose of the analysis, the type of program being costed, the study perspective adopted, and the type of costs being estimated.

As mentioned previously, the inputs to be evaluated will depend upon which aspect and delivery strategy of the immunization program will be the focus of

Ijeoma Edoka, Stephen Resch, and Logan Brenzel, *Designing a primary costing study or analysis* In: *Handbook of Applied Health Economics in Vaccines*. Edited by: David Bishai, Logan Brenzel and William V. Padula, Oxford University Press.
© Oxford University Press 2023. DOI: 10.1093/oso/9780192896087.003.0010

the study. Routine immunization programs are largely delivered within health facilities but may sometimes be delivered through outreach campaigns within the community. Supplementary immunization activities are often conducted to augment coverage of routine vaccines as well as in response to infectious disease outbreaks. Both program types have different resource use implications and, consequently, program delivery costs. For example, cost inputs such as transportation and fuel cost or per diems and travel allowances will not be included in a facility-based routine immunization program but would be counted if supervision is occurring or an outreach program is being costed. On the other hand, building costs and overheads would be counted in a routine immunization program costing exercise but may not be a cost input in a community-based outreach program.

2.3.1.2 Perspective

The perspective of a costing study identifies who is bearing the costs. Specifying the study perspective is important for setting the boundaries of the costing exercise and determining the types of data to collect and analyze. There are three main types of perspectives: provider, payer, and societal.

A healthcare provider perspective would evaluate the costs incurred directly by providers, such as those made by public or private hospitals or frontline health facilities.

A payer perspective would analyze costs from the viewpoint of the agencies that are currently financing services, or that might be financing them in the future. This could include evaluating costs from the perspective of the Ministry of Health, or that of development partners, or both.

The broadest perspective for costing is a societal perspective which includes costs borne by providers and payers, as well as costs incurred by households, such as transportation and waiting time costs. The societal perspective may include resources utilized by other government entities, such as costs to the Ministry of Education for human papillomavirus vaccination in schools.

There are some ambiguities when it comes to defining a costing perspective. Most immunization costing studies reflect costs borne by the public health sector (e.g., government or public payer). The provider perspective is also sometimes ambiguous, as private providers are not always included in studies in the same way that publicly funded providers are studied. The perspective taken for a costing study should directly pertain to the objective of the study and the requirements of the target audience. If the purpose of the study is to understand how much the government needs to plan and budget for immunization services, the correct perspective would be the payer (public sector) perspective. If donor support is expected to be taken up by a government after a time period, then the perspective of donor and partner contributions also need to be valued.

If the purpose of the study is to provide a cost estimate for a cost-effectiveness analysis, a societal perspective is the most appropriate. This may require conducting a household survey or an exit interview with households to determine the direct costs incurred by patients seeking immunization services, as well as the indirect costs of foregone productivity due to lost work time. The societal perspective broadens the scope of the cost analysis and requires more data. The Second Panel on Cost-effectiveness in Health and Medicine and the Global Health Costing Consortium recommend a societal perspective as well as the health sector perspective (i.e. a hybrid perspective of the individual patient, payer, and provider) (Sanders et al., 2016; Vassall et al., 2017).

Finally, if the interest is to be able to compare and contrast how much it costs for different types of facilities to provide services, and to ascertain whether any efficiencies could be obtained, then the provider perspective would be useful.

2.3.1.3 Time horizon

Another dimension of scope is the study time horizon. Time horizon is an important feature of a costing model since vaccination program costs vary considerably based on the type of vaccine. For instance, consider that a tetanus vaccination may be given to newborns and again several times over their lifespan, and an influenza vaccination may be an annual event. Vaccination to protect against shingles may be taken later in life. Depending on the vaccine program, the time horizon could be very different.

Costing studies are usually conducted retrospectively, such that the time period pertaining to data collection is in the past, such as for the previous year. This type of study provides an historical perspective and evaluates the total and unit cost of what was achieved in the past. One could design a prospective costing study that collects data as services are delivered. An example of this would be a study that is coupled with a clinical trial and gathers data related to resource use on a patient or provider questionnaire completed after each visit, or which measures labor with time–motion observation methods.

Cost modeling exercises that project the expected costs of future immunization services consider a time horizon that is in the future. When making projections for new program implementation, special consideration of the time horizon is warranted, as there are often large one-time costs at the start of a program, and it often takes some time for a program to reach the flat part of a learning curve and reach an efficient scale.

2.3.2 Data collection

This part of the chapter highlights useful data sources for costing studies, data collection instruments and approaches, issues with data quality, as well as incorporation of shared costs and sampling procedures.

2.3.2.1 Data sources

Retrospective costing studies often rely heavily on administrative records, such as expenditure data in cost accounting systems, claims filed by providers to bill payers, purchase orders, payroll records or human resources personnel records, activity logs, routine reports, inventory lists, and clinical records. This administrative data is typically supplemented with data gathered via interview or questionnaire from program managers and other key staff. A third type of data collection is direct observation. Although there are limitations in combining direct observation (which is necessarily prospective) with other data collected retrospectively, it can be a useful approach to measuring certain aspects of resource use—especially the allocation of shared labor resources. Guidance documents are available on how to best collect data through direct observation, which can be done as a scientific approach (Resch et al., 2020).

2.3.2.1.1 Administrative records

Accounting systems are frequently used as a source of information on expenditures such as utilities, fuel, per diems, expenses for training activities such as venue rental, catering, and travel. In order to use information from a cost accounting system, one must determine the extent to which financial transactions can be mapped specifically to immunization inputs or activities. Purchase order information can be a useful source for information on the price paid for commodities, vehicles, and equipment. Payroll records are useful for estimating average salaries for workers with different job positions and level of experience. Activity logs such as a vehicle trip log can be useful for allocating an appropriate portion of a health facility's shared vehicle pool to immunization activities. Program managers may have other logbooks with information regarding the number of training, management, or supervision events, and details regarding the duration and number of participants at such events. Routine reports will often be a source of information on the number of immunization sessions held, number of outreach activities and campaigns, number of doses used and discarded, and vaccine inventory stock levels. There may also be inventory lists for cold chain equipment and vehicles indicating information such as the make and model, location, condition, and age of capital items.

Another source of cost data is health insurance claims data and other administrative records of healthcare providers (Riley, 2009). In the US, claims data from Medicare and Medicaid and other insurers provide useful information on payments made to providers for specific services. The Medical Expenditure Panel Survey contains a wealth of data for tracking expenditures for the most prevalent conditions (Aizcorbe et al., 2012). Records from the US Veterans' Health Administration and other hospital systems generally contain information on the resource used to produce services. When using these data sources, it is important to distinguish between payments made, billed charges, and resource use.

2.3.2.1.2 Retrospective self-report of program manager and staff

Some needed information may not exist in routine records. In this case, a common solution is to conduct interviews with or administer surveys to program managers or key staff members. Interviews or questionnaires might be used for gathering information about the frequency or duration of outreach sessions, training events, supervision visits, or the use of vehicles.

An important example is labor quantity, which represents a substantial share of total immunization program cost. The share of nursing labor that is dedicated to immunization is usually not routinely tracked. Questionnaires can be used to gather information from a sample of healthcare workers and administrative staff about their time spent on a range of immunization activities. The proportion of time or absolute value of time spent by healthcare workers can be identified through a series of questions.

Several issues arise when designing questionnaires for estimating labor time allocation. First, is the choice of who will be interviewed. In some cases, the senior nurse in charge of immunization at the health facility site can be asked to estimate the number of hours (or percent of total hours) of each staff member that was spent on immunization-related activities. Probing questions can be used to explore time allocation by activity category such as vaccine administration or record keeping. A second issue is related to the period of recall for interviews. Respondents reporting labor allocation information may refer to other records to aid with recall. A shorter recall period improves reliability of responses. A variant of this approach could involve interviewing workers themselves about the allocation of their own time, but this would be far more time-consuming, and may not be much more accurate. Questions to ask about labor time should ascertain usual working hours for each cadre of staff, the usual hours for immunization services, and either the hours or proportion of time a particular health worker or cadre of worker spends on a particular activity during that day. In many countries, vaccines are given on a single day per week in an immunization session, and this will greatly facilitate data collection on time allocation to immunization. In some studies, there may be interest in allocating immunization time per staff member or cadre of staff to specific activities, such as record keeping or collecting and distributing vaccines. In these cases, additional questions will need to be asked.

One common issue with labor time allocation is deciding how to handle downtime when staff are not busy due to demand-side factors such as a lack of patients, which can often be the case for rural, remote health facilities. It is suggested that information on the proportion of downtime be collected. This type of information can be used as additional explanatory factors in the analysis. Additional guidance on how to handle downtime can be found in the reference guide by Resch et al. (2020).

2.3.2.1.3 Direct observation and other methods

Rather than collect subjective information on time allocation that may be subject to recall bias, an alternative approach is through direct observation. Time–motion studies can be conducted where the vaccination session is observed, and the time spent on various activities by individual staff is recorded and analyzed. Activities like community outreach may only happen on a single day per month. A direct observation approach should be designed to accommodate the service delivery schedule. Observing multiple immunization sessions allows the researcher to improve the quality of the time allocation estimates (Brenzel, Young, & Walker, 2015). Direct observation will necessarily be prospective, and therefore not match the exact time period of the other input data collected retrospectively for the study. An assumption must be made that the share of labor time allocated to immunization activities has not changed significantly between the study time period and the current observation time period. Direct observation methods are time-consuming and more expensive to carry out. Health workers may change their workflow if they become aware of observers.

Another approach for collecting labor time allocation is through a daily diary of activities that records the time spent. Diaries should be kept over a period of a month and may need to be reviewed for compliance in filling them out and in making any course corrections in how they are being utilized. Diaries may not be practical for facility samples where the sampled units are not in proximity to one another.

2.3.2.1.4 Data collection instruments
Data on costs, outputs, and facility characteristics should be collected using pretested, standardized questionnaire formats. Several tools exist for constructing data collection instruments. Sample questionnaires for immunization costing studies can be found at https://dataverse.harvard.edu/dataverse/ EPIC. Other costing methodologies can generate customized data collection instruments tailored to specific study requirements (Pan American Health Organization, 2019).

2.3.2.2 Addressing shared costs

Often, inputs into the delivery of immunization services will be shared with other health services and interventions. For instance, a vehicle can be used to transport a range of commodities, including vaccines. A multipurpose health worker provides different services. If shared resources will be included in immunization cost estimates, the proportion of resources used by the program will need to be estimated to correctly allocate those shared resources and their respective costs to the program.

Determining what portion of a shared resource to allocate to immunization may not be straightforward and usually requires making educated assumptions. Allocating shared resources requires developing an "allocation key" or "tracing factor" that serves as the basis for allocation. These tracing factors can also be used to allocate the cost of inputs within immunization to different program activities. Some examples of tracing factors include (1) allocating shared costs based on the proportion of immunization visits out of total outpatient visits to the facility; (2) allocating the use of a vehicle based on the share of mileage or distance traveled per week specific to immunization as a proportion of total mileage; and (3) allocating building space based on the proportion of square feet or meters. Additional sources of information exist on determining the best allocation or tracing factors for immunization programs (Brenzel, 2014; Resch et al., 2020).

2.3.2.3 Health system levels

The scope of a costing study can be framed by level of the health system. Some immunization activities may occur at levels in the health system above the point of service. Costs can be incurred at administrative levels (national, regional, provincial, or district) as well as the specific facility level. Costing studies can include "above facility costs" to determine where the balance of resource use lies—with delivery of services or with their management and administration. Evaluating administrative costs is becoming more common in the conduct of immunization costing studies (Clift, Arias, Chaitkin, & O'Connell, 2017; Vassall et al., 2017).

To evaluate costs at different health system levels, it is important to map specific activities to where the resources are being used. For example, microplanning might take place at a district health office and resources used for meetings and travel to and from that office should be mapped to that level. Vaccine supply and distribution might be the responsibility of the district health system level, while procurement of vaccines might be primarily a national level exercise. Information on inputs and prices used in a cost analysis may be aggregated and maintained at particular levels of the health system, such as information on coverage estimates or vaccine wastage rates.

Defining activities within each level of the health system is also useful for identifying where resources may be shared between levels. For example, the tender prices for a new vaccine may include not only procurement costs (freight, insurance, customs duties) and storage cost but may also include transportation costs to different administrative units of the health system, such as from national to regional storage facilities. For this reason, it is important to know in advance the types of immunization activities that occur at different levels of the health system. Data collection may require separate questionnaires for different health system levels.

2.3.3 Sampling for immunization costing studies

Immunization costing studies are based, more and more, on sampling of facilities and delivery sites. Sampling is required because of the heterogeneity

of total and unit costs across geographical areas and between and within facility types (Resch et al., 2020). In addition, inputs into unit costing are rarely
known in their entirety. For most resource inputs to vaccine programs, data
will have to be gathered from a sample of units of the immunization system,
and the total resource use will need to be extrapolated from that sample.

The extent of sampling will be determined by the budget and time available
to do the study, and whether representativeness is required and at what level
(whether national or subnational).

Care should be taken in the sample design to ensure it is representative and
sufficiently large to generate estimates with acceptable precision. Random
sampling is preferred to other approaches when the goal is to have nationally
or sub-nationally representative estimates. Random sampling can also facilitate comparisons of cost between different locations, types of sites, or service
delivery approaches. An additional benefit of random sampling is the ability
to derive unbiased estimates of sample mean cost estimates, and to calculate
confidence intervals around that estimate.

An alternative is to select units deliberately based on some features of those
units, or select units based on convenience, such as nearby or easy-to-reach
facilities (purposive or convenience sampling). Purposive sampling can help
to reduce the cost of the exercise and may also provide more control over context and variables of interest for the study. For instance, if the study aims to
evaluate the costs of accessing hard-to-reach populations in rural, remote
areas, a purposive sample of facilities located in those areas will provide more
direct evidence on costs. However, the results may be biased and it will be difficult to estimate precision for these types of studies.

Standard methods for sample size determination can be used for immunization costing studies (Leslie, Laos, Cárcamo, Pérez-Cuevas, & García, 2021;
Vassall et al., 2017). For more complex sample designs, a statistician should
be consulted. Increasing the number of units selected in a costing study
sample will improve the precision of the results, but this also becomes more
costly. Balancing precision and costs through alternative sampling frames can
be achieved with the Sample Design Optimizer (ImmunizationEconomics.
Org, 2020).

Ultimately, the sample design for an immunization costing study will depend on the objective of the study and the information available prior to data
collection. The most critical piece of information is a complete list of all sites
by type. For example, if the study is going to collect information at the central/
national level, as well as from a sample of districts and a sample of facilities
within the sampled districts, it will be important to have a list of districts and

of health facilities within those districts. This list is the sampling frame. It is this population of sites for which we can infer costs based on statistical analysis of the data collected from the sampled sites.

Other factors can be used to stratify the sample. For instance, the type of health facility (private or public hospital, clinic, health post), the location of the facility (urban or rural), or the volume of services provided in that facility (high, average, or low volumes) can be used to stratify units for selection. Stratified random sampling is more and more common in immunization costing studies since services are organized along a hierarchy of administrative levels from region to district to health facility. However, random sampling may lead to a more expensive data collection process, as facilities and health system sites may be more widely spread out geographically. There is a potential loss of precision associated with stratification.

2.3.3.1 Illustrative sampling procedure

Typically, for immunization costing studies attempting to sample a sufficient number of sites at different organizational levels, a clustered design is recommended, in order to reduce data collection cost. Below is an outline of a possible sampling procedure oriented toward a study of the cost of routine facility-based immunization delivery:

- *Geographical areas are selected.* If the country is small, the geographical area may be the entire country. If the country is large, provinces may be selected at random or purposively. For example, if the goal is to compare more developed provinces to less developed ones, at least one of each type should be included. This could be accomplished by purposive selection or by random selection from strata.
- *Subnational units are selected* below the province level. Districts or other subnational units can be randomly selected where the probability of their selection is proportional to the number of health facilities. This is done so that there is equal representation in the sample between small or larger districts.
- *Facility sampling* is based on a complete list of health facilities that are relevant for the scope of the study. For instance, a study evaluating government facilities should be based on a complete list of those facilities. Incorporating private or nongovernmental organization facilities will require complete lists of those types of facilities. If the scope of the study

considers only certain facilities that have immunization service available, then the list would be restricted to these immunization-relevant sites.

- If a *stratified sample of facilities* will be selected, additional information on the following is useful to collect for each district and facility in the sample:
  - The number of vaccine doses administered or the number of outpatient visits in the past year.
  - For each district, information on population density should be obtained.
  - Facilities could be classified as urban (urban/peri-urban) and rural/remote and also by ownership (government, nongovernment, private).
- The final stage of the sampling procedure is to *randomly select the same number of facilities from each selected district*. Healthcare costs, which are constrained to be non-negative, are generally right skewed rather than normally distributed (ImmunizationEconomics.Org, 2020; Turner, Angeles, Tsui, Wilkinson, & Magnani, 2001). Because costs tend to be right tailed (a large number of sites have low costs, with a few sites having much higher costs), oversampling those sites that may have lower costs may be desirable to more accurately represent the cost distribution in a country. These sites tend to be low-volume, rural, or remote sites rather than high-volume, urban, or peri-urban facilities. (ImmunizationEconomics.Org, 2020; Turner et al., 2001) For this reason, simple random sampling is recommended in order not to overly favor those facilities that administer a large number of doses. Oversampling of low-volume, rural, or remote facilities could be accomplished by stratifying on this basis and selecting a relatively larger sample from that stratum.
- Should a *facility be unavailable for survey*, such as for security/safety reasons or respondents being absent or preoccupied during the survey period, that facility can be replaced in the sample through random sampling. It might be useful to select the replacement facilities in advance to use as substitutes if needed while collecting data.

Each sampled unit may have a different probability of being selected into the sample. As a result, each unit in the sample may represent a different-sized portion of the sampling frame, which must be accounted for in data analysis and when generalizing from the sample to the larger population. Incorporating sample weights into the analysis (inverse of the probability of a selection) will be important. The sampling procedure will determine sample weights used in the data analysis.

References

Aizcorbe, A., Liebman, E., Pack, S., Cutler, D. M., Chernew, M. E., & Rosen, A. B. (2012). Measuring health care costs of individuals with employer-sponsored health insurance in the U.S.: A comparison of survey and claims data. *Statistical Journal of the IAOS, 28*(1–2), 43–51. doi:10.3233/SJI-2012-0743

Brenzel, L. (2014). Working Paper: Common approach for the costing and financing analyses of routine immunization and new vaccine introduction costs (EPIC). Mimeograph. Bill & Melinda Gates Foundation. www.immunizationeconomics.org/epic-info.

Brenzel, L., Young, D., & Walker, D. G. (2015). Costs and financing of routine immunization: Approach and selected findings of a multi-country study (EPIC). *Vaccine, 33*, A13–A20. doi:10.1016/j.vaccine.2014.12.066

Clift, J., Arias, D., Chaitkin, M., & O'Connell, M. (2017). *Landscape study: The cost, impact, and efficiency of above service delivery activities in HIV and other global health programs.* Results for Development. https://r4d.org/resources/landscape-study-cost-impact-efficiency-service-delivery-activities-hiv-global-health-programs

ImmunizationEconomics.Org. (2020). *Sample design optimizer.* ImmunizationEconomics.org. http://immunizationeconomics.org/sample-design-optimizer

Leslie, H. H., Laos, D., Cárcamo, C., Pérez-Cuevas, R., & García, P. J. (2021). Health care provider time in public primary care facilities in Lima, Peru: A cross-sectional time motion study. *BMC Health Services Research, 21*(1), 123. doi:10.1186/s12913-021-06117-9

Pan American Health Organization. (2019). *COSTVAC.* http://immunizationeconomics.org/recent-activity/2019/9/23/update-of-pahos-provac-e-toolkit

Resch, S. C., Menzies, N. A., Portnoy, A., Clarke-Deelder, E., O'Keefe, L., Suharlim, C., & Brenzel, L. (2020). *How to cost immunization programs: A practical guide for primary data collection and analysis.* http://www.immunizationeconomics.org/epic

Riley, G. F. (2009). Administrative and claims records as sources of health care cost data. *Medical Care, 47*(7 Suppl 1), S51–S55. doi:10.1097/MLR.0b013e31819c95aa

Sanders, G. D., Neumann, P. J., Basu, A., Brock, D. W., Feeny, D., Krahn, M., . . . Ganiats, T. G. (2016). Recommendations for conduct, methodological practices, and reporting of cost-effectiveness analyses: Second Panel on Cost-Effectiveness in Health and Medicine. *JAMA, 316*(10), 1093–1103. doi:10.1001/jama.2016.12195

Turner, A. G., Angeles, G., Tsui, A. O., Wilkinson, M., & Magnani, R. (2001). *Sampling manual for facility surveys for population, maternal health, child health and STD programs in developing countries.* MEASURE Evaluation. https://www.measureevaluation.org/resources/publications/ms-01-03

Vassall, A., Sweeney, S., Kahn, J., Gomez, G. B., Bollinger, L., Marseille, E., . . . Levin, C. (2017). *Reference case for estimating the costs of global health services and interventions.* LSHTM Research Online. https://researchonline.lshtm.ac.uk/id/eprint/4653001/1/vassall_etal_2018_reference_case_for_estimating_costs_global_health_services.pdf

2.4

Data analysis

Stephen Resch and Logan Brenzel

2.4.1 Introduction

Data analysis is the process of preparing the collected data, performing calculations, and applying statistical methods to produce results that answer research questions. A data analysis plan should typically be developed prior to data collection, so that one can be assured that the data collection includes everything needed to carry out the analysis. The data analysis process will typically start with a data cleaning step. Next, there is a standard set of adjustments applied to account for currency conversion and inflation, discounting streams of cost that occur over time—annualization of capital investments. Another analysis step pertains to allocating shared resources to activities. This allocation can be "built in" to the design of the data collection process, but is also sometimes handled in the analysis phase, after data is collected.

When data have been collected from a representative sample in which randomization was used to select sampled units, the data analysis step will include statistical methods to make inferences about the population and estimate the precision of the results. In some costing studies, classic methods of statistical inference from a representative sample may not be feasible due to lack of randomization in the sample design, or in situations where there is a policy need to extrapolate beyond the sample frame. In these cases, other methods of extrapolation may be utilized. In these situations, sensitivity analysis explores the uncertainty of cost estimates given the number of assumptions used in the analysis, and because it is not possible to estimate traditional confidence intervals.

Stephen Resch and Logan Brenzel, *Data analysis* In: *Handbook of Applied Health Economics in Vaccines*. Edited by: David Bishai, Logan Brenzel and William V. Padula, Oxford University Press. © Oxford University Press 2023. DOI: 10.1093/oso/9780192896087.003.0011

2.4.2 Discounting

In primary costing studies, it is rare to need to use discounting, as the time horizon is usually short and the study retrospective in nature. However, in costing exercises to model projected costs of some future immunization activity, discounting may be needed if a longer time horizon than 1–2 years is being considered. Discounting is a way to account for time preference and risk aversion. There is a large literature on economic theory and empirical evidence regarding discounting as it applies to cost accounting, economic evaluation, and social policy. For most economic evaluations in the health sector, guidelines recommend a discount rate of 3–5%, though some have argued for higher discount rates in low-income settings. Thus, 3% would be a common discount rate applied to high-income countries, as recommend by the US Panel on Cost-Effectiveness in Health and Medicine, whereas 5% may be a more appropriate rate specifically for low- and middle-income countries. The purpose of discounting is to convert a stream of future costs over time into their present value.

Equation 2.4.1. Discounting:

$$Present\ value\ = \frac{Future\ value}{(1+r)^t}$$

where r is the annual discount rate and t represents the number of years when the future value occurs.

2.4.3 Annualization

For program inputs that last more than 1 year, such as vehicles and cold chain equipment, the annual value of that input should be proportional to the fraction of the item's expected useful life and the opportunity cost of capital being tied up in the input and unavailable for other uses.

In an economic analysis, annualization of capital cost "smooths out" the actual stream of fiscal outlays in order to provide a better picture of the long-run average cost of an immunization program. This is important if one is considering a short time horizon such as 1 year. It would not be appropriate to allocate the total cost of the capital inputs only to the doses delivered in that year when those capital inputs are expected to be in use for several years and contribute to the delivery of many more doses over time. By annualizing the cost of capital resources, we can assign a fair proportion of the cost to the program output of a given time period and avoid idiosyncratic variations in cost estimates that might occur simply due to the timing of large capital investments.

The useful life of an asset is the period of time during which it is expected to be fully employed for its original purpose. A general rule of thumb is that useful life is equivalent to the number of years until the cost of maintaining and repairing a piece of equipment (opportunity cost of using an outdated model/make) outweighs the cost of buying a new piece of equipment. It is not uncommon to find items that have exceeded their useful life but are still in operation. However, one should not base useful life on these examples. Nor should one base useful life on the current age of an item in the inventory. Many countries have standard benchmark values for useful life of capital items. Benchmarks for useful life for immunization programs have been developed (Resch et al., 2020; World Health Organization, 2021).

The calculation of an annualized cost requires information about the purchase price (or replacement value), an annualization factor which is a function of the useful life, and a discount rate. The annualization factor is sometimes referred to as the "present worth of annuity" factor. A table of these factors can be found online (Resch et al., 2020) or in textbooks (Drummond, Sculpher, Claxton, Stoddart, & Torrance, 2015).

For financial cost analysis, the annualized cost doesn't factor in the opportunity cost of capital. In this case, the purchase price (or replacement value) is divided only by the number of years of useful life. This will generally give a similar result to annualization, unless useful life is very long. The example in Box 2.4.1 shows how annualized costs are estimated.

Equation 2.4.2. Annualization factor:

$$Annualization\ factor = \frac{(1+r)^n - 1}{\left(r \times (1+r)^n\right)}$$

where r is the discount rate (use 3% unless you have justification for using an alternative rate) and n is the number of years of useful life. This may or may not correspond with an item's actual physical or economic life.

Box 2.4.1 Example of using an annualization factor

A freezer costs $20,000 to purchase and has an estimated useful life of 10 years. Using a discount rate of 3%, the annual cost of the freezer would be $2,344.61 each year. Stated differently, a stream of payments of $2,344 per year for 10 years has a present value of $20,000.

Cost estimate: $20,000.

Discount rate: 3%.

Years of useful life: 10.

Annualization factor = $[1 - (1 + 0.03)^{10}]/0.03 = 8.5302$

Annualized cost = $20,000/8.5302 = $2,344.61

Excel formula: = -PMT (0.03, 10,$20000) = $2,344.61

Note: the PMT formula command in Microsoft Excel can be used to estimate annualized value of cost. It is important to include a minus sign ahead of that command, because Excel assumes you are using PMT to get the value of an annual payment that will be equivalent to the present value of some lump sum (such as a loan amount).

2.4.4 Evaluating costs

Once data on inputs, unit prices, and allocation factors have been collected, the analyst can assemble the estimates of total immunization costs per sampled unit. This will generally follow a standard formula:

Equation 2.4.3. Cost of input:

$$Cost\ of\ input = Quantity\ of\ input\ (by\ type) \times Unit\ price\ of\ input \\ \times Allocation\ factor$$

Costs of all inputs are summed up for each facility to estimate total immunization cost at the facility. These costs can be divided into capital and recurrent line items or by specific immunization activity. Representation of costs may be best illustrated through pie charts or bar graphs. The share of total immunization cost by line item or activity is referred to as the cost profile. Cost profiles can be compared across the sample by facility type or location. Most cost studies evaluate total or full immunization program or strategy costs, as well as unit costs (total costs divided by doses administered or total costs divided by the number of children or target population vaccinated).

2.4.5 Evaluating costs from a sample of facility sites

Facility-based cost estimates are often aggregated to reflect the total cost of the immunization program based on the sample. In doing so, it is essential to account for underlying relationships between cost and volume and to minimize bias and maximize precision of the estimates.

As mentioned previously, total immunization costs are not normally distributed across a sample of health facilities, but are right tailed, with lots of facilities providing a lower volume of services at lower costs. Taking the simple average of total immunization facility costs across the sample or within the strata of the sample will not likely represent the true value of costs, although simple averages can be used for benchmarking and for identifying and describing facilities with lower unit costs and higher volumes (higher performing, more efficient).

A recent systematic review of estimation techniques in multisite costing studies found the majority of them (52%) used a volume-weighted mean, and the remaining studies relied on simple means or medians of total and unit costs. Each of these estimators are associated with different levels of bias and precision. A simple mean cost calculation could be upwardly biased by 12% to over 100% (Clarke-Deelder, Vassall, & Menzies, 2019).

A better approach evaluates the volume-weighted mean of costs across the sample of sites. The volume-weighted mean unit cost is derived from the sum of the total costs across the sample of sites divided by the sum of doses delivered across the sample of sites. To estimate the volume-weighted total cost of the national immunization program, the mean of total costs for the sample sites is multiplied by the ratio of the total delivery volume in the overall program to the mean delivery volume in the sample. This approach requires additional information about the total delivery volume in the population. While slightly biased, this approach significantly improves precision (World Health Organization, 2021).

The calibration estimator uses additional information to reweight the data in the sample to match the true distribution of costs more closely in the population. At a minimum, auxiliary information will include the total volume of services delivered in the overall program of interest and the total number of sites in the overall program of interest. Information about other variables that drive costs can be incorporated to further improve precision. The calibration estimator has improved precision relative to the volume-weighted mean (and has a similar upward bias in small samples). However, estimation is more complex and requires the use of more advanced software than the volume-weighted mean (Rivera-Rodriguez, Resch, & Haneuse, 2018).

A regression approach improves precision by incorporating additional information, such as information related to distance between health facilities, quality of care, and other factors. One simple example is a log–log regression of costs on delivery volumes: $\log(C_i) = Q_i + i$ where C is the cost and Q is the quantity of doses. From this model, unit costs are the sum of the predicted costs divided by the number of doses delivered in the population.

2.4.6 Sample weights

As mentioned previously, sampling weights should be incorporated into estimates of total costs. The sample frame will determine the weights used. Weights are the inverse probability of selection. With stratification, there are multiple probabilities of being selected and these probabilities should be multiplied by each other, with weights being the inverse of these joint probabilities. For example, if one district is selected out of five (1/5), and five facilities are selected out of 20 (5/20), then the probability of facilities being selected in that district in the sample is ($1/5 \times 5/20 = 1/50$). The sample weight for a facility in that district would be the inverse, or 50.

2.4.7 Aggregating cost data

Researchers may be interested in aggregating total and unit cost data from one health administrative level to the next. The methods described above would be appropriate for calculating summary estimates of unit and total costs at each level of the healthcare system before aggregation. Appropriate sample weights and methods for estimation of standard errors should be used at each level of the analysis. For example, in order to estimate total costs across three levels of the health system, it is recommended that the methods previously described are utilized for each level, and the total immunization cost or unit costs for each level are combined to result in the national level costs. One caution is that if vaccine and syringe costs are estimated for facility and subnational levels, it is recommended to remove that aspect of costs in the aggregation process, and to add in the total value of vaccines and syringes obtained from the national level.

Where more complicated sampling and/or analysis methods are chosen, it is recommended to have these methods reviewed by a survey statistician or other individual with expertise in the application of these techniques. Additional guidance is available (Drummond et al., 2015).

2.4.8 Evaluating uncertainty in cost analysis

Cost analysis of immunization programs is undertaken to inform decision-making around resource allocation and use. A researcher, policymaker, or funder who understands both the heterogeneity and level of uncertainty in the cost results can make more informed decisions. In addition, decisions can be taken to mitigate the level of uncertainty.

While care is taken to generate the most robust and accurate estimates of total and unit costs of immunization services, all immunization costing studies contain some level of uncertainty in the estimates. Uncertainty means there is a range of values that cost estimates can take and the true estimate is somewhere in that range, and that there is some deviation in accuracy and precision of the estimate. Some uncertainty is derived from the study sampling process. An example is when the study sample of units (facilities) is not representative of the entire population of units. Cost estimates will have sample error and a higher degree of uncertainty. Randomization decreases sample errors; increasing the sample size will improve precision.

Sampling doesn't represent the full picture of uncertainty in cost estimates. Many inputs into the cost calculations are based on subjective assumptions which may lead to greater errors and level of uncertainty. We often don't directly observe these inputs and need to make assumptions. Measurement error may also stem from poor record keeping and recall bias. For instance, records on number of doses of vaccines administered may be sketchy, missing, or have reporting errors. Measurement of labor time allocation is often done by asking individuals how much time they spend on immunization activities. Time allocation data may be a major substantial source of measurement error in cost studies. Researchers are encouraged to verify and validate those estimates during data collection and analysis.

Uncertainty of immunization cost estimates should be estimated and reported, but this is often not undertaken as it is an additional analytical step in immunization costing studies. This is an area of methodological development that needs to be addressed. Usually, policymakers and funding agencies do not request this type of analysis so it has been conveniently avoided. Yet, given that point estimates of total or unit costs may drive policy and programmatic decisions, it is important to present the level of uncertainty to improve understanding of the estimates and quality of these decisions. The Second Panel on Cost-Effectiveness in Health Care and Medicine, the International Decision Support Initiative reference case, as well as the Global Health Costing Consortium recommend that uncertainty be appropriately characterized (Sanders et al., 2016; Vassall et al., 2017).

There are several ways that uncertainty in cost estimates can be evaluated:

1. Calculating a confidence interval is one way to represent the level of uncertainty of an immunization cost estimate. A 95% confidence interval means that we are 95% confident that the true value is found within that range of estimates.
2. Identify and document major assumptions and potential sources of measurement error in the cost estimation and conduct a one-way sensitivity analysis, testing each of those assumptions and sources. This might include re-estimating the number of doses delivered using an alternative assumption, utilizing other options for tracing factors to allocate shared costs, and examining the impact of different prices of inputs, among others. A table or tornado diagram (Fig. 2.4.1) that reports the original estimate and the new cost estimates with each change, and the percent difference in the value, highlights how easily the baseline estimates are influenced by assumptions.
3. Other statistical techniques, such as a Monte Carlo analysis, scenario analysis, and threshold analysis can be used for economic evaluation including costs. Please see Chapter 4.2 for further details.

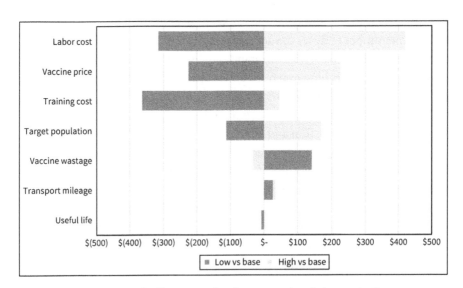

Fig. 2.4.1 Sample Tornado diagram evaluating uncertainty in immunization program costs.

2.4.9 Conclusion

This chapter describes various techniques related to immunization program delivery cost study design, data collection, and analysis. Discounting and annualization are important for evaluating the costs of capital assets that have a long useful life. Using the sampling weights to evaluate total and unit costs is another recommended approach. Finally, all cost studies should evaluate sources of uncertainty in the baseline estimates.

References

Clarke-Deelder, E., Vassall, A., & Menzies, N. A. (2019). Estimators used in multisite healthcare costing studies in low- and middle-income countries: A systematic review and simulation study. *Value in Health, 22*(10), 1146–1153. doi:10.1016/j.jval.2019.05.007

Drummond, M., Sculpher, M., Claxton, K., Stoddart, G. L., & Torrance, G. W. (2015). *Methods for the economic evaluation of health care programmes* (4th ed). Oxford: Oxford University Press.

Resch, S. C., Menzies, N. A., Portnoy, A., Clarke-Deelder, E., O'Keefe, L., Suharlim, C., & Brenzel, L. (2020). *How to cost immunization programs: A practical guide for primary data collection and analysis.* ImmunizationEconomics.org. http://www.immunizationeconomics.org/epic

Rivera-Rodriguez, C. L., Resch, S., & Haneuse, S. (2018). Quantifying and reducing statistical uncertainty in sample-based health program costing studies in low- and middle-income countries. *SAGE Open Medicine, 6*, 2050312118765602. doi:10.1177/2050312118765602

Sanders, G. D., Neumann, P. J., Basu, A., Brock, D. W., Feeny, D., Krahn, M., . . . Ganiats, T. G. (2016). Recommendations for conduct, methodological practices, and reporting of cost-effectiveness analyses: Second Panel on Cost-Effectiveness in Health and Medicine. *JAMA, 316*(10), 1093–1103. doi:10.1001/jama.2016.12195

Vassall, A., Sweeney, S., Kahn, J., Gomez, G. B., Bollinger, L., Marseille, E., . . . Levin, C. (2017). *Reference case for estimating the costs of global health services and interventions.* LSHTM Research Online. https://researchonline.lshtm.ac.uk/id/eprint/4653001/1/vassall_etal_2018_reference_case_for_estimating_costs_global_health_services.pdf

World Health Organization. (2021). *CHOosing Interventions that are Cost-Effective (CHOICE).* https://www.who.int/news-room/feature-stories/detail/new-cost-effectiveness-updates-from-who-choice

2.5

Costing new vaccine introduction

Susmita Chatterjee, Siriporn Pooripussarakul, and Logan Brenzel

2.5.1 Introduction

Since 2000, lower-income countries have been able to introduce new and underused vaccines at subsidized prices through Gavi, the Vaccine Alliance. More than 70 Gavi-eligible countries have introduced pentavalent and injectable polio vaccines. Gavi supported 60 vaccine introductions and campaigns in 2019, and the coronavirus disease 2019 (COVID-19) Vaccines Global Access (COVAX) initiative is supporting introduction of COVID-19 vaccines in over 100 countries (Gavi, 2021). Country decision-making around whether to introduce a new vaccine or not depends upon a range of factors. The introduction of new vaccines depends on a range of criteria, including clinical efficacy, safety, feasibility, policy and regulatory and economic considerations, among others (Pooripussarakul, Riewpaiboon, Bishai, Tantivess, & Muangchana, 2018). When introducing a new vaccine, there are major concerns such as the magnitude of disease burden, vaccine safety and effectiveness, and the viability and sustainability of the immunization program, among other factors (Loze et al., 2017). New and underutilized vaccine introduction (NUVI) requires substantial investment, not only in terms of vaccines and supplies but also health systems and other infrastructure inputs such as cold chain, training, and advocacy. This chapter presents methodological considerations for costing NUVI.

The costs of NUVI can be higher per dose than those for routine immunization services (Griffiths et al., 2016; Le Gargasson, Nyonator, Adibo, Gessner, & Colombini, 2015; Levin, Wang, Levin, Tsu, & Hutubessy, 2014; ThinkWell, 2020; World Health Organization: Immunization Vaccines and Biologicals, 2002). This is largely because the highest fixed costs associated with introduction are spread over fewer children being reached in the early phases. The main drivers of NUVI costs tend to be training, social mobilization, and actual service delivery.

Susmita Chatterjee, Siriporn Pooripussarakul, and Logan Brenzel, *Costing new vaccine introduction* In: *Handbook of Applied Health Economics in Vaccines*. Edited by: David Bishai, Logan Brenzel and William V. Padula, Oxford University Press. © Oxford University Press 2023. DOI: 10.1093/oso/9780192896087.003.0012

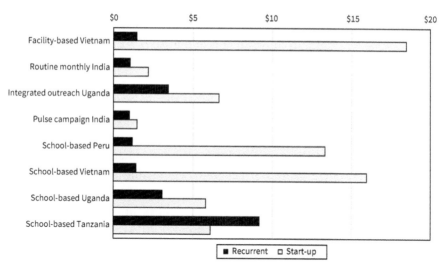

Fig. 2.5.1 Cost of delivering HPV vaccine per fully immunized girl.
Source: Levin et al. (2014).

Fig. 2.5.1 shows the variation in start-up and recurrent costs for introduction of human papillomavirus vaccine in eight countries, depending upon the strategies used. Start-up costs were generally higher than recurring costs, and school-based delivery was also larger per fully immunized girl than facility-based delivery on the whole (Griffiths et al., 2016; Le Gargasson et al., 2015; Levin et al., 2014; ThinkWell, 2020).

2.5.2 Overall approach and rationale for NUVI costing

Costing of NUVI is different from costing the routine immunization program. The main difference is that unlike in routine immunization costing which examines the total cost of the program, in NUVI costing, the focus is on incremental inputs and costs above and beyond the routine baseline costs. This approach has implications for the types of inputs evaluated and how they are measured.

The incremental cost of NUVI may be measured as a fiscal cost, a financial cost, or an economic cost, depending on the objective of the cost estimation. If the objective is to plan for the budget of the program, a fiscal cost analysis is appropriate as it measures the additional expenditures required on goods and services related to NUVI.

Economic costs are the opportunity costs, defined as resources that have been forgone for alternative investments and uses. A NUVI may require additional injections and time spent delivering a vaccine that could be used to provide other productive interventions. If the purpose is to evaluate the cost-effectiveness of a new vaccine, then the focus should be on incremental economic costs of vaccine introduction. If the result of the costing exercise is to incorporate the findings into a sustainability plan or ascertaining budget impact, the focus needs to be on evaluating incremental financial costs.

The World Health Organization generated a guideline for estimating NUVI costs into the existing program (World Health Organization: Immunization Vaccines and Biologicals, 2002). Other guidelines provide a step-by-step overview of how to estimate NUVI costs (Brenzel, 2014).

Costing of NUVI poses several additional requirements on new immunization programs (Pooripussarakul et al., 2018). The first step is to identify the quantities and prices of the additional inputs above and beyond the routine program required for NUVI and delivery. The type of new vaccine introduced will determine storage volumes, cold chain requirements, types of syringes to be used, and additional time allocated for various activities such as administration of the vaccine or record keeping. Depending upon the delivery strategy used, there may other inputs to include. Table 2.5.1 shows the various

Table 2.5.1 Costs of NUVI related to type of vaccine

New vaccine formulation	Likely additional resources required
Combination vaccines	Vaccines, syringes Additional labor time for administration, record keeping, and other activities Cold storage and distribution, including vehicles Social mobilization and advocacy Training for health workers Vaccination cards and reporting systems Disease surveillance
Monovalent vaccines	Vaccines, syringes Additional labor time for administration, record keeping, and other activities Supplies (reconstituting syringes, alcohol wipes, etc.) Waste management Additional time costs Cold storage and distribution Social mobilization and advocacy Training for health workers Vaccination cards and reporting systems Disease surveillance

additional inputs that may be required for different types of vaccines. Adding a monovalent vaccine may entail additional inputs such as syringes, training, reprinting of vaccination cards, advocacy and social mobilization, disease surveillance, and additional cold storage and waste management supplies. If the vaccine needs to be reconstituted, additional storage space and syringes are required. Combination vaccines, such as the pentavalent vaccine, may eventually save on cold storage space if replacing more than one vaccine. A combination vaccine that doesn't require additional syringes or supplies may not pose additional costs for the cold chain, inventory management, and distribution system. On the other hand, a monovalent vaccine or a combination vaccine with a different dosing schedule will require additional inputs into the existing immunization program (World Health Organization: Immunization Vaccines and Biologicals, 2002).

NUVI may require additional cold chain management, for example, the replacement of ten-dose vials of whole-cell diphtheria–tetanus–pertussis (DTwP) vaccine with single-dose vials of pentavalent (DTwP– hepatitis B–*Haemophilus influenzae* type b) vaccine. If the transportation of the new vaccine exceeds the capacity of the existing transportation system, the inclusion of additional vehicles or shorter supply intervals may be required. The increase in vaccine and supply chain volume also requires additional storage and cold chain management. These result in increasing financial investment to accommodate the larger volume of vaccines in the distribution system (Mvundura et al., 2014).

Costing of NUVI can be focused retrospectively based on historical information or can be conducted as a projection of future costs. Cost projections will require making assumptions based on expert interview and anticipated changes in the routine program.

2.5.3 NUVI cost estimation

NUVI costs should be divided into initial or start-up costs (needed to set up the program) and ongoing costs (needed to keep the program going). Investments related to NUVI can start long before the actual introduction of the vaccine and may continue after the introduction. Therefore, the time period for considering costs related to NUVI needs to be carefully demarcated to set the boundaries for NUVI costing, for example, when the introduction period begins, for start-up cost estimation, and when it ends, so costs are mapped into recurrent costs. In large countries where the NUVI will be in a phased manner, the approach to classify investment costs may require modification.

2.5.3.1 Initial or start-up costs

Investments that occur during the initial phase of the introduction or are one-off costs in the first year of the introduction are referred to as initial or start-up costs (Hidle et al., 2018; Ngabo et al., 2015). Initial costs of a new vaccine will focus on the additional activities and resources that occur when a new vaccine has been introduced, for example, microplanning, additional procurement of supplies, additional cold chain and logistics, additional transportation and per diem related to meetings and supervision, disease surveillance, development of new training materials, advocacy, and social mobilization materials (Hidle et al., 2018; Le Gargasson et al., 2015). Cost data include additional costs of capital, labor, and material of those activities. For example, the cold chain of a new vaccine may require extra cold containers and other equipment, such as refrigerators, computers, and printers. Logistic costs may increase in purchasing, storage and inventory management, and transportation of a new vaccine. A buffer stock, which is usually set at an additional 25% of doses, should be included in the estimation of initial vaccine costs (World Health Organization: Immunization Vaccines and Biologicals, 2002).

The initial costs are not only from new vaccine procurement, but also the costs of expanding the cold chain as well as increasing distribution costs, staff training costs, and expanding social mobilization and surveillance systems. UNICEF estimates that the introduction of pneumococcal conjugate vaccine, rotavirus, and human papillomavirus vaccines needs additional storage capacity of 100 cm^3 and adds a cost up to $20 per child (Chauke-Moagi & Mumba, 2012). In Thailand, 8.3% of healthcare centers required one additional refrigerator, 50% or 54.2% of the district warehouses for an additional one or two vaccines, respectively (Riewpaiboon et al., 2015). Different vaccines have consequences for cold chain storage and waste management. For instance, the cold chain volumes for pneumococcal conjugate vaccine, rotavirus, and human papillomavirus vaccines were estimated to be 55.9 cm^3, 46.3 cm^3, and 15 cm^3, respectively (Ngabo et al., 2015).

An important tool for estimating vaccine volume is the World Health Organization vaccine volume calculator (World Health Organization, 2021). This tool can help estimate the net storage volume per vaccine per child as well as the net storage volume per injection supplies and diluents per child. This will assist in the estimation of whether new cold chain equipment is required. The ratio of the share of vaccine volume for the new vaccine compared to existing storage volumes can be used to allocate cold chain cost to NUVI costs.

Capital investments made during the start-up period are usually annualized (Walker & Kumaranayake, 2002), following the same approaches outlined in Chapter 2.4. Capital investments include cold chain equipment, as well as initial training and information, education, and communication materials for social mobilization and advocacy. One approach is to allocate capital item costs that occur 6 months prior to and 6 months after introduction to NUVI costs.

2.5.3.2 Ongoing recurrent costs of NUVI

Ongoing recurrent costs for NUVI pertain to those inputs that will be continued past the initial introduction phase, and include vaccines and supplies, personnel, per diems, transportation operation and maintenance of cold chain equipment and vehicles, monitoring and evaluation, and supervision (Brenzel, Young, & Walker, 2015; Hidle et al., 2018; Levin et al., 2014; World Health Organization: Immunization Vaccines and Biologicals, 2002).

A combination vaccine with fewer injections requires fewer needles and syringes, and thus has lower administrative costs and vaccine storage costs compared to a monovalent vaccine (Hidle et al., 2018). For economic costs, donated vaccines, freight, customs, transport of vaccine and supplies, vaccine carriers, and cold packs should be factored into the estimates (Hyde et al., 2012).

For the freeze-dried vaccines, a reconstitution syringe will be required. The number of reconstitution syringes can be estimated using the number of freeze-dried vaccine doses administered per year, number of doses per vial, wastage rate, reserve stock, and price per syringe including freight rate. In case of syringes, wastage rate is generally fixed at 10%. Similar to vaccines, a reserve stock of 25% needs to be added in the first-year demand calculation at the district and state level.

NUVI will require the involvement of a wide range of staff members for planning, training, social mobilization, surveillance, monitoring and supervision, administration of the vaccine, waste management, and reporting. However, most of these staff members will not be exclusively involved in NUVI; therefore, personnel cost needs to be calculated based on time allocation for the new vaccine. The hours spent in each NUVI-related activity can be multiplied by the hourly wage (obtained from gross salary and work hours per week) to obtain the personnel cost related to NUVI.

NUVI will require extensive advocacy and social mobilization activities to inform the general public and healthcare workers about the new vaccine. It may involve displaying flyers and posters, distributing leaflets, conveying the message regarding the new vaccine through celebrities and actors, and advertisements through the media (radio/television/print). The incremental costs related to advocacy and social mobilization need to be calculated by gathering information on all such activities occurring before and during the introduction period. The majority of the social mobilization costs may be start-up costs which can be annualized.

Disease surveillance and monitoring of the new vaccine will be integrated into the existing system. The incremental costs of surveillance and evaluation include additional staff, training programs, transport, and laboratory findings. Recurrent costs associated with the new vaccine will revolve around additional personnel, transportation, and per diems (Erondu, Ferland, Haile, & Abimbola, 2019).

Table 2.5.2 provides a framework for evaluating the costs of vaccination activities related to NUVI. These are divided into start-up and recurrent costs, split into their financial or economic costs.

2.5.4 Data sources

The main data sources for calculating the incremental cost of NUVI will be immunization program managers at different levels. Information about different activities related to NUVI can be gathered through discussions with officials and the related staff using a standardized questionnaire. Financial records and other key documents related to the number of doses delivered can be obtained and reviewed at national or subnational health authority offices. To determine the time spent on new vaccine administration and other activities such as record keeping, waste management, and sensitization of the community, facility staff should be interviewed using a standardized questionnaire. Other important sources of information include the country's new vaccine application to Gavi which provides a detailed budget for NUVI. The Comprehensive Multi-Year Plan or the National Immunization Strategy may also provide useful information for NUVI costing. Records from UNICEF and World Health Organization offices in the country will be other sources of data.

Table 2.5.2 Activities and cost components of NUVI

Cost and description	Financial cost	Economic cost
Start-up costs		
Micro-planning related to new vaccine introduction, including meetings and events at different health system levels	Room rental Refreshments Per diem Printing	Financial cost + value of staff time
Training Training sessions and development of materials for a range of healthcare workers and administrators	Printing of training materials Supplies Venue rental Refreshments Per diem	Financial cost + value of staff time + value of volunteer worker time
Social mobilization and advocacy Community level and health worker sensitization to the new vaccine, including meetings, events, development and production, and materials and media	Venue rental Refreshments Supplies Printing of IEC materials Development of radio, television, social media messages, and materials Payment for securing radio/TV spots, and newspaper, internet, and social media advertising	Financial cost + value of staff time + value of volunteer worker time Financial cost of materials to be annualized
Cold chain Purchase of new cold chain equipment and/or use of existing cold storage space at various levels of the health system for storing and distributing the new vaccine	Cold chain equipment	Annualized financial cost + value of donated items + value of existing space used for new vaccine
Transport Purchase of additional vehicles, additional donated vehicles, and/or use of existing vehicles to transport vaccines and vaccinators.	Vehicle	Annualized financial cost + value of donated items + value of usage for new vaccine
Waste management Purchase of additional incinerators and/or use of existing incinerators	Incinerators	Annualized financial cost + value of existing space used for new vaccine
Recurrent costs		
Vaccines and injection supply	Cost of vaccine (excluding donor-supported vaccines) Cost of syringes Cost related to customs, receiving transport, and storage Co-financing fees for Gavi-supported vaccines	Financial cost + cost of vaccine (less co-financing fees) In case of donated vaccine: financial cost + cost of donor-supported vaccine

(continued)

Table 2.5.2 Continued

Cost and description	Financial cost	Economic cost
Service delivery Personnel time spent on administering the new vaccine, incremental per diem, and transportation costs	Per diem Travel allowance Fuel and maintenance	Financial cost + value of staff time + value of volunteer worker time
Supervision, monitoring, and evaluation Ongoing supervision and record keeping, reporting activities related to the new vaccines	Per diem Travel allowance Fuel and maintenance Printing vaccination cards and reporting formats	Financial cost + value of staff time
Disease surveillance Activities specific to identifying adverse events following immunization, and cases of disease	Refreshments Per diem Travel allowance Laboratory supplies Fuel and maintenance	Financial cost + value of staff time
Waste management Management of waste at the vaccination site	Safety boxes Hub cutters Containers Per diem Refreshments	Financial cost + value of staff time
Vaccine transport Vehicle use related to administration of the new vaccine	Vehicle	Financial cost + value of donated items + value of existing space used for new vaccine
Cold chain	Ongoing running costs related to storage of the new vaccine on a recurrent basis (energy)	Financial cost
Ongoing training	Ongoing costs associated with refresher training related to the new vaccine	Financial cost
Social mobilization and advocacy	Ongoing social mobilization and advocacy costs	Financial cost

2.5.5 Conclusion

This chapter highlights a general approach and framing for evaluating the costs of NUIV. Costs for NUVI are incremental to the existing system and can be evaluated as fiscal, financial, or economic costs depending upon the use of the results by decision makers. In addition, costs should be divided into initial/start-up costs or ongoing, recurrent costs for NUVI. Guidance documents are available to provide additional recommended approaches for data collection and analysis.

References

Brenzel, L. (2014). Working Paper: Common approach for the costing and financing analyses of routine immunization and new vaccine introduction costs (EPIC). Mimeograph. Bill & Melinda Gates Foundation. www.immunizationeconomics.org/epic-info.

Brenzel, L., Young, D., & Walker, D. G. (2015). Costs and financing of routine immunization: Approach and selected findings of a multi-country study (EPIC). *Vaccine, 33*, A13–A20. doi:10.1016/j.vaccine.2014.12.066

Chauke-Moagi, B. E., & Mumba, M. (2012). New vaccine introduction in the East and Southern African sub-region of the WHO African region in the context of GIVS and MDGs. *Vaccine, 30*(Suppl 3), C3–C8. doi:10.1016/j.vaccine.2012.05.086

Erondu, N. A., Ferland, L., Haile, B. H., & Abimbola, T. (2019). A systematic review of vaccine preventable disease surveillance cost studies. *Vaccine, 37*(17), 2311–2321. doi:10.1016/j.vaccine.2019.02.026

Gavi. (2021). *Homepage.* http://www.gavi.org/

Griffiths, U. K., Bozzani, F. M., Chansa, C., Kinghorn, A., Kalesha-Masumbu, P., Rudd, C., . . . Schutte, C. (2016). Costs of introducing pneumococcal, rotavirus and a second dose of measles vaccine into the Zambian immunisation programme: Are expansions sustainable? *Vaccine, 34*(35), 4213–4220. doi:10.1016/j.vaccine.2016.06.050

Hidle, A., Gwati, G., Abimbola, T., Pallas, S. W., Hyde, T., Petu, A., . . . Manangazira, P. (2018). Cost of a human papillomavirus vaccination project, Zimbabwe. *Bulletin of the World Health Organization, 96*(12), 834–842. doi:10.2471/BLT.18.211904

Hyde, T. B., Dentz, H., Wang, S. A., Burchett, H. E., Mounier-Jack, S., & Mantel, C. F. (2012). The impact of new vaccine introduction on immunization and health systems: A review of the published literature. *Vaccine, 30*(45), 6347–6358. doi:10.1016/j.vaccine.2012.08.029

Le Gargasson, J. B., Nyonator, F. K., Adibo, M., Gessner, B. D., & Colombini, A. (2015). Costs of routine immunization and the introduction of new and underutilized vaccines in Ghana. *Vaccine, 33*(Suppl 1), A40–A46. doi:10.1016/j.vaccine.2014.12.081

Levin, A., Wang, S. A., Levin, C., Tsu, V., & Hutubessy, R. (2014). Costs of introducing and delivering HPV vaccines in low and lower middle income countries: Inputs for GAVI policy on introduction grant support to countries. *PLoS One, 9*(6), e101114. doi:10.1371/journal.pone.0101114

Loze, P. M., Nasciben, L. B., Sartori, A. M. C., Itria, A., Novaes, H. M. D., & de Soárez, P. C. (2017). Vaccines are different: A systematic review of budget impact analyses of vaccines. *Vaccine, 35*(21), 2781–2793. doi:10.1016/j.vaccine.2017.03.088

Mvundura, M., Kien, V. D., Nga, N. T., Robertson, J., Cuong, N. V., Tung, H. T., . . . Levin, C. (2014). How much does it cost to get a dose of vaccine to the service delivery location? Empirical evidence from Vietnam's Expanded Program on Immunization. *Vaccine, 32*(7), 834–838. doi:10.1016/j.vaccine.2013.12.029

Ngabo, F., Levin, A., Wang, S. A., Gatera, M., Rugambwa, C., Kayonga, C., . . . Hutubessy, R. (2015). A cost comparison of introducing and delivering pneumococcal, rotavirus and human papillomavirus vaccines in Rwanda. *Vaccine, 33*(51), 7357–7363. doi:10.1016/j.vaccine.2015.10.022

Pooripussarakul, S., Riewpaiboon, A., Bishai, D., Tantivess, S., & Muangchana, C. (2018). Identifying important factors impacting the adoption of new vaccines in Thailand by using a best-worst scaling. *Journal of Health Systems Research, 12*(1), 137–149. https://kb.hsri.or.th/dspace/bitstream/handle/11228/4857/hsri_journal_v12n1_p137.pdf

Riewpaiboon, A., Sooksriwong, C., Chaiyakunapruk, N., Tharmaphornpilas, P., Techathawat, S., Rookkapan, K., . . . Suraratdecha, C. (2015). Optimizing national immunization program supply chain management in Thailand: An economic analysis. *Public Health, 129*(7), 899–906. doi:10.1016/j.puhe.2015.04.016

ThinkWell. (2020). *Immunization delivery cost catalogue.* http://www.immunizationeconom ics.org/ican

Walker, D., & Kumaranayake, L. (2002). Allowing for differential timing in cost analyses: Discounting and annualization. *Health Policy and Planning, 17*(1), 112–118. doi:10.1093/heapol/17.1.112

World Health Organization. (2021). *Vaccine volume calculator.* https://www.who.int/publicati ons/m/item/vaccine-volume-calculator

World Health Organization: Immunization Vaccines and Biologicals. (2002). *Guidelines for estimating costs of introducing new vaccines into the national immunization system.* https:// apps.who.int/iris/handle/10665/67342

3

ECONOMIC EVALUATION OF VACCINES AND VACCINE PROGRAMS

Edited by William V. Padula, Emmanuel F. Drabo, and Ijeoma Edoka

3.0

Section introduction: economic evaluation of vaccines and vaccine programs

William V. Padula, Emmanuel F. Drabo, and Ijeoma Edoka

Economic evaluation is increasingly used to inform decision makers about the value that various interventions deliver to health systems. Sometimes the greatest value in healthcare is achieved not by what is provided to the patient in terms of services and technology, but what is avoided. We know for a fact that prevention of infectious diseases is a win–win for patients, providers, and society as a whole. When we invest in the prevention of infectious diseases through vaccines, the relatively small costs of vaccines achieve enormous value. Providers and payers do not have to care for as many patients facing the symptoms of infectious disease. And patients do not have to deal with the personal costs of treatment, or deal with the acute and long-term fall out of infectious disease. We know that many diseases ranging from influenza to polio have impacts on well-being in ways that are detrimental to the patient and the productivity of society as a whole. Methods in economic evaluation measure impacts of these outcomes and their value.

All these aspects of value added through vaccines might be implicit, but we need to use empirical science in order to quantify value so that decision makers can make informed choices about the adoption of vaccines for entire populations of at-risk individuals. These are not small investments. Investments in vaccines that represent whole percentages of a nation's gross domestic product rely on accurate assessments of value to solidify decisions. Approaches in economic evaluation, ranging from cost-effectiveness to budget impact analysis, are tools that can be used to inform decision makers. The methods to conduct these analyses are not always easy, but we recommend starting with simple,

William V. Padula, Emmanuel F. Drabo, and Ijeoma Edoka, *Section introduction: economic evaluation of vaccines and vaccine programs* In: *Handbook of Applied Health Economics in Vaccines*. Edited by: David Bishai, Logan Brenzel and William V. Padula, Oxford University Press. © Oxford University Press 2023. DOI: 10.1093/oso/9780192896087.003.0013 intuitive models to calculate the resulting measures of value that decision makers can rely on.

This section is broken down into several chapters which are necessary steps in a progression toward achieving economic evaluation. Here, we take you through a synopsis of each chapter in order to understand what data are needed to build a value assessment.

Chapter 3.1 is an overview of decision analysis and cost-effectiveness. Here we want to understand value by defining it. Many academics have often expressed value as a function of *cost* and *quality*, but measuring vaccine value and expressing it quantitatively is not so straightforward. By focusing on cohort-level analyses of value, we can more accurately determine the impact that a certain vaccine will have for a specific population that is at risk for infectious disease. Thus, decision makers can make local, replicable decisions about investment in vaccines that protect different populations based on regional variation, age, sex, race, or ethnicity. The chapter introduces basic concepts such as the difference between cost-effectiveness and cost–benefit analysis, as well as how to derive measures of budget impact and return on investment from a single economic model.

Chapter 3.2 offers guidance on defining the scope and study design of a cost-effectiveness analysis. As mentioned earlier, healthcare involves many stakeholders ranging from payers, to providers, to integrated health systems, to patients, and ultimately to society as a whole. Economic models can range in their measurement of costs and effectiveness depending on the perspective of these stakeholders. We will explore how these perspectives impact the design and calculation of different economic model parameters. We will also highlight basic types of economic models (i.e., decision trees and Markov chains) which are used to simulate the impacts of vaccines on different types of static or time-dependent health outcomes, as well as accumulate costs and effectiveness measures.

Chapter 3.3 focuses on parameter estimation. Economic models that are used to measure vaccine value are only as strong as the data used in the model. Health economists depend on the availability of data from a number of different reliable sources in order to populate a model with parameters. These sources include some of the typical study designs that one might encounter from data on vaccine effectiveness, such as randomized controlled trials, observational studies, and so on. The chapter explores how to extract high-quality information about costs, effectiveness, and probability parameters that can be used to make an economic model functional.

Chapter 3.4 reviews the methods used to measure and evaluate health outcomes. There are a number of different measures that economists have developed over the years to quantify the effectiveness of vaccines. Two of the most commonly used in cost-effectiveness analysis are quality-adjusted life years and disability-adjusted life years, in addition to more intuitive measures such as mortality and incidence rates in an at-risk population. The chapter explores these effectiveness measurements and the types of psychometric approaches that have been developed to derive estimates of effectiveness.

Chapter 3.5 explains some of the important considerations for reporting and interpreting the results of economic evaluations. Once a model has been developed and populated with parameter information, an investigator should be prepared to understand what the results are telling them about value from the perspective of the key stakeholders. Incremental cost-effectiveness ratios, budget impacts, and return on investment results are all key statistics that one should be able to know and interpret to make recommendations about vaccine value. Furthermore, there are number of data visualization techniques that can go along with these statistics to make the results clearer to decision makers about value.

Chapter 3.6 examines other measures of economic efficiency that may be important to decision makers. Not all determinations of value end with cost-effectiveness analysis. Often, decision makers depend on budget impact analysis (BIA) to determine affordability with respect to budget constraints. In addition, return on investment (ROI) calculations give decision makers reassurance that vaccine programs are not sunken costs, but rather investments in the public's health that pay dividends over time. By becoming familiar with multiple forms of value estimation, economic modelers can be prepared to produce results that gain the attention of decision makers, whatever their preference may be for information.

Chapter 3.7 consolidates the material on economic evaluation for vaccines throughout this section with an applied case. By following along with the construction of a simple decision tree and data parameter inputs, one should be able to accurately derive and interpret key resulting statistics of value for a common example in vaccine decision-making.

3.1

Overview of decision analysis and cost-effectiveness

Emmanuel F. Drabo, Ijeoma Edoka, and William V. Padula

3.1.1 Understanding "value"

Resource allocation decisions within the health sector can be made based on the benefits or value of the vaccine program and its associated costs. Economic evaluations typically compare the benefits and costs of competing alternatives to assess whether a vaccine technology represents good value for money. Vaccines are considered one of the most effective health technologies for preventing mortality and morbidity due to infectious disease. In addition to their direct health benefits in vaccinated individuals, vaccines can lead to indirect health benefits in unvaccinated individuals due to a reduction in the transmission of disease (e.g., the herd effect) as well as broader microeconomic and macroeconomic benefits that extend beyond health.

In the economic evaluation of new vaccines, the value of vaccines is typically expressed in terms of health gains (both direct and indirect) measured using different outcomes such as the number of infections averted, deaths averted, life years gained, disability-adjusted life years (DALYs), or quality-adjusted life years (QALYs). The value of vaccines also extends beyond health benefits to include direct and indirect economic benefits to individuals and healthcare systems. Direct economic benefits include costs savings due to reductions in direct cost incurred by individuals when seeking healthcare or direct costs incurred by healthcare systems in delivering healthcare for infectious diseases. Indirect economic benefits, on the other hand, may include productivity gains to vaccinated individuals accruing from reductions in days lost from work due to illness or premature death as well as productivity gains to caregivers, also accruing from reductions in days lost from work to care for an ill individual.

Emmanuel F. Drabo, Ijeoma Edoka, and William V. Padula, *Overview of decision analysis and cost-effectiveness* In: *Handbook of Applied Health Economics in Vaccines*. Edited by: David Bishai, Logan Brenzel and William V. Padula, Oxford University Press. © Oxford University Press 2023. DOI: 10.1093/oso/9780192896087.003.0014

The microeconomic benefits of vaccines have traditionally been used for assessing the value for money of vaccines when making funding decisions. However, these benefits may underestimate the true value of vaccines and a growing body of literature has highlighted the broader value of vaccination that goes beyond the direct/indirect health and health-related economic benefits to individuals and health systems (Bärnighausen, Bloom, Cafiero-Fonseca, & O'Brien, 2014; Bärnighausen, Bloom, Canning, & O'Brien, 2008; Deogaonkar, Hutubessy, van der Putten, Evers, & Jit, 2012; Jit et al., 2015; Ozawa, Mirelman, Stack, Walker, & Levine, 2012). These broader benefits can be more important in low-resource settings where funding decisions are often made alongside broader development goals that fall outside the health sector (Deogaonkar et al., 2012). Bärnighausen et al. (2008) classify benefits of vaccines as narrow or broad. Narrow benefits include health gains, healthcare cost savings, and care-related productivity gain and broad benefits include outcome-related productivity gains, behavior-related productivity gains, and community externalities.

This framework has since been extended to incorporate other broad values that are potentially important for making resource allocation decisions on introducing new vaccines. These include broader community and health system externalities such as ecological effects, equity, financial sustainability, and household security as well as broader economic indicators such as public sector budget impact and macroeconomic impact. While the link between vaccination and the so-called narrow benefits of vaccines are well established, the causal link between vaccines and several broad benefits remains less certain (Jit et al., 2015), and may limit their incorporation into assessments of the value for money of vaccines.

3.1.2 The importance of economic evaluation of vaccines

Economic evaluations, such as cost-effectiveness analyses (CEAs), cost-utility analyses (CUAs), and cost–benefit analyses (CBAs), compare the costs and benefits of competing alternatives (e.g., preventive vaccines versus treatment of disease) to assess trade-offs that arise when inevitable choices must be made between alternative courses of action and budgets are fixed. Comparing costs to valued outcomes is useful for decision makers in order to choose health interventions that produce the highest benefits for a given cost. Valuing outcomes is simplest when health maximization is the sole policy objective.

Given the high value of vaccines in terms of their direct and indirect health and economic benefits to vaccinated and unvaccinated individuals and the relatively low costs of first-generation vaccines, vaccines have largely been shown to be a cost-effective health intervention for preventing mortality and morbidity associated with infectious diseases.

With growing innovation and technological advancements in the development of new vaccines, the costs of new and next-generation vaccines are expected to be substantially higher (Delany, Rappuoli, & De Gregorio, 2014; Tahamtan, Charostad, Hoseini Shokouh, & Barati, 2017). For example, human papillomavirus (HPV) and pneumococcal conjugate vaccines have a significantly higher price per dose compared to first-generation vaccines such as yellow fever and oral polio vaccines. The high costs of new-generation vaccines have significant budget implications for many countries, particularly for middle-income countries with limited access to external funding mechanisms. Given that decisions to fund new vaccination programs must be made in the wider context of other competing goals both within and outside the health sector, economic evaluations that capture the value of new-generation vaccines in addition to their costs are important for assessing the value for money of these vaccines and motivating to increase allocation of resources to new vaccination programs.

In addition to informing resource allocation decisions on the introduction of new vaccination programs, economic evaluations can be useful for informing the prioritization of vaccination programmatic strategies. For example, the World Health Organization recommends various programmatic strategies for eliminating rubella infection and congenital rubella syndrome within a 10–30-year timeframe (World Health Organization, 2011). These strategies range from vaccinating all children from 9 months to 4 years old to vaccinating only women of childbearing age or vaccinating all adolescents and adults between the ages of 15 and 39 years (World Health Organization, 2011). Economic evaluation has been applied in several countries, particularly in high-income countries to inform decisions on rubella elimination strategies (Babigumira, Morgan, & Levin, 2013). Other examples of the application of economic evaluation include the prioritization of HPV vaccination strategies such as decisions about when to add adolescent boys into the existing female-only HPV vaccination programs. CEAs showing higher cost-effectiveness of the HPV vaccine in girls than in in boys (Datta et al., 2019; Seto, Marra, Raymakers, & Marra, 2012) have contributed to informing this decision.

Economic evaluations can also be useful as price negotiation tools through the value-based pricing approach. This approach allows for the determination of the price of new health technologies based on the maximum price at which the technology is considered cost-effective using predefined cost-effectiveness thresholds of decision makers (see Chapter 3.5). This approach required a consensus on the type(s) of value to be measured as well as an appropriate threshold or benchmark against which this value is assessed (Claxton, 2007; Drummond & Towse, 2019). Value-based pricing approaches have been widely adopted in several countries that use CEAs to inform reimbursement decisions such as in the UK (Claxton, 2007; Drummond & Towse, 2019) and Thailand (Teerawattananon, Tritasavit, Suchonwanich, & Kingkaew, 2014), and have been instrumental in these countries for negotiating reductions in the price of new health technologies including vaccines. For example, in Thailand, data from CEA informed price negotiations resulting in a 55% reduction in the original asking price of a HPV vaccine (Teerawattananon & Tritasavit, 2015). Although value-based pricing is an instrumental tool for price negotiation of vaccines, it may not always be appropriate for setting the price of some health technologies, particularly interventions against rare conditions or interventions that cost significantly less than an existing intervention (Drummond & Towse, 2019).

3.1.3 Introduction to measures of value

Vaccines may generate both positive and negative externalities beyond the healthcare sector. These externalities can significantly influence disease patterns, as well as the impacts of disease on healthcare and society. At the same time, the procurement and the distribution of vaccines require significant resources. However, with scarce healthcare resources and multiple competing needs over these resources, cost containment is becoming important. It is critical that whenever a decision is to be made about adopting a new vaccine, the additional benefit produced by the intervention be sufficiently larger than the cost. In other words, we need to ensure that the new intervention or policy provides good value. To more accurately assess the value generated by a vaccination program or the introduction of a new vaccine, it is therefore critical that we capture the value of all its relevant economic costs and benefits. Given that vaccines may have value to a variety of non-healthcare stakeholders such as governments and households, vaccine value measurement must be broad to capture the downstream consequences of vaccine introduction, such as potential displacements in healthcare resources.

Economic evaluation can systematically determine the "value for money" of healthcare interventions, such as immunization programs. By "value for money," we mean the monetary value of the benefits of the program, that is, the maximum amount of money a payer such as a government or an insurance company, would be willing to pay to enjoy these benefits, also known as the willingness to pay. Measures of value can incorporate better outcomes as well as ideals such as increased quality, better access, and equity (Goldman & McGlynn, 2005; Padula, Lee, & Pronovost, 2017). Decisions require a comparison of value to costs, often using the ratio of value to cost (Nelson, Batalden, Godfrey, & Lazar, 2011; Porter & Advantage, 1985). By economic cost, we mean the opportunity cost of adopting the program, that is, the cost of the next best alternative use of the resources devoted to the program. Hence, economic value can be more broadly defined as the comparative analysis of the costs and consequences of an intervention, policy, or strategy against similar outcomes of its next best alternative(s).

Measurement of the cost component of the value equation is done by assigning monetary values to resources used. In contrast, measurement of outcomes, quality access, and equity is more challenging, because these goals are can be less tangible than cost, and involve multidimensional constructs (Garrison, Jansen, Devlin, & Griffin, 2019; Padula et al., 2017). Economic evaluation methods vary in their approaches to assessing the value of new and existing interventions, mainly along the types of health outcomes used. The most common types of economic evaluation analyses include cost of illness (COI) analysis, budget impact analysis (BIA), return on investment (ROI) analysis, cost comparison analysis, cost-minimization analysis (CMA), cost–consequence analysis (CCA), CEA, CUA, and CBA.

The first two methods (i.e., COI and BIA) assess the burden of disease and affordability of a new intervention. More concretely, COI analysis aims to determine the economic impact of an illness or condition, such as hepatitis B, on a given population (e.g., people with diabetes) or geographic area (e.g., region, country), including its associated treatment costs. BIA estimates the affordability, that is, the impact of adopting a new intervention, such as introducing a new vaccine, on a payer's budget (Mauskopf, Earnshaw, Brogan, Wolowacz, & Brodtkorb, 2017; Sullivan et al., 2014). The value of an intervention can therefore be determined in COI analysis and BIA by examining the *opportunity cost* of implementing that intervention.

The remaining economic evaluation methods listed above are more explicitly designed to assess value for money spent. Specifically, ROI analysis evaluates the efficiency of an intervention, by measuring the amount of return (i.e., net benefit) on the intervention in monetary terms, relative to its cost. Hence, ROI measures the value of investing in the intervention. CMA determines the least costly intervention among competing alternatives that are assumed to produce equivalent health outcomes (Berger, Bingefors, Hedblom, Pashos, & Torrance, 2003). CEA compares two or more alternative interventions in terms of their costs, expressed in monetary units, and health outcomes, expressed in "natural" health units such as mortality or morbidity. CUA is a particular case of CEA, in which the health outcomes of interventions are expressed, unlike CEA, in terms of utility and mortality, which is expressed in QALYs. CCA is a form of CEA in which costs and health outcomes are presented in disaggregated form, thus allowing the decision maker to place preference weights on the costs and health outcomes. Finally, CBA compares the costs and health benefits of an intervention, in terms of monetary units.

Because CBA, CCA, CEA, CUA, and CMA measure and compare the costs and outcomes of at least two interventions, they are referred to as full economic evaluations (Table 3.1.1). Analyses that only evaluate a single intervention or consider only one domain (e.g., cost only or effectiveness only) are known as partial economic evaluations.

Outcomes in health can be multidimensional constructs, leading to several measures, including QALYs gained, net costs, insurance value, value of hope, and so on (Garrison et al., 2019). Costing is the approach used to *evaluate* the "next best" use of scarce resources that would be needed to produce a certain health effect. Depending on the context, QALYs and DALYs are the most commonly used dimensions of value assessment in healthcare decision-making. As a composite measure which combines the length of life with preferences (health-related quality of life), QALYs provide a measure of value of health outcomes which is advantageous for evaluating health technologies and interventions.

While value assessment for vaccines can be conducted from various perspectives, the fact that vaccines generate significant externalities that can span multiple sectors implies that vaccine value assessment should be conducted at the population level rather than at the individual level. This requires using measures of value that make sense at the population level and a broader evaluation beyond the clinical focus.

Table 3.1.1 Types of economic evaluations based on costs and outcomes typologies

Type of analysis	Costs		Outcomes		Comparison of interventions
	Inclusion	Valuation	Inclusion	Valuation	
Partial economic evaluation					
Cost of illness analysis (COI)	Yes	Monetary units	No	–	None (disease-level analysis)
Budget impact analysis (BIA)	Yes	Monetary units	Yes	None or maximize various	Yes
Return on investment (ROI) analysis	Yes	Monetary units	Yes	Monetary units	Yes, ROI
Cost comparison analysis	Yes	Monetary units	No	–	Yes
Full economic evaluation					
Cost–minimization analysis (CMA)	Yes	Monetary units	Yes	None (assume unchanged)	Yes
Cost–consequence analysis (CCA)	Yes	Monetary units	Yes	Natural units	Yes
Cost–effectiveness analysis (CEA)	Yes	Monetary units	Yes	Natural units	Yes, ICER or NMB
Cost–utility analysis (CUA)	Yes	Monetary units	Yes	Utilities: QALY, DALY, healthy year equivalent	Yes, ICER or NMB
Cost–benefit analysis (CBA)	Yes	Monetary units	Yes	Monetary units	Yes, cost–benefit ratio or net benefit

3.1.4 Define methods of value analysis

Health economics provides tools for defining and measuring value for money. Tools of economic evaluation enable identification of the most efficient course of action from a set of alternative options, that is, the alternative that provides the highest value for money. CEA is one of the most widely used methods of economic evaluation; other methods include cost-finding or cost-identification analysis (CFA/CIA), CMA, COI analysis, CCA, CBA, BIA, and ROI analysis (Drummond, Sculpher, Claxton, Stoddart, & Torrance, 2015).

CFA/CIA is the process of identifying all costs and their relative importance (Berger et al., 2003). The goal of a CFA/CIA is to identify resources used to produce a particular program or intervention, and to estimate the monetary value of these resources. The cost data generated can then be used as standalone information for decision-making or integrated into decision support frameworks to inform policymakers.

Cost comparison analysis compares only the costs associated with two or more alternative healthcare interventions. Costs are typically identified through a CFA/CIA. The method consists of comparing the costs of two different treatment mixes (including medical and non-medical products and services). Cost comparison analysis is particularly useful in situations when the interventions are recurrent and complex (e.g., multiple dosage regimens), because it can help quantify and compare the differences in costs between alternative strategies (e.g., differences in costs of vaccination programs with different intensities or coverage levels). As it is essential to identify all costs related to an intervention, including the treatment costs, and costs of drugs, devices, nutritional supplements, and professional care, policymakers usually use COI analysis (described below) instead of a cost comparison analysis.

CMA aims to identify the least costly alternative among a set of options with similar expected health outcomes (Berger et al., 2003). CMA achieves this by identifying resources consumed in the provision of alternative interventions, to estimate and compare the monetary value of these resources across alternatives. In rare situations when health outcomes are extremely similar across alternative strategies, the least expensive (least costly) intervention should be prioritized. In the context of vaccine economics, one may use CMA to decide, for example, between a combination measles, mumps, rubella, and varicella vaccine to separate injections of its equivalent component vaccines (i.e., a measles, mumps, and rubella vaccine plus a varicella vaccine), provided that the health outcomes of the two options are equal. CMA is criticized for too often assuming identical health outcomes across interventions when this is hardly ever the case (Briggs & O'Brien, 2001). For example, all vaccination campaigns are not created equal, and could result in different effectiveness outcomes. Despite this criticism, CMA can be very useful in resource-constrained settings to inform cost-cutting measures when outcomes are similar across interventions of varying costs. Even in developed countries, CMA can be useful, as resources are scarce and must be efficiently allocated among interventions that yield the best value for money. For example, generic versions or cheaper bioequivalent of drugs are now more commonly preferred over costly branded drugs, to minimize costs, as these price variations are sometimes very substantial.

COI analysis, also called "burden of illness" analysis, focuses on the health status of a target population without an intervention to estimate both healthcare resources consumed and associated costs. The approach consists of measuring the medical and other costs resulting from a specific disease or condition. Unlike cost comparison analysis, which only measures the costs of different interventions, COI measures all relevant cost of the disease, including its treatment. "Burden of illness" is quantified with metrics such as the direct costs of the disease (e.g., medical costs, and non-medical costs such as travel costs), mortality (e.g., years of life lost), intangible costs of a disease or injury (e.g., disabilities, limitations on daily activity), or productivity losses such as absenteeism (being physically absent from work due to illness or caregiving) and presenteeism (being physically present at work but working at reduced capacity) costs.

CCA identifies resources consumed in the provision of alternative interventions, to estimate the cost of each alternative intervention. In addition, CCA identifies and quantifies the effects of each intervention. CCA methodology does not indicate the relative importance of the components enumerated. The weighting of these components is left at the decision maker's discretion. For complex interventions with complex outcomes, CCA can be a relatively difficult exercise to conduct, as each outcome and its costs must be assessed separately, and then evaluated.

CBA is a method derived from the economic theory that compares alternative interventions in terms of their net social cost, defined as the difference of the social cost and social benefit, expressed in monetary value. All relevant consequences for each intervention are assigned a monetary value, including survival gains, and days of disability. CBA can be used to evaluate the worthiness of adopting a single program (i.e., whether the program's net social benefits are positive) or to compare alternative interventions (i.e., determine

which program yields the greatest net social benefit). The net monetary benefit (NMB) of the intervention is then calculated as follows:
Equation 3.1.1. NMB:

$$NMB = Benefit\ of\ intervention - Cost\ of\ intervention$$

Sometime, this value assessment is done by calculating the benefit–cost ratio:
Equation 3.1.2. Benefit–cost ratio:

$$Benefit - cost\ ratio = \frac{Benefit\ of\ intervention}{Cost\ of\ intervention}$$

When the NMB is positive, or equivalently, when the benefit–cost ratio exceeds 1, the intervention is said to be cost beneficial, and to represent good value for money. In the case where two interventions are being compared, the incremental NMB can be calculated as the difference of the NMBs. The corresponding incremental benefit–cost ratio can also be calculated to aid decision-making. The CBA approach has been successfully used to estimate the benefits of *Haemophilus influenzae* type b vaccine (Bärnighausen et al., 2011).

Social ROI analysis is a pragmatic form of CBA that accounts for effects on all community stakeholders to include their perspectives on social value where appropriate. Social ROI analyses appeal to what is known as the "triple bottom line" to take account of the intervention's effects on the economy, environment, and people (Drabo et al., 2021; Then, Schober, Rauscher, & Kehl, 2018).

While CBA methodology is commonly used by economists to value programs in many sectors (e.g., environmental, transportation, education, healthcare, etc.) and is a widely accepted valuation method in public projects, it is often difficult to apply CBA in clinical decision-making, due to reluctance by many to assign a monetary value to clinical and health outcomes. Instead, alternative economic evaluation methods such as CEA and CUA (described below) are more commonly used in healthcare.

CEA is an economic evaluation methodology used to determine whether a healthcare intervention such as the introduction of a vaccine produces sufficient improvements in health to justify its costs. A CEA compares two or more alternative interventions—including the status quo—in terms of their efficiency, by relating their cost and outcomes. CEA does this by identifying and measuring the costs and health benefits of these alternative interventions. In CEA, "benefits" are measured in "natural units," such as survival or life years gained, clinical outcomes (e.g., reduction in body mass index), number of cases detected, or number of cases averted. The efficiency of each alternative is calculated as a cost per unit of benefit produced, relative to the comparator intervention. This is known as the incremental cost-effectiveness ratio (ICER), more explicitly defined as the ratio of the incremental cost and incremental health benefits of an alternative intervention, relative to its comparator intervention (see Chapter 3.5). Interventions that yield the largest units of incremental benefits per cost are more efficient. To determine whether a given intervention represents good value for money to the payer, the ICER is compared to the decision maker's willingness-to-pay threshold per unit of the outcome.

CUA is a specific type of CEA in which benefits are calculated in terms of marginal gains in both number and quality (health-related quality of life) of life years lived. These marginal gains are measured in QALYs, DALYs, or healthy year equivalent.

CEA and CUA have the promise of improving health outcomes within the constraints of available funding, given their focus on efficiency. However, efficiency may not be the only outcome that is important to a decision maker. For example, a decision maker may also care about reducing social inequalities or disparities in health that are considered unfair or unjust. Unfortunately, traditional CEA and CUA provide no information about the equity impacts of health interventions such as vaccination programs, on social inequalities. More recent and emerging methods such as extended CEA and distributional CEA extend the CEA and CUA approaches to explicitly incorporate equity impacts of healthcare interventions (Asaria, Griffin, & Cookson, 2016; Cookson, Griffin, Norheim, & Culyer, 2020; Verguet, Kim, & Jamison, 2016). For more detailed discussion of general approaches to incorporating equity the equity impacts of social investments in economic evaluation, the reader should refer to the work by Cookson, Drummond, and Weatherly (2009).

Other important methods of economic evaluation which deserve a brief discussion in this chapter and are further discussed in subsequent chapters of this textbook are BIA and ROI analysis.

BIA is an economic assessment methodology that estimates the financial consequences of adopting a new intervention. BIA methodology is concerned with the affordability of adopting a new intervention or healthcare technology to a payer (Mauskopf et al., 2017; Sullivan et al., 2014). The approach consists of measuring the cost of the intervention for all those in need in the population, on a "per capita" basis, per unit of time. BIA can be used by governments or vaccine payers to assess whether they can afford to introduce a new vaccine for a particular population subgroup or the entire population.

ROI analysis measures the value of an investment, in terms of its efficiency in use of resources to produce benefits. The approach consists of determining the net benefits (i.e., benefits minus costs) of a vaccine program in the long term over a fixed amount of time (e.g., 1 year, 5 years, or 10 years). This is done by calculating the ROI metric, which is the ratio of the net benefits of an intervention to its costs, expressed as a percentage:

Equation 3.1.3. Return on investment:

$$ROI = \frac{Benefits\ of\ investment - Cost\ of\ investment}{Cost\ of\ investment} \times 100\%$$

The ROI captures, therefore, the amount of return (profitability) on a project, relative to its cost. ROI estimates across different projects can be compared to assess their relative efficiency. It is worthwhile highlighting here that ROI analysis differs from CBA in one important way: CBA is an evaluation exercise as its results help identify a better intervention strategy in relation to alternative competing strategies, whereas ROI analysis is a valuation exercise that measures the value of an investment.

3.1.5 Understanding the incremental cost-effectiveness ratio

The ICER is the single most important interpretation of a CEA. The ICER can be represented by a formula:

Equation 3.1.4. Incremental cost-effectiveness ratio:

$$ICER = \frac{Cost\ A - Cost\ B}{Effectiveness\ A - Effectiveness\ B} = \frac{\Delta Cost}{\Delta Effectiveness}$$

The ICER provides a fundamental interpretation of the value of a vaccine program compared to its next best alternative(s), and this can be interpreted in multiple directions. For instance, the ICER can be reflective of value as a result of CEA or CUA, so it is common to see this reported with either approach. Resulting ICERs can be positive or negative from these analyses, and each sign change implies different meanings.

First, let's explore the meaning of an ICER value. If a *negative* ICER occurs with a negative numerator it implies that the cost of the vaccine program (A) is less than the cost of an alternative (B), even though a positive denominator implies that A has greater clinical effectiveness than B. A negative ICER in a case with a negative numerator offers more effectiveness at less cost. The opposite case where a negative ICER has a positive numerator would imply that the vaccine program is not in fact a cost-effective solution at the given price.

Second, ICERs can also be positive, where perhaps the vaccine program (A) is more costly than the alternative, but also arrives at a greater clinical effectiveness. In such cases, it is important to examine a community's willingness-to-pay threshold so that we can determine whether or not the vaccine program has an opportunity cost which exceeds its alternative (Padula & Sculpher, 2021).

3.1.6 Translating value into resource allocation

A typical problem is deciding if a vaccine should be allocated to the general population.

Measuring an ICER relative to the community's willingness-to-pay threshold, also termed "cost-effectiveness threshold" and symbolized by λ, is key to examining its priority to be allocated to the general population. Threshold parameter λ is defined as the maximum value of the ratio of Δ Cost/Δ Effectiveness at which an intervention is acceptable. An intervention that is better than the threshold is said to offer positive net monetary benefit which can alternatively be expressed as a positive net health benefit as shown in the equations below.

Note that in the following equations, NMB is different when interpreted from the results of a CEA or CUA, compared to the interpretation of a CBA:

Equation 3.1.5. NMB:

$$NMB = \Delta Effectiveness \times \lambda - \Delta Cost$$

Equation 3.1.6. Net health benefit:

$$NHB = \Delta Effectiveness - \frac{\Delta Cost}{\lambda}$$

In either case, net benefits that are positive imply that the vaccine program would generate value for the community of interest. Likewise, negative net benefits imply that the community would pay more money for less health benefit than current alternatives at a given willingness to pay.

When considering the value of investments, one must also consider opportunity costs. That is, the costs of forgone benefits relating to the next best option when financial resources are committed to a particular activity. For example, spending resources on expensive vaccine delivery programs can withdraw finances from other priorities, such as primary and preventive care, or treatment of infectious disease. Opportunity costs create differential consequences for stakeholders that will affect their support for an intervention that might be in the overall public interest. Payers investing in covering vaccines for some patients may have limited budgets. In the long run, payers can overcome budget constraints by increasing premiums or sharing costs with patients and providers (McGuire, 2000). Providers might not be compensated for all the costs of a new vaccine policy and they might fail to support it. Overall, these tactics place other higher-value, preventive programs such as vaccines in greater jeopardy, and therefore necessitate mindful inclusion of the various stakeholders' considerations into models of value and cost.

References

Asaria, M., Griffin, S., & Cookson, R. (2016). Distributional cost-effectiveness analysis: A tutorial. *Medical Decision Making, 36*(1), 8–19. doi: 10.1177/0272989X15583266

Babigumira, J. B., Morgan, I., & Levin, A. (2013). Health economics of rubella: A systematic review to assess the value of rubella vaccination. *BMC Public Health, 13*(1), 406. doi:10.1186/1471-2458-13-406

Bärnighausen, T., Bloom, D. E., Cafiero-Fonseca, E. T., & O'Brien, J. C. (2014). Valuing vaccination. *Proceedings of the National Academy of Sciences of the United States of America, 111*(34), 12313–12319. doi:10.1073/pnas.1400475111

Bärnighausen, T., Bloom, D. E., Canning, D., Friedman, A., Levine, O. S., O'Brien, J., ... Walker, D. (2011). Rethinking the benefits and costs of childhood vaccination: The example of the Haemophilus influenzae type b vaccine. *Vaccine, 29*(13), 2371–2380. doi:10.1016/j.vaccine.2010.11.090

Bärnighausen, T., Bloom, D. E., Canning, D., & O'Brien, J. (2008). Accounting for the full benefits of childhood vaccination in South Africa. *South African Medical Journal, 98*(11), 842, 844–846. https://pubmed.ncbi.nlm.nih.gov/19177886/

Berger, M. L., Bingefors, K., Hedblom, E. C., Pashos, C., & Torrance, G. W. (2003). *Health care cost, quality, and outcomes: ISPOR book of terms.* Lawrenceville, NJ: International Society for Pharmacoeconomics and Outcomes Research.

Briggs, A. H., & O'Brien, B. J. (2001). The death of cost-minimization analysis? *Health Economics, 10*(2), 179–184. doi:10.1002/hec.584

Claxton, K. (2007). OFT, VBP: QED? *Health Economics, 16*(6), 545–558. doi:10.1002/hec.1249

Cookson, R., Drummond, M., & Weatherly, H. (2009). Explicit incorporation of equity considerations into economic evaluation of public health interventions. *Health Economics, Policy, and Law, 4*(2), 231–245.

Cookson, R., Griffin, S., Norheim, O. F., & Culyer, A. J. (2020). *Distributional cost-effectiveness analysis: Quantifying health equity impacts and trade-offs*. Oxford: Oxford University Press.

Datta, S., Pink, J., Medley, G. F., Petrou, S., Staniszewska, S., Underwood, M., . . . Keeling, M. J. (2019). Assessing the cost-effectiveness of HPV vaccination strategies for adolescent girls and boys in the UK. *BMC Infectious Diseases, 19*(1), 552. doi:10.1186/s12879-019-4108-y

Delany, I., Rappuoli, R., & De Gregorio, E. (2014). Vaccines for the 21st century. *EMBO Molecular Medicine, 6*(6), 708–720. doi:10.1002/emmm.201403876

Deogaonkar, R., Hutubessy, R., van der Putten, I., Evers, S., & Jit, M. (2012). Systematic review of studies evaluating the broader economic impact of vaccination in low and middle income countries. *BMC Public Health, 12*(1), 878. doi:10.1186/1471-2458-12-878

Drabo, E. F., Eckel, G., Ross, S. L., Brozic, M., Carlton, C. G., Warren, T. Y., . . . Pollack, C. E. (2021). A social-return-on-investment analysis of Bon Secours Hospital's "Housing For Health" affordable housing program. *Health Affairs (Millwood), 40*(3), 513–520. doi:10.1377/hlthaff.2020.00998

Drummond, M., Sculpher, M., Claxton, K., Stoddart, G. L., & Torrance, G. W. (2015). *Methods for the economic evaluation of health care programmes* (4th ed). Oxford: Oxford University Press.

Drummond, M., & Towse, A. (2019). Is rate of return pricing a useful approach when value-based pricing is not appropriate? *European Journal of Health Economics, 20*(7), 945–948. doi:10.1007/s10198-019-01032-7

Garrison, L. P., Jansen, J. P., Devlin, N. J., & Griffin, S. (2019). Novel approaches to value assessment within the cost-effectiveness framework. *Value in Health, 22*(6), S12–S17. doi:10.1016/j.jval.2019.04.1915

Goldman, D. P., & McGlynn, E. A. (2005). *US health care: Facts about cost, access, and quality*. Santa Monica, CA: Rand Corporation.

Jit, M., Hutubessy, R., Png, M. E., Sundaram, N., Audimulam, J., Salim, S., & Yoong, J. (2015). The broader economic impact of vaccination: Reviewing and appraising the strength of evidence. *BMC Medicine, 13*(1), 209. doi:10.1186/s12916-015-0446-9

Mauskopf, J., Earnshaw, S. R., Brogan, A., Wolowacz, S., & Brodtkorb, T.-H. (2017). *Budget-impact analysis of health care interventions: A practical guide*. Cham: Springer International Publishing AG.

McGuire, T. G. (2000). Physician agency. In A. J. Culyer & J. P. Newhouse (Eds.), *Handbook of health economics* (Vol. 1, pp. 461–536). Amsterdam: Elsevier.

Nelson, E. C., Batalden, P. B., Godfrey, M. M., & Lazar, J. S. (2011). *Value by design: Developing clinical microsystems to achieve organizational excellence*. Hoboken, NJ: John Wiley & Sons.

Ozawa, S., Mirelman, A., Stack, M. L., Walker, D., & Levine, O. S. (2012). Cost-effectiveness and economic benefits of vaccines in low- and middle-income countries: A systematic review. *Vaccine, 31*(1), 96–108. doi:10.1016/j.vaccine.2012.10.103

Padula, W. V., Lee, K. K. H., & Pronovost, P. J. (2017). Using economic evaluation to illustrate value of care for improving patient safety and quality: Choosing the right method. *Journal of Patient Safety, 17*(6), e568–e574. doi:10.1097/PTS.0000000000000410

Padula, W. V., & Sculpher, M. (2021). Ideas about resourcing health care in the United States: Can economic evaluation achieve meaningful use? *Annals of Internal Medicine, 174*(1), 80–85. doi:10.7326/m20-1234

Porter, M. E., & Advantage, C. (1985). Creating and sustaining superior performance. *Competitive Advantage, 167*, 167–206.

Seto, K., Marra, F., Raymakers, A., & Marra, C. A. (2012). The cost effectiveness of human papillomavirus vaccines: A systematic review. *Drugs, 72*(5), 715–743. doi:10.2165/11599470-000000000-00000

Sullivan, S. D., Mauskopf, J. A., Augustovski, F., Caro, J. J., Lee, K. M., Minchin, M., . . . Shau, W.-Y. (2014). Budget impact analysis—principles of good practice: Report of the ISPOR 2012 Budget Impact Analysis Good Practice II Task Force. *Value in Health, 17*(1), 5–14.

Tahamtan, A., Charostad, J., Hoseini Shokouh, S. J., & Barati, M. (2017). An overview of history, evolution, and manufacturing of various generations of vaccines. *Journal of Archives in Military Medicine, 5*(3), e12315. doi:10.5812/jamm.12315

Teerawattananon, Y., & Tritasavit, N. (2015). A learning experience from price negotiations for vaccines. *Vaccine, 33*(Suppl 1), A11–A12. doi:10.1016/j.vaccine.2014.12.050

Teerawattananon, Y., Tritasavit, N., Suchonwanich, N., & Kingkaew, P. (2014). The use of economic evaluation for guiding the pharmaceutical reimbursement list in Thailand. *Zeitschrift fur Evidenz, Fortbildung und Qualitat im Gesundheitswesen, 108*(7), 397–404. doi:10.1016/j.zefq.2014.06.017

Then, V., Schober, C., Rauscher, O., & Kehl, K. (2018). *Social return on investment analysis: Measuring the impact of social Investment.* Cham: Springer.

Verguet, S., Kim, J. J., & Jamison, D. T. (2016). Extended cost-effectiveness analysis for health policy assessment: A tutorial. *PharmacoEconomics, 34*(9), 913–923.

World Health Organization. (2011). Rubella vaccines: WHO position paper. *Weekly Epidemiological Record, 86*(29), 301–316. https://pubmed.ncbi.nlm.nih.gov/21766537/

3.2

Defining the scope and study design of cost-effectiveness analysis

Joseph F. Levy and Charles E. Phelps

3.2.1 Defining the scope of an economic evaluation study

3.2.1.1 Building from basics

The scope of any analysis of the value of a vaccine begins with the incentives for individuals in a defined population to want to be vaccinated. In the purest economic terms, wanting to be vaccinated means that one's willingness to pay for the vaccine exceeds the cost that the person confronts, both monetary and personal (time, pain, fear of vaccines, etc.). Here, standard economic analysis of a "representative single consumer" comes into play, using standard models of human choices in healthcare (Phelps, 2017).

However, as Chapter 1.2 emphasized, vaccines (unlike almost all other healthcare interventions) have "spillover" benefits to others in the society who surround each "representative individual" (Phelps, 2017). While there are some "private" benefits to vaccination (reduction of disease risk, with attendant reductions in lost earnings, and even lower risk of death), there are also "public" benefits—the most important of which is increased protection for others in the community ("herd immunity"). Therefore, analysis of vaccination programs must include "everybody" in a defined population, not just those who receive the vaccine. This forms the first basis for establishing the proper scope of analysis.

3.2.1.2 The "adoption" question

Now consider a typical public health decision maker with responsibility over some specific defined population—a county, state, or nation, or a subdivision,

Joseph F. Levy and Charles E. Phelps, *Defining the scope and study design of cost-effectiveness analysis* In: *Handbook of Applied Health Economics in Vaccines*. Edited by: David Bishai, Logan Brenzel and William V. Padula, Oxford University Press.

district, division, state, or nation. The relevant "local" decision focuses on the following question:

> If a vaccine against disease X existed that had certain specific attributes (efficacy, number of injections required, side effects, cold chain storage demands, fit with existing vaccine schedules in target communities, and others), would it be cost-effective to deploy that vaccine in "my community"?

This analysis, if properly done, should account for the public good aspects of the vaccine among the community's citizens. If the disease is tetanus or rabies, there is essentially no public good issue, since the disease does not transmit from person to person. But for diseases that are spread from person to person, spillover effects are essential components of the analysis.

Just as local officials must consider spillover effects of vaccination programs among individuals in the local community, so too must national officials consider spillovers between local settings (counties, districts, shires). The "private" incentives of the director of public health in a single county or district will not fully consider the benefits conferred on surrounding counties or districts.

The same is true even as we aggregate from regional to national levels: vaccination levels in country X provide spillover benefits to nations around the world, particularly in a world with regular international travel by air and sea. The coronavirus disease 2019 (COVID-19) pandemic of 2020 highlighted this issue, since international travel rapidly spread the virus from country to country, creating a worldwide pandemic in the space of weeks.

When modeling the benefits of vaccines, local health officers will likely make decisions based on the interests and financial capacity of their own defined populations, and that is necessary, but not sufficient, in understanding the full value of vaccines for contagious diseases. Somebody—the public health officer at a higher level of government—must also evaluate the benefits from a wider perspective. Eventually, for highly contagious diseases, international modeling of the disease, and then international coordination and cooperation, are necessary to fully capture the benefits of vaccines on a worldwide basis.

An extensive software program is available for free to assist in dealing with these types of questions—the SMART Vaccines software from the National Academy of Medicine.[1] While originally designed to prioritize vaccine

---

[1] See https://nap.nationalacademies.org/smartvaccines/ to access the software and download all three reports about the project.

development choices, it readily helps guide decisions about adoption, with the ability to define various populations at all levels of analysis from "local" to "national" or even "super state" combinations of nations. Based on multi-attribute utility theory, it allows users to choose among 29 possible attributes to describe vaccines (and to add their own if desired) and to specify value weights on the attributes chosen for inclusion in the analysis.

3.2.1.3 The investment decision

We now turn to the scope of analysis that logically comes first: is it worth trying to develop the vaccine in the first place? Here, the investment decision basically adds up the potential benefit across all potential target populations, and then asks if it is worth taking the risk of investing in a vaccine, taking all the potential worldwide benefits into account as summarized by answers to all the "community" questions.

This is in some sense a business planning decision for vaccine manufacturers, adding up the presumptive demands for their product from around the world. Indeed, manufacturers can use the SMART Vaccines software to help assemble this information in a coherent fashion, and to model how different vaccine specifications (attributes) might alter the demand. However, financial return to developing vaccines can be more complicated than other pharmaceuticals as various nongovernmental organizations (NGOs) often participate in collective purchase agreements for vaccines (assuring a large quantity of sales in return for lower prices). This is discussed in Chapter 1.3.

3.2.1.4 Alternatives to vaccination

When thinking about the value of developing a new vaccine, one must always consider the alternatives available to deal with the disease in question. These fall into two main categories: treatments of the disease and non-vaccine methods to reduce disease spread. These issues affect both the desired scope of analysis and measures of value of vaccines.

3.2.1.5 Herd immunity and disease eradication

Many alternatives exist to deal with contagious diseases, but one important issue differentiates contagious diseases from other health conditions, and another related issue differentiates vaccines from other alternatives. These two concepts are herd immunity and disease eradication, respectively.

Standard economic analyses of vaccine programs invariably emphasize the difference between private gain from immunization and the public good that also comes with it. The private gain is the reduction in or elimination of the chances of getting the disease in question, saving the person the aches and pains of the disease, the lost time from work or school, and the medical costs that might be needed to treat the condition. But getting the vaccination also confers a small benefit to others in the community—their chances of getting the contagious disease fall, perhaps only by a bit, but this applies to many people. When enough people in a community become immune to the disease, any new introduction of an imported case will be unable to lead to a sustained epidemic. They have achieved "herd immunity." This issue affects the proper scope of analysis of vaccines.

Eradication of a disease takes place when the disease has no carriers in the population. Eradication has almost been completed for polio and the last known case of smallpox occurred in 1977. In some cases, vaccination alone can achieve total disease eradication.[2]

3.2.1.6 Treatment

The most obvious alternative to vaccination is medical treatment, but often, treatment and prevention go hand in hand as public health policies. They are not in opposition to one another. Some diseases have wonderful vaccines but no effective treatments, for example, polio. Others have highly effective therapies, but no viable vaccines, including HIV and gonorrhea. Some diseases have both, and disease control strategies use them in concert to combat the disease. Examples include tuberculosis, influenza, pneumococcal pneumonia, and others.

Comparing treatments with vaccines is a relatively straightforward task, with vaccines reducing the probability of disease (and hence the risk of death in some cases) and treatments reducing the consequences (severity of illness, costs of treatment, and, in some cases, the risk of death). Such comparisons must include not only the issues of medical costs but the value of reducing the illness burden on people, either by reducing the probability of disease or the consequences of contracting it.

---

[2] A counterexample is hepatitis C, where the reproduction rate, R_0, is so low that eradication through treatment of infected individuals can in concept eradicate the disease.

3.2.1.7 Social interventions

Social interventions are the earliest known methods to control infectious diseases. The ancient book of Leviticus has numerous passages devoted to the isolation (and then possible readmission to society) of lepers. When a novel pathogen appears in the modern world, often neither vaccines nor treatments are available, as evidenced (for example) in the Medieval Black Plague, the 1918 "Spanish Flu" pandemic, and the 2020 COVID-19 pandemic. These methods include forced quarantine,[3] self-isolation, physical distancing, face-mask wearing,[4] swimming pool closures (for polio), prohibitions on public gatherings, and similar restrictions on behavior. These inevitably cause economic disruption, sometimes of major magnitude, and these economic losses highlight the potential value of vaccines. In general, social interventions provide only stop-gap protections until vaccines and/or effective treatments emerge.

3.2.1.8 Vector control

Vector control will commonly enter consideration for any disease that has other animal species involved, including mosquitos, snails, and ticks, and *zoonotic* diseases that are transmitted directly from animals to humans (including rabies, hantavirus, anthrax, and numerous diseases transmitted through "wet" markets for wild animals that are desired for various alleged exotic properties). In all such cases, control of the vector (or zoonotic carrier) is an important alternative to vaccination.

3.2.1.9 Public sanitation

Simple measures of public sanitation are often important (and sometimes, sufficient) to control infectious diseases. Clean drinking water is essential for public health, often requiring investment in waste disposal systems that are distinctly separated from water supplies. Better housing, sanitation, and

---

[3] "Typhoid" Mary Mallon, an American woman, was forcibly quarantined twice over decades after she was identified as an asymptomatic carrier of typhoid fever. A cook by occupation, she was known to have infected 53 people, three of whom died. After release from quarantine, she worked as a cook using false names, and some believe that up to 50 deaths were caused by her behavior.

[4] As in the previous 1918 "Spanish Flu" outbreak, mandatory mask-wearing became highly politicized in some countries in 2020.

solid waste management are all benefits of modern public health practice. Investments in basic public health strategies should always be considered as complements if not alternatives to vaccination programs where applicable.

3.2.1.10 Comparators in cost-effectiveness analysis

We now come to the final step in this introduction to evaluation of vaccines. Every cost-effectiveness analysis model compares the *incremental* value of the intervention to the *incremental* cost. The key question, then, is "Compared to what?" In some diseases, the answer is straightforward. For many cancers, the answer will be "state-of-the-art" combinations of chemotherapy, radiation therapy, and surgery. For a badly arthritic knee, the comparison is continued pain medication (perhaps augmented by physical therapy) versus joint replacement. In some cases, with no effective treatments or vaccines, the comparison may be to "doing nothing." Finally, as we have seen earlier, for vaccines, the issues of choosing the proper alternative to vaccines can be much more complicated, particularly in cases of vector-borne diseases.

3.2.1.10.1 For adoption

For decisions about adopting a new vaccine, the obvious choice is to use the most cost-effective of *existing* and *available* alternatives. The comparison should not be something that doesn't exist yet, perhaps such as another vaccine in phase I trials or a new medication touted by the company that makes it (but without clinical trial data to support it).

The comparator must deal with the same disease. Comparing a potential zika vaccine with existing polio vaccines has no meaning. In some cases (such as zika), no meaningful preventive intervention may exist, which means that the ongoing costs of treatment in the relevant community are the only issue. Of course, in diseases with potential fatalities, their possible prevention also has major economic value, and the quality-adjusted life years saved from preventing premature deaths may be the most important part of a cost-effectiveness analysis for many infectious diseases.

As appropriate, non-medical interventions such as vector control or behavioral control are appropriate comparators for vaccines. Malaria offers the useful example where home screening, bed netting, mosquito repellants, reduction of standing water in the community, and widespread application of pesticides are viable alternatives to vaccines, and in some cases, would be the proper comparator.

3.2.1.10.2 For research and development decisions

Decisions about investing in research and development for new vaccines have similar dimensions, but innovators will likely also want to consider what they know of other innovations underway in parallel, how far along they are in development, and (as far as is known) their likelihood of scientific success. These are relatively straightforward business activities that will rely not only on the progress of the vaccine in question but also "corporate intelligence" on other alternatives.

3.2.2 Define the perspective impacted by a vaccine program

As introduced in Chapter 2.3, all decisions depend on the perspective of the decision maker. Therefore, presenting an economic model with respect to the primary perspective of interest is required to undertake an economic evaluation for a vaccine program. Here, we review perspectives again with respect to how these options impact models. The choice of a third-party payer's perspective, for instance, should align with the incentives of the intended decision maker who will utilize the results of the model. This is a methodological choice that establishes the viewpoint of the analysis — and answers the question regarding which costs and outcomes should be considered in the model.

Consider first a narrow viewpoint, that of a single insurer. For a vaccine program, an insurer will pay the costs of the vaccine, and the costs (or avoided costs) of future disease impacted by the decision. At the same time, the insurer will accumulate the health benefits (life years, quality-adjusted life years, disability-adjusted life years, burden avoided, etc.) of their insurance plan members. To that insurer, these are the only relevant costs and effects to examine, as these are relevant to their covered population. So, using this payer's perspective, if a patient were to switch insurance, the cost and benefits after switching would no longer impact the initial insurer. For this reason, narrow perspectives like a single insurer, or even a single NGO or municipality, are less frequently considered in the vaccine space, as vaccines programs tend to have wide and long-lasting impacts on entire populations.

The most common payers' perspectives considered for vaccine economic evaluations are those of (1) *the healthcare sector*, an amalgam of all the payers who remunerate providers for formal healthcare services and includes all relevant health effects to an entire population; and (2) *the societal payers' perspective*, which includes the healthcare sector costs and effects as well as broader costs beyond formal health services, informal healthcare services, and even beyond the healthcare sector that may be impacted by treatment.

3.2.2.1 The healthcare sector payers' perspective

The healthcare sector payers' perspective considers costs for direct healthcare that would emanate from the decision to vaccinate (or alternatives). This would include the costs of the vaccine itself and vaccine administration costs, costs of potential side effects, and costs associated with treatment of the disease that patients may incur or that may be avoided as a result of the vaccine program. The healthcare sector payers' perspective is agnostic about who is paying the costs; thus, it would include patients' out-of-pocket costs, costs to an NGO of running the vaccine distribution, costs to a private insurance firm to pay for treatment in the future, and costs to the government if it provides state-funded health medical services, and so on.

3.2.2.2 The societal perspective

The societal perspective is an even broader perspective that will consider non-healthcare-related costs and effects that may emanate from the decision of interest. Under this perspective, costs of any kind and to anyone that will emanate from the treatment decisions are considered. Generally, these include the informal healthcare sector costs related to treatment, such as patients' lost work time, caregivers' lost leisure/work time, and transportation costs associated with treatment, and non-healthcare sector costs, such as a patient losing work and productivity due to illness, or loss of consumption of goods (which are a benefit to society) due to mortality differences across treatment strategies. Other non-healthcare sector costs relevant for vaccine programs would be the positive spillovers effects, such as improved educational attainment due to pediatric vaccine programs. The positive societal costs emanating from that additional education attainment, for example, should be considered as costs in a societal perspective model.

3.2.2.3 Which perspective should we use?

The Second Panel on Cost-Effectiveness in Health and Medicine advocates conducting cost-effectiveness analysis from both the healthcare sector payers' and societal payers' perspective (Sanders et al., 2016). As societal perspective encompasses all healthcare sector costs and more, redoing the model with societal-only costs removed is not complicated. Further, highlighting the potential difference in results from the model using one approach may have particular interest for decision makers who weigh non-healthcare sector costs differently from others.

3.2.3 Framing the time horizon for a vaccine program

As first discussed in Chapter 2.3, time horizons of economic evaluations should be of sufficient length to capture all costs and effects that can be attributed to the decision being considered. For certain vaccines, such as seasonal flu, the effect (and thus the impact) of the disease and or immunity is short, so the benefits and costs possibly emanating from the decision will also be short too, perhaps 1 year after the decision about the program. So, a time horizon of 1 year would be reasonable to accumulate costs and effects post treatment, as we would not expect the strategies under consideration (e.g., to provide a flu vaccine or not) to produce additional differential impacts far beyond 1 year.

However, many vaccines impact mortality and/or health outcomes long in the future, sometimes over the person's remaining life. It would be preferable to track costs and health outcomes over this remaining lifetime for all individuals. In practice, however, we only observe costs and outcomes for individuals over a short time window. To extrapolate this information over the individual's lifetime, it is common to resort to economic modeling. In modeling studies, this extrapolation of costs and health effects is done by allowing the model to run until all patients (e.g., individuals or a cohort of individuals) expire. This hypothetical ideal is frequently juxtaposed with the realities of data available to inform decision-making; for instance, data for a new vaccine cannot, with certainty, predict the long-term costs and outcomes. Balancing the need for long-term results to make efficient allocation decisions with a lack of, or unreliable, data to inform these outcomes presents a challenge.

It is becoming more common to apply modeling approaches that use observed data to project beyond the period of data collection. Extrapolation of survival or time-to-event data is an important and growing field in economic evaluations. It will often be necessary to extrapolate treatment efficacy estimates beyond what has been observed (Latimer, 2013). Indeed, there is growing consensus that analyses should consider various extrapolation techniques. A standard approach is to present the model results using different extrapolation techniques to assess robustness of model results to these different assumptions.

3.2.4 Role of modeling and applicability of data inputs

Decision-analytic models are to decision makers what animal models are to a bench scientist. They can be used to construct counterfactual worlds and test the impacts of alternative interventions. They can also help overcome several challenges with the estimation of the impacts of health interventions, by systematically combining the best available data (e.g., epidemic, clinical, economic) from multiple sources (e.g., individual clinical trials, pooled results of multiple clinical trials, i.e., meta-analysis, observational studies, or primary data collected), to permit comparisons of the current and future epidemiological, clinical, and economic impacts of multiple alternative interventions or strategies, and for different population subgroups. They are particularly useful in situations where there are multiple strategies that need to be evaluated, when strategies vary in "intensity" of implementation, when strategies combine multiple interventions, and, importantly, when it is impractical and costly to evaluate strategies within a single randomized controlled trial. Even in situations where randomized controlled trials can be conducted, models can be useful in extrapolating the effect sizes observed the short time frame of the randomized controlled trial over a longer time horizon, such as a lifetime.

Decision models are particularly relevant in the evaluation of vaccine interventions, where the benefits can be long-lasting, and where the externalities (mostly positive) are considerable. A common critical input parameter to a vaccine economic evaluation is the hazard ratio of infection rate among those vaccinated (compared to the unvaccinated). Ideally, estimates from multiple phase III clinical trial studies would inform this hazard ratio and the estimates would be weighted using meta-analytic methods. Nonetheless, many countries may only necessitate one large individual study of a population for targeted vaccine use in order to obtain regulatory approval; however, there remains the question as to whether information conducted between countries is exchangeable. Thus, external validity remains an important consideration for the interpretation of results between countries. Overall, the influence of results from alternate communities should be explicitly considered for decision making.

For example, using results from a different context, say, the hazard ratio of the efficacy of a vaccine in a phase III trial conducted in a developed country, may not be the perfect analogue to a similar trial conducted in a low- or middle-income setting. This could be due to several reasons, including differences in adherence or the prevalence of comorbid conditions across these settings. Transparency about the limitations of applying data from one context into another is therefore critical. This is why conducting sensitivity analyses (discussed in detail in Chapter 3.5) is a critical topic in economic evaluation, as it allows the modeler and decision maker to probe how one assumption (that may not be the perfect analogue) can potentially impact the recommended decisions by the model. Careful consideration about the inputs from other studies and context applies to cost and effects estimates as well.

References

Latimer, N. R. (2013). Survival analysis for economic evaluations alongside clinical trials—extrapolation with patient-level data: Inconsistencies, limitations, and a practical guide. *Medical Decision Making, 33*(6), 743–754. doi:10.1177/0272989x12472398

Mutapi, F., Billingsley, P. F., & Secor, W. E. (2013). Infection and treatment immunizations for successful parasite vaccines. *Trends in Parasitology, 29*(3), 135–141. doi:10.1016/j.pt.2013.01.003

Phelps, C. E. (2017). The demand for medical care: Conceptual framework. In *Health economics* (6th ed., pp. 82–111). New York, NY: Routledge Press.

Sanders, G. D., Neumann, P. J., Basu, A., Brock, D. W., Feeny, D., Krahn, M., . . . Ganiats, T. G. (2016). Recommendations for conduct, methodological practices, and reporting of cost-effectiveness analyses: Second Panel on Cost-Effectiveness in Health and Medicine. *JAMA, 316*(10), 1093–1103. doi:10.1001/jama.2016.12195

3.3

Parameter estimation

Emmanuel F. Drabo and David W. Dowdy

3.3.1 Introduction

The quality of an economic evaluation is only as good as the data that comprises it. Therefore, it is important to accurately translate data from primary and secondary resources in order to supply a vaccine model with appropriate estimates of probability, cost, and effectiveness. Investigators must typically estimate both a point estimate and an uncertainty distribution for each parameter. In order of quality, these estimates generally derive from empirical data, the scientific literature, or assumptions (e.g., "expert opinion"). Most economic evaluations will additionally require some parameter estimates based on assumption (i.e., where empiric data or scientific literature do not exist); it is therefore important to evaluate the influence of all parameter estimates on the primary results and conclusions of any economic evaluation.

The materials covered in this chapter are intended to provide a strong foundation for students interested in conducting basic, yet highly impactful work in vaccine economics. There are more advanced methods available to handle the topics covered in this chapter that are beyond the scope of this text. Readers interested in these more advanced methodologies are encouraged to undertake more advanced study or collaborate with peers with such advanced training. Several reference textbooks in the Handbooks in Health Economic Evaluation series (Briggs, Sculpher, & Claxton, 2006; Glick, Doshi, Sonnad, & Polsky, 2014) are good starting points.

3.3.2 Ways to derive model input parameters

Parameters for vaccine economics applications should be estimates from high-quality data wherever possible. The "gold standard" for parameter estimation

Emmanuel F. Drabo and David W. Dowdy, *Parameter estimation* In: *Handbook of Applied Health Economics in Vaccines*.
Edited by: David Bishai, Logan Brenzel and William V. Padula, Oxford University Press. © Oxford University Press 2023.
DOI: 10.1093/oso/9780192896087.003.0016

is to collect all data empirically in the context of a combined effectiveness–economics study of primary or secondary data, such as a clinical trial or observational study. Ideally, parameters used in vaccine economics model—or any health economics model—would be estimated from carefully designed randomized controlled trials (RCTs).

For example, in estimating the cost-effectiveness of *Haemophilus influenzae* type b vaccine, one could theoretically perform a cluster-randomized trial of vaccine effectiveness with long-term follow-up while also directly collecting data on costs of implementation, delivery, and sustainability. Unfortunately, such studies are typically large and resource intensive. In addition, it is also not always possible to track all necessary parameters within a single reported RCT. Simply put, the authors of RCT reports seldom think, "I bet that an economist is going to want to put together a health economic model of this intervention." Even if they did, clinical trial reports would still differ according to specific research questions, types of health states, study population, effectiveness measures, time step, and so on.

Furthermore, the costs of delivering a vaccine in the context of a clinical trial may be very different from those of programmatic delivery. As such, this "gold standard" is rarely—if ever—fully achieved. Hence, it is often the responsibility of the economist to find data in the literature and translate those data into meaningful parameters to inform vaccine economics models.

3.3.2.1 Types of parameters that may need to be estimated

Depending on the type and complexity of model being considered, different types of parameters may need to be estimated. For example, for a decision tree model such as the one in our hepatitis B vaccination example (see Chapter 3.7), we would need to estimate probabilities of changes in the risk of contracting *H. influenzae* type b with or without a vaccine, which relies heavily upon the efficacy of the vaccine. For a Markov model, parameters that are typically estimated for each health state are:

- Initial distributions of the cohort, costs, and health outcomes.
- Costs and effectiveness per cycle.
- Transition probabilities.
- Transition costs.
- Fixed probabilities in non-Markov nodes of a semi-Markov model.
- Fixed costs (e.g., infrastructure costs) and fixed effectiveness measures (e.g., payoffs).

Consider the example of hepatitis B vaccination (more details are provided in Chapter 4.6), the relevant parameters include disease state transition probabilities, disease state utilities, costs, and pharmacological effectiveness measures. It is also important to consider, as noted above, that not all costs and effectiveness outcomes are time dependent, and not all health state transition models are full Markov models (e.g., semi-Markov models).

3.3.2.2 Sources of data for parameter estimation

Parameters should be estimated from empiric, scientific data, whenever possible. These empiric data can come from a single source (albeit rarely) or multiple sources. Indeed, data from multiple sources are typically combined to inform the estimation of model parameters for a particular decision problem such as the decision whether to introduce a new vaccine.

Hence, when relying on existing empirical data or the scientific literature to estimate parameters, it is important to understand and appreciate whether the evidence generated emanates from a single study or is synthesized from multiple studies.

3.3.2.2.1 Estimating parameters using existing empirical data from a single study

On very rare occasions, and most likely for simpler decision problems, one may identify a high-quality peer-reviewed journal article reporting precisely the type of information needed to estimate one, multiple, or all parameters in a health economic model. In this simplest scenario, the challenge is to utilize that single source of data to estimate the model's parameters.

Suppose all the evidence is available in the form of summary results of a single published study. In that case, we can use these data "as they are" to estimate the relevant parameter(s) for the model. For example, a single published study of a single (three-arm) trial can provide head-to-head effectiveness and cost data for a decision model assessing the value of three coronavirus disease 2019 (COVID-19) vaccines. There are currently single-shot and double-shot vaccines, as well as vaccines structured using antibodies or messenger RNA (mRNA) delivery. Because the resulting measures of relative effectiveness (e.g., odds ratios, log-odds ratios, or relative risk ratios) between the arms of the trial are inherently correlated, parameters estimated from these data will also be correlated. So, it is critical to explicitly model these correlations whenever possible, in order to best assess uncertainty in the model, and correctly estimate each vaccine's expected costs and benefits.

Occasionally, individual patient data may be available to aid in estimating single or multiple parameters in a model. A reanalysis of these data can help derive appropriate model input parameters and explore and answer clinical and economic research questions in the most flexible manner. For example, we can use the individual-level data from a trial comparing the efficacy, safety, costs, and health outcomes of two vaccines to estimate the parameters for a vaccine economics model (e.g., cost, effectiveness) by using a range of statistical models. It is also easy to construct the correlation structure between the correlated input model parameters.

The availability of individual-level data can also aid in the analysis, or reanalysis, of time-to-event data, thereby allowing the extrapolation of a trial's results (e.g., fatal and non-fatal events) beyond its short observation period. It is common to use parametric distributions to model the outcomes of interest, which are typically governed by a combination of two or more correlated ancillary parameters, such as the mean and the standard deviation in the case of the Weibull distribution. Other popular examples of parametric distributions include the log-logistic, and generalized gamma distributions for the analysis of time-to-event outcomes (Collett, 2015).

3.3.2.2.2 Estimating parameters by synthesizing existing data from multiple studies

In most situations, the evidence base is represented by multiple studies, which may report results on the same parameter. In this case, it is common to combine these into a single quantitative estimate for use in health economic models. The exercise of combining multiple values for a parameter, derived from different sources, must be conducted with great care in order to minimize bias. Approaches for synthesizing and combining results from multiple studies rely on meta-analytic methods such as meta-analysis, meta-regression, and mixed treatment comparison. These approaches are intended to help eliminate, or at least minimize, bias.

Bias can be defined in multiple ways but can be more generally characterized as a systematic tendency that prevents unprejudiced consideration of the available evidence about a question (Pannucci & Wilkins, 2010). There are different types of bias, including publication bias (i.e., the tendency for studies with similar results to be published or unpublished, incomplete or selective reporting of outcomes, etc.), truncation bias (i.e., tendency for studies to be published in a briefer form with less details), time-lag bias (i.e., tendency for delayed publication of findings), language bias (i.e., tendency for studies being more likely to be published in a particular language such as English), citation bias (i.e., tendency for certain research findings to be cited more or less), selective outcome reporting bias (i.e., tendency for selective report or non-report of certain study outcomes), location bias (i.e., tendency for certain studies to be published in journals with different ease of access or levels of indexing in standard databases), duplication bias (i.e., tendency for multiple or duplicate publications), or database bias (i.e., tendency for some databases to be are more likely to index certain languages or journals).

Meta-analysis
It is recommended and common, in economic evaluation studies such as cost-effectiveness analysis, to use estimates of relative treatment effects derived from a meta-analysis of multiple studies (Gold, Siegel, Russell, & Weinstein, 1996; Neumann, Ganiats, Russell, Sanders, & Siegel, 2016). For example, in their cost-effectiveness analysis of routine and campaign use of typhoid Vi-conjugate vaccine in Gavi-eligible countries, Bilcke et al. (2019) used meta-analytic methods to synthesize and combine the available evidence on typhoid disease and its burden (e.g., hospital admission rates, typhoid treatment costs, vaccine delivery costs, length of stay in hospital, duration of illness).

There are at least two commonly used types of meta-analyses. The first is the *fixed-effect meta-analysis* in which it is assumed that every study included in the analysis is estimating the same statistic (most often an odds ratio), and that a single common and fixed effect characterizes every study included in the analysis, so that only within-study variations can influence the uncertainty in the results (Higgins et al., 2021). However, it is not uncommon to also observe between-study variations in the estimates of treatment effects (e.g., heterogeneous treatment effects). This gives rise to a second type of model, the *random-effects meta-analysis*. The random-effects model assumes that individual studies are estimating different treatment effects, but that these effects derive from a common distribution with some measure of central tendency such as the mean or median and some measure of dispersion, such as the variance (Higgins et al., 2021). Bilcke et al. (2019) used random-effects models to estimate the probability that an infected patient is admitted to the hospital, the length of stay (in days) in the hospital, the probability of death after admission to the hospital for typhoid infection, and the duration of illness in inpatient and outpatient settings. For a more in-depth review of meta-analytic methods, the reader can refer to the articles by Rosenthal and DiMatteo (2001) and Sutton and Higgins (2008).

While one of the critical tenets of good meta-analysis is the consideration of all the available evidence, it is clear that all evidence is not created equal.

Some studies are stronger than others. Doing a perfect meta-analysis based only on badly designed biased studies will still produce a biased combined statistic. Analysts must therefore face the difficult task of assessing the quality of each study, and account for it in the meta-analysis. In addition to needing to account for the quality of the evidence, analysts must also deal with other related biases that may be present in each study, some of which are detectable and addressable (Sutton, Song, Gilbody, & Abrams, 2000).

For example, study-level features, such as the characteristics of participants, may contribute to between-study variability in effects. In the meta-analytic framework, this can be accommodated through a *meta-regression* approach in which study-level covariates are included in the meta-analysis. Rather than excluding weaker and low-quality studies from a meta-analysis, it may be preferable to use the meta-regression approach with all studies included while controlling for study-level covariates which reflect the methodological quality of the studies. This approach can then permit the assessment of the impact of study quality on the pooled effect size. Unfortunately, it is often impossible to control for all biases, as there are various sources and manifestations of bias across studies. For example, meta-regression approaches a number of weaknesses that have been discussed elsewhere (see Thompson & Higgins, 2002), including yielding significantly lower statistical power over individual patient data methods, due to the use of mean study-level covariate values, and, importantly, potentially leading to "ecological fallacy," that is, an incorrect inference at the individual level of the relationships observed at the aggregate variable level (Berlin, Santanna, Schmid, Szczech, & Feldman, 2002; Lambert, Sutton, Abrams, & Jones, 2002; Piantadosi, Byar, & Green, 1988). However, when one has access to individual-level data from each study, the relationships between the parameter of interest and the individual covariates can be more rigorously examined across the pooled studies (Wakefield, 2008). When individual-level data are available for each study to permit a meta-regression, such analysis is called a *mega-analysis* and is considered the "gold-standard" in evidence synthesis (Higgins, Whitehead, Turner, Omar, & Thompson, 2001; Sutton, Abrams, Jones, Sheldon, & Song, 2000).

It is possible to incorporate between-study variability in decision-analytic models, such as those for vaccination decision, whenever possible, and strategies for doing so have been previously discussed extensively (Ades, Lu, & Higgins, 2005). Intuitively, the approach consists of using the heterogeneity parameter from the meta-regression to derive the parameters for the decision-analytic model. Hence, three types of parameters are derived: the random-effect estimate of the treatment effect, the variability of the random-effect estimate, and a measure of heterogeneity.

Multivariate meta-analysis model
Sometimes, multiple outcomes are of interest, such as costs and quality of life measures. A *multivariate meta-analysis* model can help with the joint estimation of these outcomes, as well as any potential correlation between them. Similar to the univariate meta-analytic model, multivariate meta-analysis models can be fixed-effects or random-effects models. The random-effects meta-analysis model is often used in applications due to its ability to capture both the within- and between-study correlation structures of the multiple outcomes of interest.

Mixed treatment comparison
When comparing two alternative vaccines or vaccination strategies, say, in term of their efficacy in preventing infections, we would ideally want data on their head-to-head comparison for that efficacy outcome. Unfortunately, RCTs rarely compare all relevant intervention strategies, head to head, and most only compare the new intervention to placebo or standard of care. Indeed, a common feature of the evidence base used to inform health economic models is the absence of head-to-head trials comparing all relevant comparators. This can pause various statistical challenges to estimation of, for example, the relative efficacy of the two interventions.

When patient-level data are available, these can be pooled across all studies to permit the estimation of the relative effects of comparator interventions, through a mega-regression. However, mega-regressions are rarely feasible. Alternatively, one might naively be tempted to use the differences in effect sizes across studies. That approach would only be valid if the studies included in the meta-analysis involved similar numbers and types of participants in terms of characteristics and behaviors, and if the endpoints (clinical or economic) were measured at the same time intervals. This wishful scenario is also hardly the case in the real world. We must therefore resort to alternative methods.

When multiple comparators are involved, more complex forms of meta-analytic evidence synthesis (indirect and mixed treatment comparison) are needed to handle the comparisons and combinations of evidence on multiple surrogate or intermediary endpoints (Baker, 2006). These complex methods, sometimes referred to as *multiparameter evidence synthesis*, include *indirect treatment comparisons* and *network meta-analysis*, which are simple extensions of the pairwise meta-analysis method, in which parameters are related to one another by a definable structure. These models have been primarily developed within the Bayesian framework, both for computational reasons, and for its natural connection to decision making (see Ades et al., 2006; Dias, Ades, Welton, Jansen, & Sutton, 2018; Hasselblad & McCrory, 1995; Lu & Ades, 2004; Lumley, 2002).

It should be noted that the multiparameter evidence synthesis framework relies on exactly the same assumption made under the pairwise meta-analytic method. Hence, depending on the analyst's assumptions about the between-study heterogeneity, a fixed- or random-effects analysis may be conducted.

3.3.2.3 Types of input data available from the literature

Many types of inputs data may be available from the literature, including probabilities or risk (e.g., probability of infection), rates (e.g., mortality rate from chronic hepatitis B infection), relative risks (e.g., relative risk of infection among vaccinated individuals, compared to unvaccinated susceptible individuals), odds ratios, risk differences, means, medians, and so on. Depending on the specific vaccine economic modeling context, any of these input data types may be relevant. Before we proceed with a more in-depth overview of each type of input data, it is worthwhile settling on some definitions.

3.3.2.3.1 Definitions
Probability is the numerical likelihood of occurrence of an event or outcome for a single individual in a given time period, and ranges from a value of 0 to 1. The *risk* of occurrence of an event (e.g., infection after vaccination) is the *probability* that the outcome will differ from an expected outcome. In that sense, risk and probability refer to the same concept.

Proportion represents the number of individuals who experienced an event, out of a population of interest; it is the number of people who had an event, divided by the total number of individuals at risk of the event in the population. Typically, the experience of the event is cumulative and the timing of when the event occurred is any time in the past. Prevalence of a long-duration disease like hepatitis B is often expressed as a proportion. The denominator of a proportion is always a count of a number of people.

In contrast, a *rate* is an instantaneous (or velocity) measure of the number of events that occur per unit time (or person-time), and ranges from a value of 0 to infinity. So, hepatitis B *incidence* is a rate, that is, the number of new individuals who acquire hepatitis B infection (hepatitis B cases) during a given time period, divided by the total person-time at risk of infection over the observation period. Similarly, the *annual vaccination rate* is the number of persons vaccinated over the course of a year, divided by the number of persons at risk of infection during that year.

Rates are typically scaled and can be expressed, for example, per 100 person-years. They differ from probabilities in many ways, the most important of which relates to the role of time. Specifically, in the calculation of a rate, time is directly included in the denominator. In contrast, time is not included in the denominator in the calculation of a probability. In the hepatitis B example, an estimate of the probability would be the number of hepatitis B cases divided by the total number of individuals at risk of infection over the relevant observation period. The denominator of a rate is always expressed in people units × time units most often person-years.

To further illustrate the concept of rate, suppose that after following 36 people with diagnosed type 2 diabetes and acute hepatitis B infection for 3 years to observe new cases of chronic hepatitis B infection, we found that exactly three, two, and one person(s) developed a chronic hepatitis B infection, exactly at the end of year 1, year 2, and year 3, respectively (so six people in total). Hence exactly 30 people (36 − 6) spent the entire 3 years without infection, and thus contributed 90 (30 × 3) person-years. One person spent 3 years without infection and became infected exactly at the end of year 3; this person thus contributed 3 (1 × 3) person-years. Two persons spent 2 years without infection and became infected exactly at the end of year 2, thus contributing collectively 4 (2 × 2) person-years. Finally, three persons spent exactly a year without infection and became infected exactly at the end of year 1, thus contributing collectively 3 (3 × 1) person-years. In total, individuals in this sample contributed 100 (90 + 3 + 4 + 3) person-years at risk of chronic hepatitis B infection (i.e., the event). The incidence rate of compensated cirrhosis in this population is 6/100 person-years = 0.06 per person-year, or 6 per 100 person-years.

It is worthwhile noticing that, in this particular example, the annual incidence rate is decreasing over time, as the rate in year 1 is 8 per 100 person-years (3/36 person-years); the rate in year 2 is 6 per 100 person-years (2/33 person-years), and the rate in year 3 is 3 per 100 person-years (1/31 person-years).

A *cumulative incidence* is the fraction of individuals in a population who experience an event over a specified time in a closed population, that is, one in which no new individual enters, no individual is lost to follow-up, and there are no competing events. In our example above, the 1-year cumulative incidence of acute hepatitis B infection is 8.3% (3/36 = 0.083); the

2-year and 3-year cumulative incidences are 13.9% (5/36 = 0.139%) and 16.7% (6/36 = 0.167), respectively. These calculated cumulative incidences are proportions, not rates. Notice here that these proportions increase at a decreasing rate, since the annual incidence rates are also declining in time.

Rates additionally possess several convenient mathematical properties that probabilities do not. They can be added and subtracted for the same time interval. They can also be multiplied or divided by a scalar, which may reflect, for example, risk factors. Rates can additionally be divided by the number of patients, or by time (Hunink, Glasziou, Siegel, & Weeks, 2001).

Furthermore, the rate varies with the distribution (i.e., the time) of the event over the observation period; the probability does not. For example, suppose that in a population of 100 individuals observed over a period of 4 years, one person died of a vaccine-preventable disease after the first year, another person died after the second year, and another died after the third year, and the other persons survived. So, a total of three persons died over this period. The probability of death from the vaccine-preventable disease over the 4-year period in this population is 0.03 (3/100), and the death rate is 0.76 per 100 person-years (3/[100 + 99 + 98 + 97] = 3/394, since 97 persons contributed 4 person-years each, and three persons contributed 1, 2, and 3 person-years each, respectively). Now, suppose instead, that the same population was observed over the same period of 4 years, but that all three deaths occurred at the end of the first year. Then the probability of death is still 0.03, but the death rate is now 0.77 per 100 person-years (3/[100 + 3 × 97] = 3/391, since 97 persons contributed 4 person-years each, and the three deceased persons contributed 1 person-year each).

The *odds* of an event are the ratio of the probability that the event will occur to the probability that it will not occur. If we denote by p the probability of the event occurring, then the probability that the event will not occur is $1-p$, since the event can either occur or not occur, and the occurrence and non-occurrence of the event are two *mutually exclusive* events, that is, they cannot both occur at the same time for the same subject. The mathematical expression of the odds of an event that occurs with probability p is:

Equation 3.3.1. Odds:

$$Odds = \frac{p}{1-p}$$

For example, if the probability of progression from an acute hepatitis B infection to a chronic hepatitis B infection is 0.06 (6%), then the probability of not progressing to a chronic infection is $1 - 0.06 = 0.94$ or 94%. Hence, the odds of progressing to a chronic hepatitis B infection are $0.06/0.94 = 0.064$.

The odds can take values ranging from 0 to infinity. For example, when the probability of occurrence of the event is 0, its odds are also 0 $(0/[1 - 0] = 0)$. Similarly, when the event occurs with certainty (i.e., probability 1), its odds are infinity. When the odds equal 1, it is referred to as even odds, since both the occurrence and non-occurrence of the event have an equal probability of 0.5. When the odds are larger than 1, say 5, it is common to hear people referring to it as 5 to 1. It is also worthwhile noting that when the probability of occurrence of an event is low, as is the case in our hepatitis B example above, the odds will be very similar to the probability.

The *odds ratio* is a statistic used to compare the odds of occurrence of an event among the exposed and unexposed groups. It is particularly useful in the case–control design in which there is no follow-up period, and the odds ratio is the only measure of association that can be computed.

In contrast, in cohort-type studies characterized by following exposure groups to compare the incidence of an outcome, it possible to calculate both a *relative risk* and an odds ratio. The relative risk is much easier to interpret than the odds ratio. It is a direct comparison of risks across exposure groups in terms of their ratio and is used to quantify the strength of association between an observed outcome and the exposure.

Using the hypothetical data in Table 3.3.1, we can calculate both the odds ratio and relative risk of the outcome for the two exposure groups. To calculate the odds ratio, we need the odds for the outcome among the two exposure groups (exposed, e, and unexposed, u). The odds for the outcome among the exposed are:

Equation 3.3.2. Odds for exposed individuals:

$$Odds_e = \frac{p_e}{1 - p_e}$$

Table 3.3.1 Illustrative 2×2 table from a hypothetical cohort study

	Outcome	No outcome	Total
Exposed	a	b	$a + b$
Unexposed	c	d	$c + d$
Total	$a + c$	$b + d$	$a + b + c + d$

where $P_e = \dfrac{a}{a+b}$ denotes the probability of the outcome among the exposed.

Similarly, the odds for the outcome among the unexposed are:

Equation 3.3.3. Odds for unexposed individuals:

$$Odds_u = \frac{P_u}{1-P_u}$$

where $P_u = \dfrac{c}{c+d}$ denotes the probability of the outcome among the unexposed.

The formula for the odds ratio is simply:

Equation 3.3.4. Odds ratio:

$$OR = \frac{Odds_e}{Odds_u} = \frac{a \times d}{b \times c}$$

Notice that the denominator is the odds for the outcome in the unexposed group, consistent with the convention.

The calculation of the relative risk ratio is also straightforward from the data in Table 3.3.1. As the relative risk is the ratio of the probability for the outcome among the two exposure groups, its formula is simple:

Equation 3.3.5. Relative risk ratio:

$$RRR = \frac{P_e}{P_u} = \frac{a \times (c+d)}{c \times (a+b)}$$

When the odds or risk of occurrence of the outcome is lower in the exposed group compared to the unexposed group, the odds ratio and relative risk ratio are less than 1. When the odds ratio or relative risk ratio is 1, the odds or risk of the outcome do not differ across exposure groups. Finally, when the odds or risk of the outcome are higher in the exposed group compared to the unexposed group, the ratios are above 1.

We can also calculate confidence intervals around these statistics. As neither the odds ratio nor the relative risk ratio follows a normal distribution, they need to be transformed before any confidence interval can be constructed. The odds and relative risk ratios are more characterized by log-normal distribution, so a logarithmic transformation is required to promote normality. Because of this, the confidence interval for an odds or relative risk ratio involves two steps. First, a confidence interval of the natural logarithm of the statistic is calculated. Second the antilog of the upper and lower limits of the constructed confidence interval for the natural logarithm of the statistic are calculated by taking their exponents, in order to derive the upper and lower limits of the confidence interval for the statistic.

Formulas for calculating the confidence interval for the natural logarithm of the odds ratio and relative risk ratios are given in the equations below:

Equation 3.3.6. Confidence interval of the natural logarithm of the odds ratio:

$$Ln(\widehat{OR}) \pm z\sqrt{\frac{1}{a} + \frac{1}{b} + \frac{1}{c} + \frac{1}{d}}$$

Equation 3.3.7. Confidence interval of the natural logarithm of the relative risk:

$$Ln(\widehat{RR}) \pm z\sqrt{\frac{b/a}{a+b} + \frac{d/c}{c+d}}$$

where Ln denotes the natural logarithm, and z denotes the standard score for the normal distribution. For each statistic, the second step consists of taking the exponent of the lower and upper limits of this constructed confidence interval in these equations.

To illustrate these concepts, consider the following hypothetical 2 × 2 table (Table 3.3.2) from a study by Massoudi and Mohit (2021), which used the cohort design to calculate the odds and odds ratio of receiving the 2019 influenza vaccine, experiencing pulmonologist-confirmed COVID-19 symptoms, and testing positive for COVID-19, among healthcare workers in a hospital setting in Iran. Table 3.3.2 presents summary counts of the numbers of healthcare workers, by vaccination status (exposure) and experience of COVID-19 symptoms (outcome). The probabilities of incident COVID-19 related symptoms (outcome) among vaccinated (exposed) and unvaccinated (unexposed) healthcare workers are 0.03 (i.e.,

Table 3.3.2 Association between vaccination status and COVID-19 symptoms

	Symptomatic	Asymptomatic	Total
Vaccinated	3	87	90
Unvaccinated	77	94	171
Total	80	181	261

3/90) and 0.45 (77/171), respectively. The corresponding odds of symptoms the two exposure groups are 0.03 (0.03/[1 − 0.03]) and 0.82 (0.45/[1 − 0.45]). The odds ratio for symptoms among vaccinated healthcare workers relative to unvaccinated workers is 0.04 (0.03/0.82). The 95% confidence interval for the odds ratio is 0.01–0.14, suggesting that the observed association between vaccination and incidence of COVID-19 symptoms is statistically significant. Massoudi and Mohit (2021) also report associations between the 2019 influenza vaccine exposure and confirmed COVID-19 cases.

For example, using data from Massoudi and Mohit (2021) (Table 3.3.2), we can also calculate the relative risk of experiencing COVID-19 symptoms among vaccinated and unvaccinated individuals; that relative risk is 0.07 (0.03/0.45), with a 95% confidence interval of 0.02–0.21, thus suggesting the observed association was still statistically significant, suggesting that vaccinated individuals have a significantly much lower risk of experiencing symptoms, relative to their unvaccinated counterparts.

Notice that the relative risk is not too far apart from the odds ratio. However, notice also that the implied treatment effect is different (larger in this case) when measured by the relative risk, compared to the odds ratio. This is because the comparison of risk ratios produces a stronger measure of the potential association between the exposure and the outcome than odds ratios do. In general, when the outcome of interest is relatively uncommon, its odds in the exposure group will be similar to its probability in the same group. As a result, the odds ratio provides a relative measure of the treatment effect for case–control studies, as well as an estimate of the risk ratio in the source population when the outcome is uncommon.

Despite the many attractive features of the relative risk ratio, it is worthwhile pointing out that the odds ratio has better statistical properties than the relative risk ratio. For example, the odds ratio of experiencing COVID-19 symptoms is the inverse of the odds ratio of experiencing no symptoms. This is not the case for the relative risk ratio: the relative risk of experiencing symptoms differs from the inverse of the relative risk of experiencing no symptom. Because of these favorable statistical properties of odds ratios, much of the data in the literature are reported as odds ratios.

Table 3.3.3 summarizes and describes some of the most commonly reported statistics in the published literature, which may be relevant to the estimation of parameters for vaccine economics models.

Table 3.3.3 Statistics commonly reported in published scientific studies that are relevant to vaccine economics models

Statistic	Definition
Probability/risk/ prevalence	$$\frac{Number\ of\ events\ ocurring\ in\ a\ time\ period}{Number\ of\ persons\ at\ risk\ in\ the\ population\ over\ that\ time\ period}$$
Rate	$$\frac{Number\ of\ events\ ocurring\ in\ a\ time\ period}{Number\ of\ persons\ at\ risk\ in\ the\ population\ over\ that\ time\ period}$$
Odds	$$\frac{Probability\ of\ outcome}{1-Probability\ of\ outcome}$$
Odds ratio	$$\frac{Odds\ of\ outcome\ in\ exposed}{Odds\ of\ outcome\ in\ unexposed}$$
Relative risk /risk ratio/hazard ratio	$$\frac{Probability\ of\ outcome\ in\ exposed}{Probability\ of\ outcome\ in\ unexposed}$$
Risk difference	Difference in probability of event among exposed and unexposed
Survival curve	Number of people alive at time $(t-1)$ who are alive at time t
Mean	$$\frac{Sum\ of\ all\ observations\ in\ a\ sample\ (or\ population)}{Total\ number\ of\ observations\ in\ the\ sample\ (or\ population)}$$

3.3.2.3.2 Types of input parameters needed in health economics models

The odds ratio, relative risk (or risk ratio and hazard ratio), and risk difference statistics in Table 3.3.3 are *comparative statistics*, as they compare risks or odds of an outcome (e.g., infection) among two different population subgroups (e.g., vaccinated versus unvaccinated). All other statistics in Table 3.3.3 are *non-comparative* statistics.

Inputs for health economic models require non-comparative parameters. For example, in the example of hepatitis B vaccination, we need the probability of acquiring an acute infection without vaccination. Hence, comparative data such as odds ratios, relative risk, or risk difference must be transformed, or combined with non-comparative data to be informative in a vaccine economics model. Furthermore, for the simplest types of models such as decision tree or Markov models, we need parameters in the form of probabilities. In more complex models (e.g., dynamic transmission models), rates might be more desirable.

3.3.3 Data quality for parameter estimation in vaccine economics applications

In practice, most parameter estimates can be judged according to two criteria: quality of the underlying data ("internal validity") and appropriateness or generalizability to the analysis ("external validity"). This principle holds whether or not the specific application relates to vaccine economics or health economics more broadly. In evaluating the quality of underlying data, a commonly used hierarchy may be applied from the principles of evidence-based medicine (Guyatt, Rennie, Meade, & Cook, 2015). These principles of evidence-based medicine include using all available evidence, not selectively relying on just one source, avoiding bias when using observational sources, and using formal evidence synthesis techniques. Certain study designs are better equipped than others to minimize certain forms of biases. In the hierarchy of evidence-based medicine, often depicted as a pyramid, quality of evidence can be assessed based on study design (listed from lowest to highest quality): case series, case–control studies, cohort studies, RCTs, systematic reviews, and meta-analyses. When considering two different RCT studies of vaccines, for example, the analyst should first ask whether the two vaccines were studied in a head-to-head trial. All things equal, priority should be given to evidence generated through head-to-head comparison trials. Study design is not the only determinant of data quality, however; investigators must also assess studies— and their corresponding parameter estimates—for their level of precision (e.g., sample size) and risk of bias.

3.3.4 Appropriateness of data to the analysis

In addition to underlying data quality, parameter values must also be evaluated for their appropriateness to the analysis at hand. For example, a high-quality cluster randomized trial successfully delivered the hepatitis B vaccine to 97.6% of eligible neonates in Qidong, China (Qu et al., 2014). However, applying this probability of vaccination in an economic evaluation of a real-world program in sub-Saharan Africa would be inappropriate. Often, investigators must identify parameter estimates from the scientific literature and consider how to adjust or modify these values (and corresponding estimates of uncertainty) for their analysis. In making any such modifications, it is important to be transparent about the assumptions made, so that analyses can be replicated and appropriately judged by readers in terms of both quality and appropriateness of parameter estimates.

3.3.5 Data conversion into a format consistent with the analytic structure of the model

One additional consideration is that parameter estimates from the scientific literature are often not presented in the form required by an economic evaluation. For example, in the context of vaccine economics, some parameters may be reported as incidence rates, but the analysis may involve a Markov model with a finite time step (for example, 1 month)—thereby requiring the parameters to be estimated as a 1-month probability (or "cumulative incidence"). To the extent possible, investigators should attempt to structure their analyses (e.g., age categories of hepatitis B infection risk) in a fashion that reflects the underlying data structure. However, the natural history of the disease, disease staging, or the clinically and economically meaningful health states associated with the condition may not necessarily coincide with how the data are reported in the literature. When this is the case, mathematical conversions may be required. For example, a 6-month probability of infection may be what is reported in the literature. However, the vaccine economics model might have a 1-year cycle length, requiring the analyst to extrapolate beyond the 6-month estimate, since a 1-year probability is needed for the model. Furthermore, and as we have noted earlier, probabilities cannot be manipulated as easily as other parameters such as rates; we cannot simply multiply or divide them. For example, a 100% probability at 5 years does not mean a 20% probability at 1 year; likewise, a 30% probability at 1 year does not mean a 120% probability at 4 years, and fortunately so, because if it did, a fundamental property of probabilities—that they cannot exceed 1—would be violated.

Data from the literature may also be reported as incidence rates or cumulative incidence. To calculate the probability of an event from incidence rates or cumulative incidence requires information on the duration of the follow-up. If the duration of the follow-up is known, the probability of the event occurring in each time step is simply the cumulative incidence per time step. Going from the incidence rate to the probability involves, however, more assumptions and steps, further described below.

3.3.5.1 Translating rates to probabilities

If the incidence rate (rate per unit time) is constant, the cumulative incidence follows what we call an exponential decay. In that case, we can convert the constant incidence rate into a probability, using the exponential decay formula:

Equation 3.3.8. Rate of decay:

$$p_t = 1 - e^{-rt}$$

where p_t is the probability of remaining event free at time t, r is the incidence rate, and t is the duration of time, with the same unit of time used in both. Thus, for example, to convert a constant incidence rate of 0.4/year to a 1-month (0.083 year) cumulative probability, one could solve for $p_{0.083} = 1 - e^{-(0.4)*(0.083)} = 0.0327$. This equals the 1-month probability of an event that occurs at an underlying constant incidence rate of 0.4/year.

3.3.5.2 Translating probabilities to rates

We can also translate rates into probabilities. To do this, it suffices to do some rearrangements of the exponential decay formula so that $e^{-rt} = 1 - p_t$.

Then, taking the natural logarithm of both sides of this equality, we have $-rt = \ln(1 - p_t)$. After some additional rearrangement, we derive our desired relationship between the rate, time, and the transition probability:

Equation 3.3.9. Probability of decay:

$$r = -\frac{\ln(1 - p_t)}{t}$$

Thus, for example, to translate the 1-month cumulative probability derived above to a constant annual rate, one could solve for $r = -\dfrac{\ln(1 - p_{0.083})}{0.083} = 0.4$/year.

3.3.5.3 Changing time frames of probabilities derived from the literature

Now that we have established the relationship between rates, probabilities, and time, we can leverage these properties to manipulate probabilities, including translating them to rates, and translating back rates into probabilities. This is extremely useful when one needs to change the time frame of probability from data derived from the literature. For example, in our hepatitis B example, we found from the literature that 30% of people have controlled diabetes at 5 years, suggesting that the 5-year probability of controlled diabetes is 0.3. However, our model runs on a 1-year cycle, so we need to convert this probability into the relevant time frame. To do this, we first convert the reported probability from the literature into a rate, using Equation 3.3.9. So, the annual rate is $-\dfrac{\ln(1-0.3)}{5} = 0.071/\text{year}$. Next, we convert back the calculated rate into an annual probability, using Equation 3.3.8: the resulting annual probability is 0.069.

3.3.5.4 Translating odds to probabilities

As we have seen earlier, the odds of an event occurring is the ratio of the probability of occurrence of that event, divided by the probability of that event not occurring, and is expressed mathematically as $odds = \dfrac{p}{1-p}$, where p denotes the probability of occurrence of the event. From this relationship, it is straightforward to express the probability in terms of the odds: the probability becomes the odds divided by 1 plus the odds:

Equation 3.3.10. From odds to probability:

$$p = \frac{odds}{1+odds}$$

3.3.5.5 Translating relative risk or risk ratios to probabilities

Translating relative risk or a risk ratio into a probability is reasonably straightforward, provided that one has the probability for one of the groups. For example, if one knows the probability of infection in the unvaccinated population, we can calculate the probability of infection among vaccinated individuals by multiplying this known parameter (probability of infection in the unvaccinated population) with the relative risk or risk ratio of infection between the two groups.

3.3.5.6 Translating risk difference to probabilities

Risk difference is risk in one group minus risk in the comparator group. Since we have defined a probability to be a measure of risk, then risk difference is simply the difference of the probabilities of events occurring. More concretely, the risk difference in adverse events between the two double-dose mRNA vaccines approved for use against COVID-19 under an Emergency Use Authorization, namely BNT162b2 (developed by BioNTech, Fosun Pharma, and Pfizer) and mRNA-1273 (developed by Moderna and NIAID), is the difference in the probabilities of adverse events for the two vaccines:

Equation 3.3.11. Risk difference:

$$Risk\ difference = P_{AE\ of\ Pfizer} - P_{AE\ of\ Moderna}$$

If a study reports the risk difference between two events or outcomes, it should and will often report one of the probabilities. In modeling applications, we are often interested in estimating the treatment effect, that is, how the intervention affects outcomes, or the risk of occurrence of certain outcomes or events. For example, in the case of vaccination we would want to know how the introduction of a new vaccine affects the risk of infection among the vaccinated individuals, and in the broader population. Analysts should therefore directly use the probability of the outcome or events of interest for the treatment (intervention) group, whenever reported in the study. If, instead, the study reports the probability of occurrence of the outcome or events of interest for the control group, we can use that information along with the risk difference to derive the probability of the outcome for the treatment group.

3.3.5.7 Translating odds ratios to probabilities

Odds ratios are more likely to be reported in the literature than relative risk ratios. Hence, it is important to understand how one can leverage this information to inform vaccine economics models. If the outcome is rare (i.e., ≤10%), it may be reasonable to assume, as we have seen earlier, that the odds ratio approximates the relative risk. In this case, the probability of the outcome (e.g., infection) in the exposed group (e.g., vaccinated) can be calculated as the odds ratio multiplied by the probability of the outcome in the unexposed group (e.g., unvaccinated). However, if the outcome is not rare, one needs to consult a statistician about how to translate odds ratio statistics into probabilities.

Whether it is reasonable to assume that the odds ratio approximates risk ratios depends on the probability of the outcome in the unexposed group. This probability should be and is often reported in the published study. In situations where the probability of the outcome in the unexposed group is conveniently reported in the study from which the odds ratio was extracted, this can be used, in combination with the odds ratio, to derive the probability of the outcome in the exposed group. It suffices to notice that the probability of the outcome in the unexposed group can be used to derive the odds for the outcome in that group (use Equation 3.3.1). Next, we can use Equation 3.3.2 to derive the odds for the outcome in the exposed group. Finally, Equation 3.3.10 can be used to derive the probability of the outcome in the exposed group. When the probability of the outcome in the unexposed group is not reported in the study, the next reasonable step is to return to the literature to find this value for a similar group of patients or population being studied.

3.3.5.8 Using survival data to estimate probabilities

In the previous sections, the probabilities are treated as constant throughout the model. But they need not be constant. For example, the risk of death is not, and should not be assumed to be, constant over time. In a more realistic model, and depending on the time horizon of the model, the probability of death will change with age. Hence, there would be multiple probabilities of death, one for each age, or cycle of the model. But how does one estimate or derive such data?

Probabilities of death are typically derived from survival curves, which are constructed from survival data largely derived from vital statistics databases. For example, in the US, these data are maintained by the Centers for Disease Control and Prevention's National Vital Statistics System, which tracks important statistics, including birth, mortality, and life expectancy data. Mortality data are reported by cause of death, and in aggregate, for any cause. These cause-specific mortality estimates can be age, sex, and race adjusted.

These mortality databases known as *life tables* or *actuarial tables* summarize the vital experiences of the individuals in the population, from birth to death. Life tables are widely used in the insurance industry to estimate beneficiaries' life expectancy, and to set insurance premia. A *cohort life table* or *follow-up life table* is a type of life table which summarizes the experiences of participants over a predefined follow-up period in a cohort study or a clinical trial, until the outcome of interest or the end of the study, or lost-to follow-up, or death, whichever comes first. For example, reported survival rates in life tables may be *death rates* (generally expressed per 100,000 population in a specified group). To translate survival rates to probabilities, we can leverage the formula for the rate to probabilities conversion discussed in Equation 3.3.8: $p_t = 1 - e^{-rt}$, where p_t is the probability of remaining event free (e.g., death) at time t, r is the incidence rate of deaths, and t is the duration of time.

Condition- or treatment-specific survival data can also be derived from the literature, where they may be reported as *probability of death at a given time*, t, or as *survival curves*. A survival curve (also known as survival function or survival distribution) represents the probability that a person "survives," that is, remains free of the outcome of interest, beyond a certain time point, where, conventionally, time is shown on the x-axis and survival (i.e., the proportion of people at risk for the outcome) is shown on the y-axis.

These condition- or treatment-specific survival data can be estimated both parametrically and non-parametrically. Common parametric methods in applications include the exponential, Weibull, Gompertz, and log-normal distributions (Cox & Oakes, 1984). The most popular of them is arguably the exponential distribution, which assumes that the likelihood of an outcome occurring in an individual is independent of the duration of that individual being event free. The other distributions make different assumptions about the probability of the outcome being realized for an individual, such as the probability increasing or decreasing over time. For more details on parametric methods for estimating survival curves, the reader should see publications by Hosmer and Lemeshow (1999) and Lee and Wang (2003).

Non-parametric methods, unlike parametric methods, make no assumption about how the probability of the outcome for a person changes with time. They typically involve estimating and plotting the survival distribution (i.e., survival curve) from the empirical data, using *Kaplan–Meier curves* which report unadjusted survival data from RCTs, or *Cox proportional hazard curves* which report adjusted survival data for observational studies (Cox & Oakes, 1984; Crawley, 2005; Gehan, 1965; Greenwood, 1926; Hosmer & Lemeshow, 1999; Kalbfleisch & Prentice, 2002; Kleinbaun & Klein, 2005; Lee & Wang, 2003; Mantel, 1966; Peto & Peto, 1972).

The evaluation of vaccination interventions often requires estimates of the survival curve of the intervention. When individual patient-level data are available, the parametric and non-parametric methods described above can be used to estimate the survival rates, which can then be used to derive the probabilities. However, as individual patient-level data are often unavailable, survival curves are typically calculated by fitting a nonlinear least squares model to the Kaplan–Meir plots available from the published literature. Unfortunately, this approach does not account for the uncertainty associated with the Kaplan–Meir curve and can produce biased estimates. In addition, Kaplan–Meier curves may only provide survival data up to a few months or years, when the analyst is interested in the life course of those affected by the intervention. Extrapolation to a lifetime horizon is therefore required.

3.3.5.9 Deriving probabilities from means of continuous distributions

Deriving probabilities from means is very challenging and should be applied with great care. There are at least two important challenges when considering this approach. First, one needs a validate method to generate a binary variable from a continuous distribution (e.g., a threshold), in order to characterize discrete events. For example, when using HbA1c to define controlled diabetes, one may want to use a threshold value of, say, 7, so that all individuals in the population with a HbA1c value below this threshold of 7 are classified as having controlled diabetes.

The second challenge is that we need an estimate of variation around the mean (e.g., standard deviation or variance) or median (interquartile range).

3.3.6 Characterize parameters by both a point estimate and an uncertainty distribution

Parameters used in models are typically not known with certainty; if they were, decision-making would be considerably simplified. Because of uncertainty in parameters, it is important to characterize parameters by both a point estimate, and an uncertainty distribution, and explore the implications of this uncertainty for the results of the analysis. Fortunately, standard statistical methods for estimation generate a point estimate, as well as some measure of precision such as standard errors (SEs) or 95% confidence intervals. In a multivariable framework, a measure of covariance between the estimated parameters is also available. Information about uncertainty should be used in economic models to characterize parameter uncertainty and inform uncertainty analyses. The link to the underlying evidence base should also be made clear. See Chapter 4.3 for more details on handling uncertainty in economic analysis.

3.3.6.1 Choosing distributions for parameters

Decision-analytic model parameters are summary representations of the average population-level experiences of potential individuals affected by an intervention or a program. Because of this, the relevant uncertainty to capture when choosing the distribution for a parameter is the second-order uncertainty of the parameter's sampling distribution, as opposed to the first-order uncertainty, which relates to the variability in the values observed in the population (Stinnett & Paltiel, 1997). The assumption of normality, which is a property of large samples, is commonly used in statistics, and is grounded in the central limit theorem. But this assumption may be unrealistic for many health economic applications. For example, normally distributed parameters can assume any value between minus infinity and positive infinity. But in reality, parameters in most applications will have logical bounds on possible values they can assume, so the normal distribution may be inappropriate, and it is critical to carefully chose the appropriate distribution.

At least five different types of parameters are used in vaccine economics models. They include probabilities, resource items, unit costs, relative risks, and effectiveness parameters. In what follows, we briefly discuss the nature of the data that can be used to inform the estimation of these parameters, the logical bounds on the parameters, and the ways in which one can reasonably select their distributions.

3.3.6.1.1 Probability parameters

Probabilities for vaccine economic models can be estimated using observed proportions of the outcome of interest (e.g., infection incidence). At the individual level, the data can be classified as success (e.g., infected) or failure (e.g., uninfected), and can be considered to be independent Bernoulli trials, so that the binomial distribution can be considered. So, it may be convenient to naturally use the proportion of successful cases (i.e., proportion of individuals infected) as an estimate of the probability of infection. However, the binomial distribution, which is a discrete distribution highly dependent on the sample size, may be inappropriate for modeling the distribution of probabilities, which are continuous measurements. To overcome these limitations the beta distribution, which is a conjugate of the binomial distribution and a continuous distribution on the time interval of 0 to 1, may be more appropriate (Briggs, 2005).

3.3.6.1.2 Resource items parameters

Full economic evaluation analyses are collectively concerned with the efficient, affordable, profitable, and equitable use of scarce health resources. The number of resource items (e.g., number of vaccine doses) needed for a particular vaccination program is a count variable and can be modeled using the Poisson distribution with constant mean-variance parameter λ. We can therefore use the Poisson estimate of the variance (λ) to calculate the SE for the mean resource use (e.g., average number of vaccine doses in a population of interest) to characterize its distribution. This SE is simply the squared root of the variance. In large samples, we can even use the estimated SE and mean, in combination with the central limit theorem, to derive a normal sampling distribution. However, as the underlying assumption of large sample is often violated, this approach is rarely recommended. In smaller samples, there is a non-zero probability that the normal distribution could take a value less than 0; this would clearly be inappropriate for resource use parameters, as they must be 0 or strictly positive. To overcome this limitation, a Bayesian framework is often recommended. Under this approach, we can use the gamma distribution to characterize the uncertainty distribution for the mean resource use parameter, without concerns of generating inconsistent values. The gamma distribution, which is constrained to be positive and is fully continuous, is a conjugate to the Poisson distribution, meaning that the two distributions belong to the same parametric family of distributions (i.e., set of distributions with the same functional form, but differing only by the value of the finite-dimensional parameter).

3.3.6.1.3 Unit cost parameters

To assign monetary values to resource use items, it is common to multiply the units of resource use with the unit cost of each resource item. This can be, for example, the cost per dose of a vaccine. If the values of the unit cost parameters had no uncertainty, they would not contribute to the broader uncertainty in the cost of resources used. Indeed, in economic evaluations alongside clinical trials, unit costs are often treated as fixed parameters. But in reality, unit costs are uncertain; for example, they may vary over time, or across vendors. The unit cost is a strictly non-negative continuous variable, unlike data for resource use, which we discussed above. Therefore, a gamma distribution could be used to represent uncertainty in unit costs (Briggs et al., 2006). If the unit cost is not more variable than the resource use it will be applied to, it may be appropriate to use a normal distribution instead.

Sometimes, costs data are presented as an aggregate value for resource use, weighted by unit costs. In this case, a log-normal distribution or a gamma distribution may be appropriate for approximating the uncertainty distribution of costs.

3.3.6.1.4 Relative risk parameters

Relative risk parameters are commonly used in economic evaluation models to derive probabilities for other groups, as we have discussed in section 3.3.2.3. For vaccine economics models, relative risk parameters are particularly important, as they can inform us about the difference in the risk of exposures, or outcomes between, say those who have been vaccinated and those who have not. Relative risk is also a common primary outcome measure in clinical trial studies. The calculation of confidence intervals for relative risk parameters in these studies often assumes, based on the central limit theorem, that the natural logarithm of the relative risk parameter is normally distributed, so that the confidence intervals can be calculated using standard techniques. As we have discussed in section 3.3.2.3, the confidence interval for the relative risk parameter is simply obtained by exponentiating the calculated confidence intervals on the logarithmic scale. This suggests that uncertainty for relative risk parameters may be characterized by the log-normal distribution.

3.3.6.1.5 Effectiveness parameters

Health outcomes are represented in health economic models by effectiveness parameters, which have inherent uncertainties. In what follows, we discuss how these uncertainties can be characterized and incorporated in vaccine economics models. Choosing the appropriate distribution of these parameters is of a paramount importance to obtain a balance between accuracy of fit to the data—which improves model precision—and simplicity—which provides ease of use.

Health outcomes are typically measured as natural units, or utilities (e.g., quality-adjusted life years, disability-adjusted life years, etc.). When the effectiveness parameter is expressed in natural units, the main source of uncertainty is other model parameters, such as probabilities, and relative risk. However, when the health outcomes are measured in utilities, additional sources of uncertainties need to be taken into account.

Utilities are preference weights applied to the length of time spent in each health state to construct the composite measure of quality-adjusted life years.

These weights, also called health-related quality of life (HRQoL), capture an individual's or population's perceived physical and mental health over time, and are measured using multi-attribute utility instruments such as the EuroQol five-dimensional (EQ-5D)—the most widely used instrument—or other instruments such as the SF-6D. HRQoL data are collected through surveys. Hence, they have uncertainties, due to measurement errors and other types of biases, so, it is critical to capture the impacts of these uncertainties in models. HRQoL data are continuous integers anchored and censored at 0 (death) and 1 (full health), but with a lower bound of minus infinity (i.e., states worse than death). For many widely used instruments, the lower bound is censored at −1. Hence, there is no single distribution which matches these characteristics (Brazier, Roberts, & Deverill, 2002; Dolan, 1997; Feeny et al., 2002). As a result, any distribution chosen to characterize HRQoLs will be an approximation. The distributions most widely used to approximate uncertainties in HRQoLs include the beta, gamma, log-normal, and normal distributions.

A related measure is the disutility, which is the disability weight associated with a health state and is used in the calculation of disability-adjusted life years. Similar to the HRQoL, the disability weights also have uncertainties, and are continuous integers on the range of 0 (full health, no disability) and 1 (disability level in a state such as death), so that their uncertainties can also be characterized with the beta distribution.

3.3.6.2 Estimating model parameters from the mean and standard error

As we have already noted, parameters are typically characterized with certain measures of variation around their mean values, and the underlying distributions of their uncertainty. The measure of variation is typically reported as a SE, 95% confidence interval, or 25% and 75% quartiles. With this information, we can fit the model's input parameters to appropriate probability distributions by estimating the parameters of the corresponding (approximate) probability distributions (Westwood et al., 2017).

For some model input parameters (e.g., utilities for chronic hepatitis B states), the literature may already report the probability distributions' parameters so that they can be included directly in the model. However, when they are not reported, the analyst must estimate them, sometimes using nonlinear fitting techniques (Westwood et al., 2017). For example, when the mean and

SE of a parameter is available, the parameters of the corresponding beta distribution can be obtained from the mean and SE as:

Equation 3.3.12. Beta distribution:

$$\alpha = mean \times \left(\frac{mean \times (1 - mean)}{SE^2} - 1 \right)$$

$$\beta = (1 - mean) \times \left(\frac{mean \times (1 - mean)}{SE^2} - 1 \right)$$

where α and β are strictly positive real numbers denoting the shape parameters (Westwood et al., 2017).

3.3.6.3 Estimating model parameters from a confidence interval or an interquartile range

When a mean, and confidence interval or any other uncertainty range, is reported, parameter estimation is not as straightforward as in the approaches mentioned above. In these situations, more complex numerical procedures may be required. For example, it may be necessary to use more advanced software packages such as R, Stata, SPSS, Python, Julia, Matlab, Mathematica, and so on, and more advanced nonlinear multivariate fitting techniques to estimate the parameters of the probability distribution function.

Sometimes, it is necessary to resort to expert opinion to obtain information on the most likely value of a parameter, its range of uncertainty, and potentially the underlying distribution of the parameter. Multiple experts may need to be consulted under this approach. In most applications, including vaccine economics applications, it is common to use the beta or PERT distributions to characterize this distribution.

3.3.7 Assessing the influence of parameter uncertainty, assumptions, and data quality and appropriateness

Sensitivity analyses should also be conducted to assess the impacts of uncertainties in model parameters, model assumptions, data quality, and data appropriateness on the model's results and conclusions. These analyses should be guided by the same sets of principles involved with parameter estimation.

These may include one-way sensitivity analyses which can help identify parameters that are most influential in the model. Multivariate and probabilistic sensitivity analyses can help assess the joint impact of parameter uncertainties on the results and can be used to construct credible confidence intervals around the model's predicted outcomes. See Chapter 4.3 for more details.

3.3.8 Concluding remarks

Ultimately, for each parameter estimate in an economic evaluation, investigators should strive to (1) include both a point estimate and an uncertainty distribution; (2) incorporate empiric data (or estimates from the scientific literature) when available, minimizing the number of assumptions; (3) utilize data of high quality; (4) assess data for appropriateness for the particular analysis; (5) convert data into a format that is consistent with the analytic structure; and (6) evaluate the influence of these decisions on the main results and conclusions. Economic evaluations that carefully follow these steps in parameter estimation are more likely to produce results that are both epidemiologically valid and meaningful to decision makers.

References

Ades, A. E., Lu, G., & Higgins, J. P. (2005). The interpretation of random-effects meta-analysis in decision models. *Medical Decision Making*, 25(6), 646–654. doi:10.1177/0272989x05282643

Ades, A. E., Sculpher, M., Sutton, A., Abrams, K., Cooper, N., Welton, N., & Lu, G. (2006). Bayesian methods for evidence synthesis in cost-effectiveness analysis. *PharmacoEconomics*, 24(1), 1–19. doi:10.2165/00019053-200624010-00001

Baker, S. G. (2006). A simple meta-analytic approach for using a binary surrogate endpoint to predict the effect of intervention on true endpoint. *Biostatistics*, 7(1), 58–70. doi:10.1093/biostatistics/kxi040

Berlin, J. A., Santanna, J., Schmid, C. H., Szczech, L. A., & Feldman, H. I. (2002). Individual patient- versus group-level data meta-regressions for the investigation of treatment effect modifiers: Ecological bias rears its ugly head. *Statistics in Medicine*, 21(3), 371–387. doi:10.1002/sim.1023

Bilcke, J., Antillón, M., Pieters, Z., Kuylen, E., Abboud, L., Neuzil, K. M., . . . Pitzer, V. E. (2019). Cost-effectiveness of routine and campaign use of typhoid Vi-conjugate vaccine in Gavi-eligible countries: A modelling study. *Lancet Infectious Diseases*, 19(7), 728–739. doi:10.1016/s1473-3099(18)30804-1

Brazier, J., Roberts, J., & Deverill, M. (2002). The estimation of a preference-based measure of health from the SF-36. *Journal of Health Economics*, 21(2), 271–292. doi:10.1016/s0167-6296(01)00130-8

Briggs, A. (2005). Probabilistic analysis of cost-effectiveness models: Statistical representation of parameter uncertainty. *Value in Health, 8*(1), 1–2. doi:10.1111/j.1524-4733.2005.08101.x

Briggs, A., Sculpher, M., & Claxton, K. (2006). *Decision modelling for health economic evaluation.* Oxford: Oxford University Press.

Collett, D. (2015). *Modelling survival data in medical research.* New York, NY: Chapman and Hall/CRC.

Cox, D. R., & Oakes, D. (1984). *Analysis of survival data.* New York, NY: Chapman and Hall/CRC.

Crawley, M. J. (2005). *Statistics: An introduction using R.* New York, NY: John Wiley & Sons.

Dias, S., Ades, A. E., Welton, N., Jansen, J. P., & Sutton, A. (2018). *Network meta-analysis for decision-making.* New York, NY: John Wiley & Sons.

Dolan, P. (1997). Modeling valuations for EuroQol health states. *Medical Care, 35*(11), 1095–1108. doi:10.1097/00005650-199711000-00002

Feeny, D., Furlong, W., Torrance, G. W., Goldsmith, C. H., Zhu, Z., DePauw, S., . . . Boyle, M. (2002). Multiattribute and single-attribute utility functions for the health utilities index mark 3 system. *Medical Care, 40*(2), 113–128. doi:10.1097/00005650-200202000-00006

Gehan, E. A. (1965). A generalized Wilcoxon test for comparing arbitrarily singly-censored samples. *Biometrika, 52,* 203–223. https://pubmed.ncbi.nlm.nih.gov/14341275/

Glick, H. A., Doshi, J. A., Sonnad, S. S., & Polsky, D. (2014). *Economic evaluation in clinical trials.* New York, NY: Oxford University Press.

Gold, M. R., Siegel, J., Russell, L., & Weinstein, M. (1996). *Cost-effectiveness in health and medicine.* New York, NY: Oxford University Press.

Greenwood, M. (1926). *A report on the natural duration of cancer.* London: HMSO.

Guyatt, G., Rennie, D., Meade, M. O., & Cook, D. J. (2015). *Users' guides to the medical literature: A manual for evidence-based clinical practice* (3rd ed.). New York, NY: American Medical Association/McGraw-Hill.

Hasselblad, V., & McCrory, D. C. (1995). Meta-analytic tools for medical decision making: A practical guide. *Medical Decision Making, 15*(1), 81–96. doi:10.1177/0272989x9501500112

Higgins, J., Thomas, J., Chandler, J., Cumpston, M., Li, T., Page, M., & Welch, V. (Eds.) (2022). *Cochrane handbook for systematic reviews of interventions,* version 6.3 (updated February 2022). Cochrane. http://www.training.cochrane.org/handbook

Higgins, J. P., Whitehead, A., Turner, R. M., Omar, R. Z., & Thompson, S. G. (2001). Meta-analysis of continuous outcome data from individual patients. *Statistics in Medicine, 20*(15), 2219–2241. doi:10.1002/sim.918

Hosmer, D. W., & Lemeshow, S. (1999). *Applied survival analysis: Regression modeling of time to event data.* New York, NY: John Wiley & Sons.

Hunink, M., Glasziou, P., Siegel, J., & Weeks, J. (2001). *Decision making in health and medicine: Integrating evidence and values.* New York, NY: Cambridge University Press.

Kalbfleisch, J. D., & Prentice, R. L. (2002). *The statistical analysis of failure time data* (2nd ed.). New York, NY: John Wiley & Sons.

Kleinbaun, D. G., & Klein, M. (2005). *Survival analysis: A self-learning text.* New York, NY: Springer Science + Business Median, Inc.

Lambert, P. C., Sutton, A. J., Abrams, K. R., & Jones, D. R. (2002). A comparison of summary patient-level covariates in meta-regression with individual patient data meta-analysis. *Journal of Clinical Epidemiology, 55*(1), 86–94. doi:10.1016/s0895-4356(01)00414-0

Lee, E. T., & Wang, J. W. (2003). *Statistical methods for survival data analysis* (3rd ed.). New York, NY: John Wiley & Sons.

Lu, G., & Ades, A. E. (2004). Combination of direct and indirect evidence in mixed treatment comparisons. *Statistics in Medicine, 23*(20), 3105–3124. doi:10.1002/sim.1875

Lumley, T. (2002). Network meta-analysis for indirect treatment comparisons. *Statistics in Medicine, 21*(16), 2313–2324. doi:10.1002/sim.1201

Mantel, N. (1966). Evaluation of survival data and two new rank order statistics arising in its consideration. *Cancer Chemotherapy Reports, 50*(3), 163–170. https://pubmed.ncbi.nlm.nih.gov/5910392/

Massoudi, N., & Mohit, B. (2021). A case–control study of the 2019 influenza vaccine and incidence of COVID-19 among healthcare workers. *Journal of Clinical Immunology, 41*(2), 324–334. doi:10.1007/s10875-020-00925-0

Neumann, P., Ganiats, T., Russell, L., Sanders, G., & Siegel, J. (2016). *Cost-effectiveness in health and medicine.* New York, NY: Oxford University Press.

Pannucci, C. J., & Wilkins, E. G. (2010). Identifying and avoiding bias in research. *Plastic and Reconstructive Surgery, 126*(2), 619–625. doi:10.1097/PRS.0b013e3181de24bc

Peto, R., & Peto, J. (1972). Asymptotically efficient rank invariant test procedures. *Journal of the Royal Statistical Society, 135*(2), 185–207. http://www.jstor.org/stable/2344317

Piantadosi, S., Byar, D. P., & Green, S. B. (1988). The ecological fallacy. *American Journal of Epidemiology, 127*(5), 893–904. doi:10.1093/oxfordjournals.aje.a114892

Qu, C., Chen, T., Fan, C., Zhan, Q., Wang, Y., Lu, J., . . . Sun, Z. (2014). Efficacy of neonatal HBV vaccination on liver cancer and other liver diseases over 30-year follow-up of the Qidong hepatitis B intervention study: A cluster randomized controlled trial. *PLoS Medicine, 11*(12), e1001774–e1001774. doi:10.1371/journal.pmed.1001774

Rosenthal, R., & DiMatteo, M. R. (2001). Meta-analysis: Recent developments in quantitative methods for literature reviews. *Annual Review of Psychology, 52*, 59–82. doi:10.1146/annurev.psych.52.1.59

Stinnett, A. A., & Paltiel, A. D. (1997). Estimating CE ratios under second-order uncertainty: The mean ratio versus the ratio of means. *Medical Decision Making, 17*(4), 483–489. doi:10.1177/0272989x9701700414

Sutton, A. J., Abrams, K. R., Jones, D. R., Sheldon, T. A., & Song, F. (2000). *Methods for meta-analysis in medical research* (Vol. 348). Chichester: Wiley.

Sutton, A. J., & Higgins, J. P. (2008). Recent developments in meta-analysis. *Statistics in Medicine, 27*(5), 625–650. doi:10.1002/sim.2934

Sutton, A. J., Song, F., Gilbody, S. M., & Abrams, K. R. (2000). Modelling publication bias in meta-analysis: A review. *Statistical Methods in Medical Research, 9*(5), 421–445. doi:10.1177/096228020000900503

Thompson, S. G., & Higgins, J. P. (2002). How should meta-regression analyses be undertaken and interpreted? *Statistics in Medicine, 21*(11), 1559–1573. doi:10.1002/sim.1187

Wakefield, J. (2008). Ecologic studies revisited. *Annual Review of Public Health, 29*, 75–90. doi:10.1146/annurev.publhealth.29.020907.090821

Westwood, M., Corro Ramos, I., Lang, S., Luyendijk, M., Zaim, R., Stirk, L., . . . Kleijnen, J. (2017). Faecal immunochemical tests to triage patients with lower abdominal symptoms for suspected colorectal cancer referrals in primary care: A systematic review and cost-effectiveness analysis. *Health Technology Assessment, 21*(33), 1–234. doi:10.3310/hta21330

3.4

Measuring and valuing health outcomes

Y. Natalia Alfonso, Stéphane Verguet, and Ankur Pandya

The impact of vaccines and immunization programs on populations can be measured with the use of a range of outcome measures, including (1) process and intermediate outputs (e.g., number of children fully immunized, vaccination coverage); (2) natural unit outcomes specific to vaccine-preventable diseases (e.g., cases or deaths associated with measles or rotavirus averted); (3) constructed summary measures of population health (e.g., incorporating both mortality or morbidity outcomes like disability-adjusted life years (DALYs) or quality-adjusted life years (QALYs)); and (4) equity metrics, such as the distribution in health outcomes and non-health benefits such as financial risk protection (prevention of medical impoverishment). A comparison of the strengths and weaknesses of all such measures in vaccine economics is described in detail elsewhere (Bärnighausen et al., 2014; Jit et al., 2015; Walker, Hutubessy, & Beutels, 2010). This chapter introduces some measures pertaining to (3) and (4) and their use in the economic evaluation of vaccines.

3.4.1 Preference elicitation

To quantify the full impact of vaccines on the health of populations, both improvements in the length of life and health-related quality of life (HRQoL) should ideally be measured. Constructed summary measures of population health that incorporate both components into a single unified metric are generally categorized as "health-adjusted life years" or HALYs. To understand how to estimate HALYs, it is important to distinguish between measuring and valuing health outcomes:

Y. Natalia Alfonso, Stéphane Verguet, and Ankur Pandya, *Measuring and valuing health outcomes* In: *Handbook of Applied Health Economics in Vaccines.* Edited by: David Bishai, Logan Brenzel and William V. Padula, Oxford University Press.
© Oxford University Press 2023. DOI: 10.1093/oso/9780192896087.003.0017

- Measuring refers to counting the number of events. For example, the number of deaths, infections averted, disability cases averted, and so on.
- Valuing refers to the subjective appreciation of avoiding a disease that is not fatal. For example, how does one compare the value of living 10 additional years without post-polio paralysis versus 5 years with post-polio paralysis?

It is difficult to define a single value that can accurately represent the reduced quality of life or enhanced disability associated with the experience of being in one specific disease state, such as post-polio paralysis. Preference-based measures provide one approach to the valuation of health states (Feeny, 2005; Rowen et al., 2020). The basic idea is to ask people to state their preferences for specific health states. For example, on a scale from 0 to 100, where 0 is death and 100 is the best health state imaginable, how would you rate your or someone else's quality of life during a year experiencing measles?

Robust methods for eliciting an individual's preferences (i.e., "patient preferences") for the HRQoL value of various health states require a rational decision-making process. This process includes understanding what is at *risk* with or without a vaccine-preventable disease, the *trade-offs* at stake, and the *uncertainty* of those risks and trade-offs. In other words, this process requires that the individual doing the quality-of-life assessment has complete information and understanding of the short-term and long-term risks and uncertainty with and without a vaccine-preventable disease. See Box 3.4.1 for an example of a preference-based valuation scenario that incorporates these aspects. This scenario presents a case in which an individual considers both the health and economic attributes that influence their decisions. Ideally, HRQoL valuation techniques would incorporate both attributes while also assessing risk, trade-offs, and uncertainty. However, it may be difficult for a single valuation technique to incorporate all these characteristics. In fact, most HRQoL techniques focus on health attributes, excluding economic attributes, and incorporate one or two of the requirements for eliciting a rational decision-making process. Another aspect to consider is that the best vaccine choice is subjective based on the individual eligible to receive it and what health or economic conditions they prefer to avoid. As such, quality-of-life valuations are likely to vary by conditions such as age, sex/gender, race, income, and other factors.

The three most common techniques used to elicit patient preferences include the visual analog scale (VAS), time trade-off (TTO), and standard gamble (SG) approaches (Feeny, 2005; Torrance, 1982; Torrance, Feeny, & Furlong, 2001).

Box 3.4.1 Example of preference-based evaluation for the
***Hemophilus influenzae* type b vaccine**

Rational decision-making for patients requires trade-offs like the following:
Short-term common-side effects of the vaccine:

- Pain, muscle aches.
- Fever in children.
- Costs of vaccine.

Long-term health benefits:

- Avoid *H. influenzae* type b sequelae (e.g., pneumonia).
- Avoid indirect consequences like lost productivity.

The decision to proceed with the *H. influenzae* type b vaccine depends on the trade-off between short-term treatment of vaccine and flu symptoms and longer-term treatment risks.

These techniques are used to design survey questions that facilitate a rational decision-making process. The focus is to assess an individual's preferences for both the length and quality of life based on vaccine usage. To do this, these techniques incorporate one or more of the following types of preference measures: (1) value, (1) risk, and (3) time. See Box 3.4.2 for a description of each of these three preference measures. Likewise, see Drummond, Sculpher, Claxton, Stoddart, and Torrance (2015a) for details and comparisons between the VAS, TTO, and SG techniques.

The overall objective of these measures is estimating HRQoL values for different health states in a given population. When quality valuations reflect preferences then the value is known as a "utility weight," "index," or "score." Utility weights are a quantifiable index of health captured on a scale ranging from 0.0 to 1.0 to inform a HALY metric such as a QALY gained or DALY averted (Drummond et al., 2015a). While many instruments use the VAS, TTO, and SG to generate HALYs, there is a hierarchy in terms of each item's fidelity to capturing value, risk, time, and uncertainty. The VAS is easy to use and interpret but it is not considered a true preference-based measure given that it does not specify aspects of risk and time to generate a utility value

---

Box 3.4.2 Preference-based measures

Value preference

How do you feel about one certain outcome relative to another certain outcome?

Risk preference

How do you feel about one certain outcome versus a gamble on another outcome?

Time preference

How do you feel about a certain outcome today versus the same outcome in the future?

(Torrance et al., 2001). The TTO and SG incorporate both a time horizon and value preferences, but only the SG incorporates measurement for risk and uncertainty. As such, the hierarchy of preference between these measures is the SG, followed by TTO, followed by VAS (Drummond et al., 2015a; Gold, Stevenson, & Fryback, 2002). See Box 3.4.3 for an example of the SG technique used to elicit patient preferences.

For more details about patient preferences and utilities see the video on "Introduction to effectiveness, patient preferences, and utilities" (Jacobs, 2018).

The most prominent survey instruments designed to elicit preference-based valuations of quality of life include the Quality of Well-Being Scale, the Health Utilities Index, and the EuroQol Group's EQ-5D questionnaires (Drummond, Sculpher, Claxton, Stoddart, & Torrance, 2015b; Mortimer & Segal, 2008). The EQ-5D questionnaires are widely used in many high-income countries and some low- and middle-income countries (LMICs) and are translated into more than 200 languages (e.g., English, Mandarin, Thai, Amharic) (Brooks, Boye, & Slaap, 2020; Herdman et al., 2011; Shaw, Johnson, & Coons, 2005). The questionnaires are designed using the TTO preference-based technique and consist of five domains that assess an individual's health, including mobility, self-care, usual activities, pain/discomfort, and anxiety/depression (e.g., the EQ-5D-5L questionnaire) (van Reenen & Janssen, 2015). A child-friendly version is also available (i.e., EQ-5D-Y) (Brooks et al., 2020; Devlin & Brooks, 2017; Kind, Klose, Gusi, Olivares, & Greiner, 2015). See Box 3.4.4 for an example of a HRQoL valuation of post-polio syndrome (PPS). The scores from these questionnaires are converted to utility weights using country-specific value sets

Box 3.4.3 Standard gamble examples

Imagine that you have recovered from acute measles and later begin to develop hearing loss. You can hear well today; you are not deaf. You have occasional hearing loss in both ears. Doctors say you will become totally deaf in the next year. But there is a potential cure . . . Successful surgery would prevent symptoms indefinitely. But there is an X% chance that you die from the surgery.

What X% chance of death would you be willing to risk for possibility of cure?

- 10%.
- 25%.
- 50%.
- 75%.
- 90%.

At the point of indifference, the relative value of the health state of post-measles deafness is 1.0 – X.

Imagine that you have early-stage symptoms of paralysis after recovering from acute polio. You can walk today; you are not paralyzed. You have occasional weakness in legs. Doctors say you will become completely paralyzed from the waist down in the next year. But there is a potential cure . . . Successful surgery would prevent symptoms indefinitely. But there is an X% chance that you die from the surgery.

What X% chance of death would you be willing to risk for possibility of cure?

- 10%.
- 25%.
- 50%.
- 75%.
- 90%.

At the point of indifference, the relative value of the health state of post-polio paralysis is 1.0 – X.

(i.e., that incorporate country-specific preferences). For a quick summary of this survey tool see the "Explaining the EQ-5D in about two-and-a-half-minutes" video (EuroQol Research Foundation, 2019). For details on how to calculate utility weights using the EQ-5D descriptive system, see R package "valueEQ5D" (Manchira Krishnan, 2020).

Box 3.4.4 Example of health-related quality of life valuation using the EQ-5D-5L

A study is recruiting participants to estimate HRQoL values for PPS, a vaccine-preventable disease. Participants are either recruited from a population of patients with PPS or from the general population without PPS. In the latter case, participants are provided a vignette describing what it feels like to have PPS.

Each participant is asked to rate his/her health status with PPS regarding their pain/discomfort by selecting one out of the five health state options below:

- I have no problems in walking about.
- I have slight problems in walking about.
- I have moderate problems in walking about.
- I have severe problems in walking about.
- I am unable to walk about.

The individual repeats this exercise for the four remaining health domains: mobility, self-care, usual activities, and anxiety/depression.

3.4.2 Measures of vaccine effectiveness

Underlying any measure of vaccine effectiveness is a strong causal study design that compares use of the vaccine to a relevant alternative (or set of alternatives). These alternatives could include strategies such as usual care or status quo coverage when evaluating vaccine scale-up policies, for example. Strong causal study designs include randomized controlled trials or rigorous quasi-experimental designs, such as controlled interrupted time series and regression discontinuity designs (Lopez Bernal, Andrews, & Amirthalingam, 2019). The outcomes from such studies, such as cases of disease averted from the vaccine, are the starting point for any measure of vaccine effectiveness. These disease-specific outcomes might not be comparable across health conditions, however (how would one value 50 cases of measles averted from one vaccine to 50 cases of high-risk human papillomavirus from another vaccine?), thus motivating the use of HALY metrics (such as QALYs or DALYs) that combined length of life and quality of life into a single number, allowing for comparisons across health conditions.

When used in economic evaluation, QALYs are an expectancy measure in a similar way that life expectancy is an expectancy measure. Life expectancy is the expected number of years that an individual will live based on relevant life tables for that individual. Quality-adjusted life expectancy, or expected QALYs, is similar to life expectancy in that it captures length of life, but QALYs also capture quality of life. Quality of life is measured on a 0.0–1.0 scale, where 0.0 indicates death and 1.0 indicates perfect health. Although perfect health is an abstract concept, one way it can be described is by using the EQ-5D framework where someone in perfect health must have no limitations with mobility, self-care, usual activities, pain/discomfort, or anxiety/depression. All values between 0.0 and 1.0 represent time spent in less-than-perfect health, and can be elicited using direction approaches or indirect approaches (such as the EQ-5D). Negative QALYs imply worse-than-death health states, for outcomes such as terminal diseases. QALYs are calculated as:

Equation 3.4.1. QALY:

$$QALYs = \sum_i years\ spent\ in\ health\ state\ i \times utility\ value\ for\ health\ state\ i$$

DALYs are similar to QALYs in that they are HALYs that combine length of life and quality of life into a single number, but are different in that DALYs are a gap measure, whereas QALYs are an expectancy measure. Put simply, more DALYs are bad; DALYs averted are good. Furthermore, more QALYs are good. Gap measures represent how far off a given individual's life experience is from ideal health in terms of length and quality of life. Ideal length of life is calculated using a synthetic life table that is constructed using the best annual survival probabilities across countries and sexes (the 2016 Global Burden of Disease analyses used a synthetic life table that resulted in an ideal life expectancy of 92 years, for example). Any premature death (i.e., any death before age 92 years) contributes to years of life lost, calculated as the ideal life expectancy minus the year of premature death. Disability weights for DALYs are measured on a 1.0–0.0 scale, where 1.0 indicates a state of disability that is no more functional than death, and 0.0 implies perfect health (i.e., zero disability). Researchers have published standard DALY weights that can be used when country- or population-specific estimates are lacking (Salomon et al., 2015). The number of years lost due to disability is calculated as the product of years lived with a certain health condition and the disability weight for that health condition. DALYs are calculated as the sum for years of life lost and years lost due to disability.

QALYs are typically used more in economic evaluations for high-income countries, while DALYs are typically used more for LMICs. The Tufts Cost-Effectiveness Registry catalogs all health utility values used in cost-per-QALY cost-effectiveness analyses, and the Tufts Global Health Cost Effectiveness Registry includes a DALY calculator that can be customized by country, health condition, and other variables (Tufts Medical Center, 2021). Other studies containing "off-the-shelf" sources have been published for QALY (Sullivan & Ghushchyan, 2006) and DALY (Salomon et al., 2015) utility values, although analysts should pay close attention to whether or not the populations and conditions that were assessed to derive those specific values match the populations of interest for their own studies.

Fig. 3.4.1 shows how the QALYs gained and DALYs averted from a vaccine can be estimated for a given individual. In an economic evaluation, the QALYs gained (or DALYs averted) would be calculated for each individual (or cohort) using a simulation model (which would project estimated QALYs or DALYs) or (less typically) from empirical observation (from a randomized controlled trial that collected quality-of-life and mortality follow-up data, for example).

Although the equations used to calculate QALYs and DALYs are straightforward and have intuitive appeal (each can be represented as areas under the curve in Fig. 3.4.1), these metrics have important limitations that should be understood by analysts and policymakers who use QALYs and DALYs. The additive nature of the QALY and DALY constructions requires certain theoretical assumptions, such as mutual utility independence and constant proportional time trade-off, which are often violated in surveys of the general public (Box 3.4.5) (Hammit, 2002; Pliskin, Shepard, & Weinstein, 1980). HALY formulations that do not require these assumptions and are usable for analyses that span interventions or populations are lacking, however, which is one reason why QALYs and DALYs are the prevailing metrics in economic evaluations of health programs (Carlson, Brouwer, Kim, Wright, & McQueen, 2020).

QALYs and DALYs imply certain value judgments that can lead to problematic ethical issues (Brock, 1995, 1998, 2004). The standard QALY formula gives no weight to distributional issues, for example, "a QALY is a QALY is a QALY" in standard economic evaluations that use QALYs gained (or DALYs averted) as the effectiveness measure (Weinstein, 1988), which can lead to potential policy recommendations that might focus interventions on already advantaged populations (richer, literate, urban) if they are easier to reach and more likely to take advantage of services. Another issue relates to discriminatory issues with the QALY or DALY for life-saving interventions; lives saved for disabled individuals (or any individuals in less than perfect health) would result in fewer QALYs gained compared to the same number of lives saved

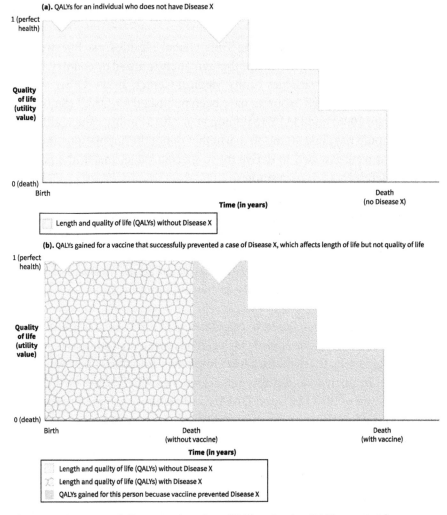

(a). QALYs for an individual who does not have Disease X

1 (perfect health)

Quality of life (utility value)

0 (death)

Birth

Time (in years)

Death (no Disease X)

☐ Length and quality of life (QALYs) without Disease X

(b). QALYs gained for a vaccine that successfully prevented a case of Disease X, which affects length of life but not quality of life

1 (perfect health)

Quality of life (utility value)

0 (death)

Birth

Death (without vaccine)

Death (with vaccine)

Time (in years)

☐ Length and quality of life (QALYs) without Disease X
☐ Length and quality of life (QALYs) with Disease X
☐ QALYs gained for this person becuase vacciine prevented Disease X

Fig. 3.4.1 Conceptual diagrams that show QALYs gained or DALYs averted from a hypothetical vaccine. (a) The life trajectory for a hypothetical individual in a counterfactual scenario without Disease X. This person ended up starting life in perfect health (utility value of 1.0), then experienced lower quality of life later in their life before dying. (b) The life trajectory for the same individual in a counterfactual scenario where they have Disease X, which affects the length of their life (premature death from Disease X) but not quality of their life (which remained at a utility value of 1.0 in early years), and the QALYs gained for this individual from a vaccine that prevents Disease X. (c) The QALYs gained for this individual from a vaccine that prevents Disease Y, which affects both length and quality of life. (d) The DALYs for this individual in a counterfactual scenario without Disease Y (or Disease X). (e) The DALYs averted from a vaccine that prevents Disease Y, which happen to be equal to the QALYs gained from the same vaccine. In practice, it is possible that DALYs averted can be different from QALYs gained for the same intervention (if the utility weights used to calculate QALYs or DALYs are not equal, for example), but these differences will usually be small.

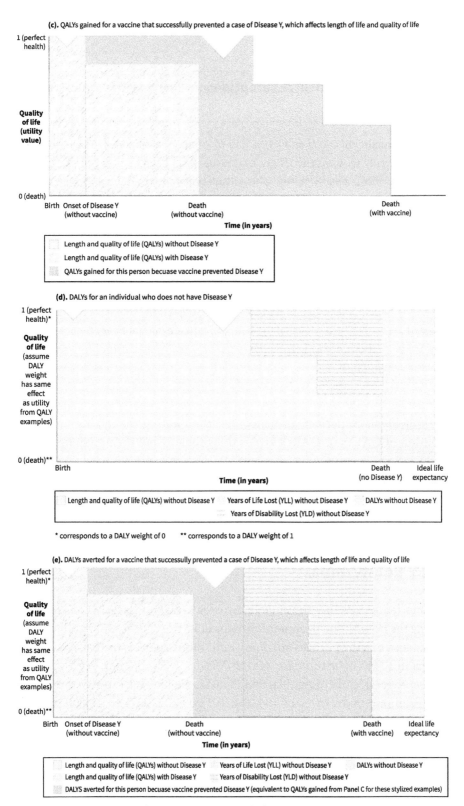

(c). QALYs gained for a vaccine that successfully prevented a case of Disease Y, which affects length of life and quality of life

Quality of life (utility value)

1 (perfect health)

0 (death)

Birth / Onset of Disease Y (without vaccine) / Death (without vaccine) / Death (with vaccine)

Time (in years)

- Length and quality of life (QALYs) without Disease Y
- Length and quality of life (QALYs) with Disease Y
- QALYs gained for this person becuase vaccine prevented Disease Y

(d). DALYs for an individual who does not have Disease Y

Quality of life (assume DALY weight has same effect as utility from QALY examples)

1 (perfect health)*

0 (death)**

Birth / Death (no Disease Y) / Ideal life expectancy

Time (in years)

- Length and quality of life (QALYs) without Disease Y
- Years of Life Lost (YLL) without Disease Y
- DALYs without Disease Y
- Years of Disability Lost (YLD) without Disease Y

* corresponds to a DALY weight of 0   ** corresponds to a DALY weight of 1

(e). DALYs averted for a vaccine that successfully prevented a case of Disease Y, which affects length of life and quality of life

Quality of life (assume DALY weight has same effect as utility from QALY examples)

1 (perfect health)*

0 (death)**

Birth / Onset of Disease Y (without vaccine) / Death (without vaccine) / Death (with vaccine) / Ideal life expectancy

Time (in years)

- Length and quality of life (QALYs) without Disease Y
- Years of Life Lost (YLL) without Disease Y
- DALYs without Disease Y
- Length and quality of life (QALYs) with Disease Y
- Years of Disability Lost (YLD) without Disease Y
- DALYS averted for this person becuase vaccine prevented Disease Y (equivalent to QALYs gained from Panel C for these stylized examples)

* corresponds to a DALY weight of 0   ** corresponds to a DALY weight of 1

Fig. 3.4.1 Continued

> **Box 3.4.5 Theoretical assumptions underlying the QALY and DALY**
>
> The construction of QALYs and DALYs has an intuitive "area under the curve" property that only requires the length of time spent in health states and the utility values for those health states. This calculation requires several assumptions (mutual utility independence, constant proportional trade-offs, and risk neutrality over life years), however, that are often violated by individuals in surveys of the general public. Mutual utility independence implies that an individual's preferences between lotteries over the length of life are independent of the quality of life. A constant proportional trade-off implies there is a constant exchange rate between length of time in a health state and time in perfect health. Risk neutral over life years means individuals are indifferent to length of life trajectories that have the same expected value of life years, even if the risks of death are different over time. Without these assumptions, the QALYs and DALYs cannot be calculated using an "area under the curve" approach.

for individuals in perfect (or better) health. Ignoring the quality-of-life dimension of QALYs or DALYs avoids this problem, but then gives no weight to quality of life-improving interventions. Newer metrics, such as the health years in total measure (Basu, Carlson, & Veenstra, 2020), have been developed to reconcile these competing forces, but they are not yet commonly used as complements or substitutes for QALYs or DALYs.

3.4.3 Equity impact

The burden of vaccine-preventable diseases (VPDs) is largely concentrated among the poorest socioeconomic groups in LMICs. As a case in point, pneumonia and diarrhea deaths still constitute about 20–30% of total under-five deaths in LMICs (Institute for Health Metrics & Evaluation, 2020). For instance, Nigeria, India, Ethiopia, and Pakistan would face estimated diarrhea deaths among under-fives of 104,000, 103,000, 32,000, and 29,000, respectively, in 2017, which is about 50% of total diarrhea deaths in that age group (Institute for Health Metrics & Evaluation, 2020). Under-five mortality is far greater among the poorest wealth quintiles than the richest quintiles in LMICs (Chao, You, Pedersen, Hug, & Alkema, 2018); and rotavirus-related deaths could be several times higher among the poor than the rich in those emerging economies (Rheingans, Atherly, & Anderson, 2012; Verguet et al., 2013). Vaccine coverage also remains unequally distributed across the socio-economic gradient, as documented by the Demographic and Health Surveys. For example, in Ethiopia, inequalities in vaccine access persist and the coverage of the first dose of measles vaccine was 42% in the poorest wealth quintile as opposed to 83% in the richest wealth quintile in 2019 (Central Statistical Agency (Ethiopia) & ICF, 2019; Memirie, Nigus, & Verguet, 2021).

Furthermore, with the onset of VPDs comes financial consequences and potentially financial risks for households in LMICs. VPDs can lead to large amounts of (1) out-of-pocket (OOP) direct medical costs (e.g., costs of physician consultations, drugs, hospitalizations for severe VPD cases); (2) OOP direct non-medical costs associated with transport (and potentially housing) costs to seek care in health facilities; and (3) indirect costs tied to time losses and wages lost associated with seeking care. As a case in point, inpatient visits for severe pneumonia and diarrhea could cost up to $50–$100 to affected households in Ethiopia (Memirie et al., 2017). In this respect, VPDs can substantially contribute to the burden of medical impoverishment in LMICs (World Health Organization, 2019a).

As a result, vaccines can promote equity in two ways, by (1) reducing disparities in the burden of VPDs across the socioeconomic gradient and by (2) preventing the burden of impoverishment associated with the onset of VPDs (Verguet, 2018). More generally, beyond immunization programs, there has been a long-standing attention to how investing in the health sector could participate in reducing and redressing inequalities in society. Specifically, improving the levels and distributions of health outcomes and financial risk protection (the prevention of medical impoverishment) are core objectives of health systems (Roberts, Hsiao, Berman, & Reich, 2019). Therefore, extended cost-effectiveness analysis methods were developed to evaluate health interventions—like immunization programs—along four dimensions: (1) the health benefits (e.g., deaths averted or QALYs gained); (2) the household costs averted (e.g., OOP direct costs and indirect costs averted) by intervention and the financial risk protection gains procured to individuals; (3) the equity impact across socioeconomic status (e.g., poorest versus richest income groups); and (4) the intervention costs (Center for Health Decision Science, 2020; Verguet et al., 2016).

Using extended cost-effectiveness analysis, analysts can study the likely equity impact—both distributional impact across income quintiles and poverty reduction impact of immunization programs (Chang, Riumallo-Herl, Perales, et al., 2018; Chang, Riumallo-Herl, Salomon, et al., 2018; Riumallo-Herl et al., 2018). Vaccines can prevent the majority of deaths among the poorest income quintiles of LMICs, as the poorest often have the most to gain in the first place, due to both greater VPD burden and smaller vaccine coverage. One can also demonstrate that vaccines can substantially reduce poverty, as the poorest would face higher VPD-related OOP costs compared with their disposable income (Chang, Riumallo-Herl, Perales, et al., 2018).

References

Bärnighausen, T., Bloom, D. E., Cafiero-Fonseca, E. T., & O'Brien, J. C. (2014). Valuing vaccination. *Proceedings of the National Academy of Sciences of the United States of America, 111*(34), 12313–12319. doi:10.1073/pnas.1400475111

Basu, A., Carlson, J., & Veenstra, D. (2020). Health years in total: A new health objective function for cost-effectiveness analysis. *Value in Health, 23*(1), 96–103. doi:10.1016/j.jval.2019.10.014

Brock, D. W. (1995). Justice and the ADA: Does prioritizing and rationing health care discriminate against the disabled? *Social Philosophy & Policy, 12*(2), 159–185. doi:10.1017/s0265052500004714

Brock, D. W. (1998). Appendix E: Ethical issues in the development of summary measures of population health status. In M. J. Field & M. R. Gold (Eds.), *Summarizing population health: Directions for the development and application of population metrics* (pp. 73–81). Washington, DC: National Academies Press.

Brock, D. W. (2004). Ethical issues in the use of cost effectiveness analysis for the prioritization of health resources. In G. Khushf (Ed.), *Handbook of bioethics: Taking stock of the field from a philosophical perspective* (pp. 353–380). Dordrecht: Springer Netherlands.

Brooks, R., Boye, K. S., & Slaap, B. (2020). EQ-5D: A plea for accurate nomenclature. *Journal of Patient-Reported Outcomes, 4*(1), 52. doi:10.1186/s41687-020-00222-9

Carlson, J. J., Brouwer, E. D., Kim, E., Wright, P., & McQueen, R. B. (2020). Alternative approaches to quality-adjusted life-year estimation within standard cost-effectiveness models: Literature review, feasibility assessment, and impact evaluation. *Value in Health, 23*(12), 1523–1533. doi: 10.1016/j.jval.2020.08.2092.

Center for Health Decision Science. (2020). *Resource pack: Extended cost-effectiveness analysis.* https://repository.chds.hsph.harvard.edu/repository/collection/resource-pack-extended-cost-effectiveness-analysis/

Central Statistical Agency (Ethiopia), & ICF. (2019). *Ethiopia mini demographic and health survey 2019.* https://dhsprogram.com/publications/publication-FR363-DHS-Final-Reports.cfm

Chang, A. Y., Riumallo-Herl, C., Perales, N. A., Clark, S., Clark, A., Constenla, D., . . . Verguet, S. (2018). The equity impact vaccines may have on averting deaths and medical impoverishment in developing countries. *Health Affairs (Millwood), 37*(2), 316–324. doi:10.1377/hlthaff.2017.0861

Chang, A. Y., Riumallo-Herl, C., Salomon, J. A., Resch, S. C., Brenzel, L., & Verguet, S. (2018). Estimating the distribution of morbidity and mortality of childhood diarrhea, measles, and pneumonia by wealth group in low- and middle-income countries. *BMC Medicine, 16*(1), 102. doi:10.1186/s12916-018-1074-y

Chao, F., You, D., Pedersen, J., Hug, L., & Alkema, L. (2018). National and regional under-5 mortality rate by economic status for low-income and middle-income countries: A systematic assessment. *Lancet Global Health, 6*(5), e535–e547. doi:10.1016/S2214-109X(18)30059-7

Devlin, N. J., & Brooks, R. (2017). EQ-5D and the EuroQol Group: Past, present and future. *Applied Health Economics and Health Policy, 15*(2), 127–137. doi:10.1007/s40258-017-0310-5

Drummond, M., Sculpher, M., Claxton, K., Stoddart, G. L., & Torrance, G. W. (2015a). Measuring and valuing effects: Health gain. In *Methods for the economic evaluation of health care programmes* (pp. 133–143). Oxford: Oxford University Press.

Drummond, M., Sculpher, M., Claxton, K., Stoddart, G. L., & Torrance, G. W. (2015b). *Methods for the economic evaluation of health care programmes* (4th ed.). Oxford: Oxford University Press.

EuroQol Research Foundation. (2019). *Explaining the EQ 5D in about two-and-a-half minutes.* https://www.youtube.com/watch?v=qhZ6goeTSLI&feature=youtu.be

Feeny, D. (2005). Preference-based measures: Utility and quality-adjusted life years. In P. Fayers, & R. Hays (Eds.), *Assessing quality of life in clinical trials* (pp. 405–431). Oxford: Oxford University Press.

Gold, M. R., Stevenson, D., & Fryback, D. G. (2002). HALYs and QALYs and DALYs, oh my: Similarities and differences in summary measures of population health. *Annual Review of Public Health, 23*(1), 115–134. doi:10.1146/annurev.publhealth.23.100901.140513

Hammit, J. K. (2002). QALYs versus WTP. *Risk Analysis, 22*(5), 985–1001. doi:10.1111/1539-6924.00265

Herdman, M., Gudex, C., Lloyd, A., Janssen, M. F., Kind, P., Parkin, D., . . . Badia, X. (2011). Development and preliminary testing of the new five-level version of EQ-5D (EQ-5D-5L). *Quality of Life Research, 20*(10), 1727–1736. http://www.jstor.org/stable/41488243

Institute for Health Metrics & Evaluation. (2020). *GBD compare.* https://vizhub.healthdata.org/gbd-compare/

Jacobs, J. (2018). *Introduction to effectiveness, patient preferences, and utilities.* https://www.hsrd.research.va.gov/for_researchers/cyber_seminars/archives/video_archive.cfm?SessionID=2400

Jit, M., Hutubessy, R., Png, M. E., Sundaram, N., Audimulam, J., Salim, S., & Yoong, J. (2015). The broader economic impact of vaccination: Reviewing and appraising the strength of evidence. *BMC Medicine, 13*(1), 209. doi:10.1186/s12916-015-0446-9

Kind, P., Klose, K., Gusi, N., Olivares, P., & Greiner, W. (2015). Can adult weights be used to value child health states? Testing the influence of perspective in valuing EQ-5D-Y. *Quality of Life Research, 24*(10), 2519–2539. doi:10.1007/s11136-015-0971-1

Lopez Bernal, J. A., Andrews, N., & Amirthalingam, G. (2019). The use of quasi-experimental designs for vaccine evaluation. *Clinical Infectious Diseases, 68*(10), 1769–1776. doi:10.1093/cid/ciy906

Manchira Krishnan, S. (2020). *valueEQ5D: Scoring the EQ-5D descriptive system.* The R Project for Statistical Computing. https://CRAN.R-project.org/package=valueEQ5D

Memirie, S. T., Metaferia, Z. S., Norheim, O. F., Levin, C. E., Verguet, S., & Johansson, K. A. (2017). Household expenditures on pneumonia and diarrhoea treatment in Ethiopia: A facility-based study. *BMJ Global Health, 2*(1), e000166. doi:10.1136/bmjgh-2016-000166

Memirie, S. T., Nigus, M., & Verguet, S. (2021). Cost-effectiveness and equitable access to vaccines in Ethiopia: An overview and evidence synthesis of the published literature. *Journal of Global Health Reports, 5*, e2021008. doi:10.29392/001c.19354

Mortimer, D., & Segal, L. (2008). Comparing the incomparable? A systematic review of competing techniques for converting descriptive measures of health status into QALY-weights. *Medical Decision Making, 28*(1), 66–89. doi:10.1177/0272989x07309642

Pliskin, J. S., Shepard, D. S., & Weinstein, M. C. (1980). Utility functions for life years and health status. *Operations Research, 28*(1), 206–224. doi:10.1287/opre.28.1.206

Rheingans, R., Atherly, D., & Anderson, J. (2012). Distributional impact of rotavirus vaccination in 25 GAVI countries: Estimating disparities in benefits and cost-effectiveness. *Vaccine, 30*(Suppl 1), A15–A23. doi:10.1016/j.vaccine.2012.01.018

Riumallo-Herl, C., Chang, A. Y., Clark, S., Constenla, D., Clark, A., Brenzel, L., & Verguet, S. (2018). Poverty reduction and equity benefits of introducing or scaling up measles, rotavirus and pneumococcal vaccines in low-income and middle-income countries: A modelling study. *BMJ Global Health, 3*(2), e000613. doi:10.1136/bmjgh-2017-000613

Roberts, M. J., Hsiao, W., Berman, P., & Reich, M. R. (2019). *Getting health reform right, anniversary edition.* Oxford: Oxford University Press.

Rowen, D., Rivero-Arias, O., Devlin, N., & Ratcliffe, J. (2020). Review of valuation methods of preference-based measures of health for economic evaluation in child and adolescent populations: where are we now and where are we going?. *Pharmacoeconomics, 38*(4), 325–340. doi:10.1007/s40273-019-00873-7

Salomon, J. A., Haagsma, J. A., Davis, A., de Noordhout, C. M., Polinder, S., Havelaar, A. H., . . . Vos, T. (2015). Disability weights for the Global Burden of Disease 2013 study. *Lancet Global Health, 3*(11), e712–e723. doi:10.1016/S2214-109X(15)00069-8

Shaw, J. W., Johnson, J. A., & Coons, S. J. (2005). US valuation of the EQ-5D health states: Development and testing of the D1 valuation model. *Medical Care, 43*(3), 203–220. https://journals.lww.com/lww-medicalcare/Fulltext/2005/03000/US_Valuation_of_the_EQ_5D_Health_States_.3.aspx

Sullivan, P. W., & Ghushchyan, V. (2006). Preference-based EQ-5D index scores for chronic conditions in the United States. *Medical Decision Making, 26*(4), 410–420. doi:10.1177/0272989x06290495

Torrance, G. W. (1982). Preferences for health states: A review of measurement methods. *Mead Johnson Symposium on Perinatal and Developmental Medicine, 20*, 37–45. http://europepmc.org/abstract/MED/6927515

Torrance, G. W., Feeny, D., & Furlong, W. (2001). *Visual analog scales: Do they have a role in the measurement of preferences for health states?* Thousand Oaks, CA: Sage Publications.

Tufts Medical Center. (2021). *Global health cost-effectiveness analysis registry.* http://ghcearegistry.org/ghcearegistry/

van Reenen, M., & Janssen, B. (2015). *EQ-5D-5L user guide: Basic information on how to use the EQ-5D-5L instrument.* Rotterdam: EuroQol Research Foundation.

Verguet, S. (2018, July 21). The equity and poverty reduction benefits of vaccines. *Harvard Health Policy Review.* http://www.hhpronline.org/articles/2018/7/21/the-equity-and-poverty-reduction-benefits-of-vaccines

Verguet, S., Kim, J. J., & Jamison, D. T. (2016). Extended cost-effectiveness analysis for health policy assessment: A tutorial. *PharmacoEconomics, 34*(9), 913–923. doi:10.1007/s40273-016-0414-z

Verguet, S., Murphy, S., Anderson, B., Johansson, K. A., Glass, R., & Rheingans, R. (2013). Public finance of rotavirus vaccination in India and Ethiopia: An extended cost-effectiveness analysis. *Vaccine, 31*(42), 4902–4910. doi:10.1016/j.vaccine.2013.07.014

Walker, D. G., Hutubessy, R., & Beutels, P. (2010). WHO guide for standardisation of economic evaluations of immunization programmes. *Vaccine, 28*(11), 2356–2359. doi:10.1016/j.vaccine.2009.06.035

Weinstein, M. C. (1988). A QALY is a QALY—or is it? *Journal of Health Economics, 7*(3), 289–290. doi:10.1016/0167-6296(88)90030-6

World Health Organization. (2019a). *Global monitoring report on financial protection in health 2019.* https://www.who.int/healthinfo/universal_health_coverage/report/fp_gmr_2019.pdf?ua=1

3.5

Reporting and interpreting results of economic evaluation

Ijeoma Edoka, Carleigh Krubiner, Andrew Mirelman, R. Brett McQueen, Mark Sculpher, Julia F. Slejko, and Tommy Wilkinson

3.5.1 Understanding a cost-effectiveness analysis plane

A cost-effectiveness analysis (CEA) plane is a common way to visualize the results of a vaccine CEA. A CEA plane is a graph where each intervention in the analysis can be plotted with costs on the vertical (y) axis and effects on the horizontal (x) axis. While the incremental cost-effectiveness ratio (ICER) is the key summary metric of interest when reporting results, a CEA plane can display the expected costs and effects of all included interventions relative to a common comparator and is a useful way of communicating results to a nontechnical audience.

To populate a CEA plane, each intervention is plotted according to calculated costs and effects. The effects are the outcomes generated by the CEA and can be natural units (e.g., infections averted) or generalizable units (e.g., the disability-adjusted life year (DALY) averted or quality-adjusted life year (QALY) gained). Using a generalizable outcome measure is the most common approach and allows a CEA plane to be interpreted relative to a cost-effectiveness threshold (CET) and other competing health systems investments. The costs reflected for each intervention are "net" and incorporate costs incurred from implementation of the intervention and any costs savings.

An example results table is shown (Table 3.5.1) with the corresponding CEA plane (Fig. 3.5.1). The costs and effects in Table 3.5.1 are relative to the status quo or existing treatment, and status quo is represented at the origin of the CEA plane in Fig. 3.5.1.

Ijeoma Edoka, Carleigh Krubiner, Andrew Mirelman, R. Brett McQueen, Mark Sculpher, Julia F. Slejko, and Tommy Wilkinson, *Reporting and interpreting results of economic evaluation* In: *Handbook of Applied Health Economics in Vaccines*. Edited by: David Bishai, Logan Brenzel and William V. Padula, Oxford University Press. © Oxford University Press 2023. DOI: 10.1093/oso/9780192896087.003.0018

Table 3.5.1 Hypothetical results table for a corresponding case study of results for cost-effectiveness analysis of vaccines and competing public health strategies

Alternative	Costs ($)	Effectiveness (QALYs)
Vaccine A	10	3.0
Vaccine B	20	4.0
Vaccine C	50	5.0
Intervention D	−40	3.0
Intervention E	−20	−3.0
Intervention F	10	−5.0

The CEA plane typically consists of four quadrants, called the North West (NW), North East (NE), South West (SW), and South East (SE). As the origin of the CEA plane represents the status quo, interventions plotted in the NE quadrant (Vaccines A, B, and C) are more expensive and more effective than current treatment, whereas an intervention plotted in the SE quadrant

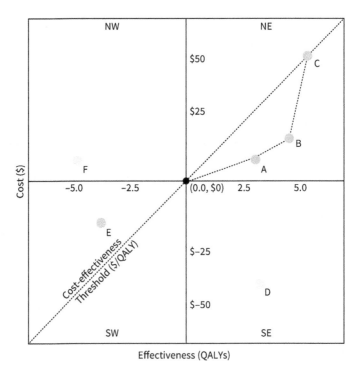

Fig. 3.5.1 Cost-effectiveness plane of a sample vaccine case.

(Intervention D) is expected to be more effective and less costly than current treatment. An intervention that is plotted in the SW quadrant (Intervention E) is expected to be less costly and less effective than current treatment; and an intervention that is plotted in the NW quadrant (Intervention F) is expected to be more costly and less effective than current treatment.

In Table 3.5.1, Vaccine A achieves three units of health for $10 compared to current treatment, while Vaccine B achieves an additional unit of health for an additional $10 compared to Vaccine A, and Vaccine C achieves an additional unit of health for an additional $30 compared to Vaccine B. Plotting a line from the origin (status quo) to Vaccine A, to Vaccine B, and to Vaccine C is called the cost-effectiveness frontier (gray dotted lines). In Fig. 3.5.1, the cost-effectiveness frontier is becoming steeper as we move from Vaccine A to B to C indicating that the incremental cost per unit of health gain (the ICER) is increasing. The CET can also be plotted on a CEA plane and is shown in as a dotted diagonal line in Fig. 3.5.1 at a hypothetical vale of $10 per unit of health gain. Where the cost-effectiveness frontier is shallower than the CET then an intervention would be considered cost-effective, and an intervention with a CEA frontier steeper than the CET would not be considered cost-effective. A policy recommendation based on cost-effectiveness would recommend an intervention with the highest ICER that remained at or equal to the CET to achieve optional spending across the health system.

In Fig. 3.5.1, the CEA frontier moving from the origin to Intervention A is shallower than the CET, the CEA frontier moving from Vaccine A to Intervention B is the same as the CET, and the CE frontier moving from Vaccine B to Vaccine C is steeper than the CET. The interpretation is that Vaccine C is not cost-effective, and that Vaccines A and B represent potential policy options. As the ICER for Vaccine B is equal to the CET, Vaccine B would be the recommended policy option based on cost-effectiveness criteria. As it is common for a CEA to be conducted on interventions that are expected to cost more but will be more effective than current treatment, frequently only the NE quadrant of a CEA plane will be reported in a published CEA. However, many CEA results will involve interventions that are plotted in the other quadrants of the CEA plane.

The interpretation of results for interventions plotted in either the SE or NW quadrants are generally straightforward. As Intervention D is less costly and more effective than current treatment, it can be considered cost-effective regardless of any CET or willingness to pay for health gain. Conversely, Intervention F would not be considered cost-effective even at a very high CET as it achieves less health compared to status quo at a higher cost.

Interventions in the SW quadrant often represent a challenging area for health policy decision makers. In Fig. 3.5.1, Intervention E is both less costly but less effective than status quo. This means that Intervention E represents a "disinvestment" option where implementing Intervention E and stopping provision of the status quo would lead to lower direct health for the immediate patient population. However, this could be considered a cost-effective disinvestment decision if the money saved (or yielded) by investing in Intervention E relative to status quo could be invested elsewhere in the health system, thereby generating more population health overall. The point at which a vaccine would yield more population health than is lost as a result of disinvesting the status quo is also informed by the CET, where interventions below the CET would yield positive overall population health and would be considered a cost-effective treatment option. In Fig. 3.5.1, Intervention E is above the CET and would not be considered a cost-effective option as the health losses associated with implementation would not be fully offset by the population health gains achievable from cost savings reinvestment in the health system. CEA can be an extremely useful tool in informing health system disinvestments; however, the policy decision would need to take further non-efficiency factors into consideration including the rights of patients to continue therapies from which they are benefiting and the feasibility, uncertainty, and risks of implementing a known less effective therapy.

Fig. 3.5.1 displays deterministic results of a CEA and each intervention is represented as a single point plotted on the graph. A CEA plane is also effective as visualizing the results of probabilistic sensitivity analysis (see Chapter 4.3), where each intervention is represented by a field of plotted points, each point representing a single simulation within the probabilistic sensitivity analysis. Viewing probabilistic sensitivity analysis results on a CEA plane shows the range of uncertainty associated with an intervention relative to the CET and other mutually exclusive interventions.

This section has introduced the CEA plane and described how results plotted on the CEA plane can be interpreted for vaccine value. The CEA plane remains the standard approach for reporting CEA results and is a powerful mechanism for communicating results of an analysis to policymakers and nonexpert audiences.

3.5.2 Cost-effectiveness thresholds for vaccine economics

3.5.2.1 Background and principles

In the process of conducting CEAs for vaccines (or other health technologies and interventions), a CET can provide guidance on whether an investment or disinvestment in that intervention is cost-effective or not. CETs can be used by analysts, or in decision-making processes such as health technology assessment, which are established to make investment and disinvestment decisions for packages of health services across a health system.

In its basic form, a CET can be conceptualized in a fraction format of the value per health benefit gained, which represents a level above or below that something is considered cost-effective. The value in the numerator is a commonly understood currency, while the value in the denominator is a summary measure of health such as a QALY gained or a DALY averted. CET is used interchangeably with another term introduced earlier, the willingness-to-pay threshold (see Chapter 3.1).

When the incremental costs per QALY or DALY of a new intervention compared to its next best alternative, expressed as an ICER, falls below the CET, then the intervention is regarded as representing good value for money and is recommended for funding. However, an ICER that falls above the threshold implies that investing in the new intervention does not constitute good value. CETs are therefore an important element for making resource allocation decisions and have been widely used in several countries. They are generally viewed as a means for improving efficiency in the allocation of scarce resources as well as for ensuring consistency, transparency, and public support in the decision-making process. This is particularly important when unpopular decisions must be made.

3.5.2.2 What do cost-effectiveness thresholds represent?

The two perspectives of what CETs should represent are often referred to as the demand-side and supply-side perspectives. Demand-side thresholds reflect the monetary value society places on additional health gains while forgoing gains from the consumption of non-health goods. In other words, this perspective suggests that thresholds should represent society's willingness to pay for additional health gains, thus reflecting consumer demand for healthcare services. Many commonly used thresholds typically reflect this perspective and are either based on value judgments or derived empirically by estimating society's willingness to pay for additional health gains (Vallejo-Torres, García-Lorenzo, & Serrano-Aguilar, 2018). One common example that had been in favor until recently was the Commission on Macroeconomics and Health's rule of thumb threshold of one to three times gross domestic product (GDP) per capita, based on value judgments on economic gains accruing from averting a DALY (Hutubessy, Chisholm, & Edejer, 2003). In Thailand, the CET used for reimbursement decisions is based on empirical estimates of society's willingness to pay for a QALY (Teerawattananon, Tritasavit, Suchonwanich, & Kingkaew, 2014; Thavorncharoensap et al., 2013).

Supply-side thresholds on the other hand, reflect the opportunity costs resulting from funding decisions when health budgets are constrained. Proponents of the supply-side perspective argue that when health budgets are fixed, decisions to introduce a new intervention should be made based on health gains displaced elsewhere in the system in order to free up resources for the new intervention. When the health displaced elsewhere in the system out-weighs health gained from funding the new intervention under evaluation, the new intervention is not worth doing. The CET should therefore reflect the value of health given up or the health opportunity cost of health spending. This perspective explicitly takes into account the budget available to the health system and/or the efficiency with which the health system is capable of pro-ducing health. Thresholds can be useful tools, and when they are explicitly set, decision-making can also be held accountable to this explicit component.

However, CETs should not be applied as the sole decision-making criteria. One reason could be that the CET itself could be inaccurate or not fully reflect different consequences of a decision. For example, the GDP multiplier-based thresholds, have been widely criticized as not suitable for health decision-making. Alternatively, a threshold estimate based on the supply-side op-portunity cost would needs extensive data to be identified, or else it would be difficult to reflect the health consequences of the decision being made. Therefore, an appropriate CET is only helpful as an aid to decision-making if it reflects the best available evidence and is incorporated in a broader decision-making process that is both transparent and accountable.

3.5.2.3 Identifying cost-effectiveness thresholds

A CET may be estimated with several techniques. One approach is to use mathematical modeling to maximize the health objective function subject to the budget constraint (Stinnett & Paltiel, 1996). More commonly, a causal link between expenditure and health is identified using either cross-country var-iation, or within-country variation to estimate the impact of relative amount of health that is given up (or gained) when there is new investment (or dis-investment). Estimating a threshold using within-country data can be inten-sive. This is because data are needed that establish the opportunity cost of the system with the causal link between expenditure changes and health changes.

Table 3.5.2 Examples of cost-effectiveness thresholds identified with quantitative approaches

Example country	Income group	Threshold estimated	Explicit threshold used	Source
Thailand	Middle-income country	Baht 240,000 per QALY	Baht 160,000	Nimdet & Ngorsuraches (2015)
England	High-income country	£5,000—£15,000 per QALY	£20,000—£30,000 NICE recommendation	Lomas et al. (2019)
US	High-income country	US $100,000 per QALY	US $50,000—$150,000 per QALY No exact threshold recognized	Vanness et al. (2021)

Within country approaches have been used in the UK and Spain, and there have been attempts to use within-country approaches in low- and middle-income countries (LMICs) as well, such as South Africa (Claxton et al., 2015; Edoka & Stacey, 2020; Vallejo-Torres et al., 2018; Vanness, Lomas, & Ahn, 2021). However, given the need for high-quality within-country data for these approaches, other approaches have been used that incorporate cross-country data (Ochalek, Lomas, & Claxton, 2018; Woods, Revill, Sculpher, & Claxton, 2016).

Table 3.5.2 provides information to shows three examples of countries with explicitly defined thresholds used in health decision-making. With the exception of the US, the other countries—Thailand and England—are two of the few with explicitly defined thresholds (Lomas, Martin, & Claxton, 2019; Schwarzer et al., 2015). The estimated values of the thresholds that are estimated in studies can vary from those that are used in practice.

3.5.2.4 Alternative approaches?

A review of CEA studies in LMICs identified that thresholds related to GDP per capita are the most widely used in cost-effectiveness studies in LMICs (Leech, Kim, Cohen, & Neumann, 2018). However, while these types of thresholds are widely cited in cost-effectiveness studies, they are often mis-used and overused. The current recommendation is to rely on context-specific thresholds that are not based on GDP per capita to inform decision-making (Bertram et al., 2016).

Given that it may either be difficult to identify a CET with quantitative approaches, or that other across-country CETs may not be suitable for national health decision makers, a recent paper convened by a group of experts at Bellagio identified other approaches to making decisions when an explicitly defined CET is not possible. These approaches include looking at decisions in other settings, looking at evidence of affordability (budget impact analysis), and developing league tables (Chi et al., 2020). One should note, however, that these approaches do not necessarily substitute for using CETs, and many of the mentioned approaches can be part of a broad-based decision-making process.

3.5.2.5 Cost-effectiveness thresholds and vaccines

Vaccines, in principle, are the same as any other health intervention. They have a cost, an associated health impact, and decisions need to be made about whether they should be introduced or removed. Vaccines, however, can also have important multisectoral impacts outside of the health sector (Bärnighausen et al., 2014). This means that in addition to considering a health-specific CET, such as the ones referred to above, one would also need to consider decision rules in other non-health sectors. This is not a straightforward task given that there may be trade-offs between sectors that are important to consider and that the measures of impact between sectors may differ.

In the UK, the Joint Committee on Vaccination and Immunisation makes decisions around vaccine introduction, and it uses the same threshold as that used by the National Institute for Health and Care Excellence (NICE). However, there have been recommendations to bring this value lower so it is supported by an evidence-based value of opportunity cost (Table 3.5.2) (O'Mahony & Paulden, 2019).

In LMICs, there are still many studies that use GDP per capita-based thresholds when making conclusions about cost-effectiveness (Fesenfeld, Hutubessy, & Jit, 2013). Another approach is to consider many different types of thresholds and to let decision makers make an assessment based on what they consider to be appropriate. Loganathan et al. (2018) do this in a study of rotavirus vaccination in Malaysia. Regardless of the threshold used, it is important to remember that economic evaluations for vaccines (and indeed other interventions) should encompass the principles of timeliness, integration, quality, and ownership/institutionalization (Jauregui et al., 2015). See Box 3.5.1.

Box 3.5.1 Applying CETs in an unequal world: is it ethical to have different thresholds for different global contexts?

CEA remains a critical tool to navigate the complexities of priority setting for health and ensure that limited resources are used effectively and efficiently to protect and promote well-being. Yet, the use of CEA and health economics more broadly has been subject to various criticisms, including that it commodifies health in ways inconsistent with conceptions of health as a human right and that it reinforces inequities in health (Farmer, 2015; Meyer, 2013). However, properly understood, the realization of the right to health is unattainable without explicit priority setting subject to resource availability (Rumbold et al., 2017). Moreover, inefficient allocations often favor the interests of the privileged few while diverting resources away from cost-effective services that would most improve the health of the politically and economically disadvantaged. Lastly, it is worth underscoring that cost-effectiveness alone cannot capture all morally relevant considerations to guide decision-making (Krubiner & Faden, 2017; Norheim et al., 2014; World Health Organization, 2014a). In any context, there may be compelling and principled reasons why a health intervention that fails to meet a CET should still be covered. The use of a threshold, however, ensures that health opportunity costs are considered in the priority-setting process and that allocations resulting in lesser aggregate health gains are reasonably justified by competing moral claims.

Regarding CETs that vary based on the resource constraints in a given country, one can understand the perception that, on its face, this approach calculates the "value of life" differently in rich versus poor settings. However, this interpretation fails to recognize that the true aim of a CET is not to set a price on the value of individuals' health, but rather to help avoid morally relevant health opportunity costs in which more people suffer from ill health and premature death as a result of a short-sighted investment in an expensive health technology with clinical benefits for a limited proportion of the population (Chi et al., 2020; Ochalek et al., 2018; Revill et al., 2014). Countries must operate within a set health budget, and make tough decisions about how to allocate domestic resources. A CET can help policymakers identify the set of health interventions that will produce the greatest health gains for their populations for a set of budget constraints.

Consider, for example, policy decisions about seasonal influenza immunization, including which vaccines to procure and which populations should be included in annual vaccination campaigns (Clements, Chancellor, Nichol, DeLong, & Thompson, 2011; Hendriks et al., 2018; Jit, Newall, & Beutels, 2013). National immunization strategies vary widely across global contexts, with some high-income countries like the US electing for universal flu immunization while most LMICs opt for targeted strategies, typically focused on populations at greatest risk of bad outcomes (e.g., those who are elderly, pregnant, or have underlying conditions) or on those who contribute most to influenza transmission (e.g., children) (Principi, Camilloni, & Esposito, 2018). Yet, cross-country variability of influenza immunization policy is not necessarily a sign of inequity, and contextualized CEA can help policymakers appropriately take into account the actual burden of influenza in their countries, the costs of influenza-like illness for those affected, and the associated costs and benefits of expanding vaccination program coverage (World Health Organization, 2016, 2020c). What may be a cost-effective strategy in the US or UK in light of the epidemiological and economic burden of influenza, the expected impact of the vaccination strategy, and the overall available resources for domestic health, could be entirely inappropriate in other country settings, where significant health gains can be realized through targeting immunization while reserving the additional funds and resources it would take to reach wider coverage for alternative investments in more cost-effective health interventions (Edoka et al., 2021). There have also been recent debates about the comparative cost-effectiveness of different influenza vaccine products, namely the value for money of moving from tetravalent to quadrivalent influenza vaccines, in LMICs—where the incremental cost and budget impact may not be justified by corresponding health gains, not to mention feasibility concerns given supply-side constraints and the need for seasonal timeliness of delivery (Teerawattananon et al., 2014). The case of seasonal influenza vaccination strategies illustrates the need for context-specific economic evaluation and consideration of the epidemiological, economic, and health system realities to guide local policy.

Additionally, that richer nations can afford to spend more on health is not a problem of thresholds—it is a reflection of the larger backdrop of global and structural injustice, which would not be solved by setting a universal threshold for what is considered "good value for money" across different country settings. Instead, an appropriate threshold for poorer countries to optimize domestic health spending could more clearly shape where global health aid from bilateral and multilateral partners is most needed to supplement national spending. With domestic resources reserved for the most cost-effective interventions, global health aid could be prioritized for expanding coverage to less affordable interventions, both those that are high priorities within countries and for donor objectives that may not align perfectly with countries' most dire needs. For example, in the context of vaccination programs, this could translate to greater development assistance for costly vaccines crucial to global health security efforts (e.g., safeguarding against pathogens with pandemic potential like coronavirus disease 2019 (COVID-19) or Ebola through contributions to Gavi and the COVID-19 Vaccines Global Access (COVAX) facility), while enabling LMICs to allocate domestic resources for more cost-effective, affordable vaccines addressing persistent endemic threats.

   It should also be noted that CETs can play an instrumental role in facilitating afford-able and equitable introduction of new vaccine products into lower-income markets, whether through bilateral price negotiations using the threshold as a reference point (Glassman, Cañón, & Silverman, 2016; Teerawattananon & Tritasavit, 2015) or through more innovative approaches that leverage tiered pricing models (Berkley, 2014). and other market-shaping mechanisms like benefits-based advanced market commit-ments (Chalkidou, Kettler, Ramakrishnan, Silverman, & Towse, 2020). So rather than being contrary to the aims of global health equity, context-appropriate CETs can pro-mote earlier introduction of new vaccines into LMICs in ways that are more affordable and sustainable.

3.5.3 Incremental cost-effectiveness ratio calculation, incremental ratios, and dominance

The ICER and related calculations such as net health benefit (NHB) and net monetary benefit (NMB) aid decision makers in determining which vaccine program or treatment strategy in question is the most "cost-effective." ICERs and related net benefit calculations depend on monetary estimates in the numerator and a common effectiveness or benefit measure in the denomi-nator. Researchers often use ICERs in practice as a pairwise measure, com-paring a new treatment to a baseline comparator regardless of the number of strategies available to clinicians and decision makers. The ICER is a ratio measure and interpretation requires a reference to a certain willingness-to-pay threshold to determine whether the additional health purchased with the intervention in question is of good value. ICER calculations differ slightly in reference to whether there are two strategies being compared to each other or more than two strategies compared to a baseline comparator (Gray, Clarke, Wolstenholme, & Wordsworth, 2011).

3.5.3.1 Two or more vaccine strategies, treatment programs, and so on

In the case of two strategies, the ICER calculation is as simple as it appears in Equation 3.1.4 in Chapter 3.1, such as in a classic example of a vaccine

(A) versus a treatment (B). In the numerator, the cost of A and B are measured and incrementally compared based on direct and non-direct medical costs, along with indirect costs such as lost productivity in cases where a societal perspective is relevant for the decision problem. In the denominator, the benefit of A and B are often measured and incrementally compared in terms of the QALYs as it is a common metric that can be compared across disease states.

However, there are other measures of benefit depending on the decision problem. In the case of two strategies, the ICER interpretation depends on the sign (+ or −) of both the numerator and denominator along with a willingness-to-pay threshold. In the case of more than two strategies, ICERs are often still compared to a baseline comparator which is often determined from clinical guidelines and real-world utilization, among other factors. Interpretation for two or more comparators is informed by various visual displays of ratio estimates such as the CEA plane, explained in detail in section 3.5.1 and again in section 3.5.5. However, interpreting the cost-effectiveness of more than two strategies involves consideration of dominance and extended dominance.

3.5.3.2 Dominance and extended dominance

When considering more than two strategies, certain treatments may be less or more effective and less or more costly than other treatments. Certain treatments may be "dominated" in that they have either higher costs and smaller or equal benefit than at least one other treatment being considered; or smaller benefits and higher or equal costs than at least one other strategy being considered (Gray et al., 2011; Paulden, 2020). For example, consider the polio vaccine, which prevents a condition that could cost tens of thousands of dollars to manage and severely depletes a patient's health utility, whereas the cost of the polio vaccine is relatively low—a few dollars per dose to administer—and provides lifelong immunity against this debilitating disease. Thus, the polio vaccine *dominates* disease management since it comes at a lower cost for increased clinical benefit. Similarly, "extended dominance" is an important concept since it rules out any intervention that has an ICER that is greater than that of a more effective alternative.

To illustrate dominance and extended dominance, consider the following example with three vaccines (A, B, and C) compared to a reference standard of care (Table 3.5.3).

Table 3.5.3 Evaluating dominance

Alternative	Cost ($)	Effectiveness (QALY)	ICER ($/QALY)
Vaccine A	40	3.0	20
Vaccine B	50	4.0	10
Vaccine C	5	2.0	−5
Standard of care	10	1.0	Reference

First, Vaccine C dominates standard of care since it comes at a reduced cost compared to the reference standard of care, −$5, and improves QALYs gained by +1.0. For LMICs with limited financial bandwidth, Vaccine C provides an appealing solution to the infectious disease outbreak at hand. For countries in a better financial position, they may be willing to pay more to gain more QALYs, making both Vaccines A and B attractive since they deliver superior QALYs to standard of care. However, we can still use extended dominance to rule out Vaccine A since it has an ICER of $20 per QALY, whereas Vaccine B provides greater QALYs at a lower ICER. Since Vaccine B generates fewer opportunity costs per QALY, it represents an efficient option for communities that have the budget to invest in it.

The general steps to calculate ICERs and determine the most cost-effective strategy involves the following:

- Step 1: rank strategies by cost or benefit.
- Step 2: rule out dominated strategies (less effective, more costly than other treatments).
- Step 3: calculate incremental estimates.
- Step 4: rule out extendedly dominated strategies.
- Step 5: recalculate incremental values.
- Step 6: rule out final extendedly dominated strategies.

While a detailed discussion of each step in context to an example is out of the scope of this handbook, interested readers can review literature in this area that provides helpful examples (Paulden, 2020).

3.5.4 Defining uncertainty of value

The assessment of uncertainty in reference to a decision problem is a standard and expected step in economic evaluation. There are a wide range of terms used interchangeably given the interdisciplinary nature of economic evaluation. In this section of this chapter, we will define uncertainty in context to other terms used in the field and provide examples of appropriate assessment of uncertainty.

3.5.4.1 Defining uncertainty

As many economic evaluations are designed to assist decision makers with maximizing health gains subject to economic constraints, assessing uncertainty is important for revealing potential deviations from the "best" course of action (Briggs et al., 2012). Specifically, uncertainty assessment informs two potential useful criteria for decision makers: (1) the confidence in selecting a particular treatment strategy; and (2) the value of collecting additional information, such as an additional trial or study on the treatment in question (Briggs et al., 2012). While there are different concepts related to uncertainty, the assessment of uncertainty should always be taken in context with the decision maker's perspective to best inform present and future decision-making.

3.5.4.2 Distinguishing between uncertainty, heterogeneity, and variability

The joint International Society for Health Economics and Outcomes Research (ISPOR)–Society for Medical Decision Making task force defines four different distinguishable terms related to uncertainty: stochastic uncertainty, parameter uncertainty, heterogeneity, and structural uncertainty. Stochastic uncertainty relates to random variability in outcomes between the same patients which is also known as first-order uncertainty. For example, the response of one treatment may differ among patients with very similar demographic characteristics. Parameter uncertainty or second-order uncertainty is the uncertainty in estimation of a particular input parameter itself. Parameter uncertainty often arises when data to generate an input parameter differs in terms of sample size, study population, external validity, and so on.

Heterogeneity is defined by the variability between patients that can be defined through measured characteristics such as age, sex, history of co-morbid conditions, and so forth. Finally, structural uncertainty refers to the underlying assumptions of the decision analysis model. In other words, does the analysis reflect the clinical plausibility and course of outcomes both with and without the treatment in question? Structural uncertainty may require input from clinicians and a literature review of the possible course of action for those with and without a disease.

3.5.4.3 Uncertainty analyses

While a researcher may assess concepts such as heterogeneity and variability in specific cases, all decision analysis modeling exercises require parameters that must be estimated and varied in uncertainty analyses. This step involves varying parameters across a plausible or evidence-based range and analyzing the impact on both cost and effectiveness outcomes. There are multiple uncertainty analyses but most economic evaluations include the following: one-way sensitivity analyses, two-way sensitivity analyses, and probabilistic sensitivity analyses.

One-way sensitivity analyses vary individual parameters while holding all other parameters constant. This exercise is useful to identify individual parameters that have a large impact on model results. The presentation of one-way sensitivity analyses most commonly comes in the form of a tornado diagram (Fig. 3.5.2). A tornado diagram presents each input parameter separately starting with the parameter that has the most impact on the model results. Lower in the tornado diagram, each input's impact on the economic evaluation results becomes smaller leading to a tornado or funnel format. It may also be useful to include a description of how conclusions may change with large uncertainty around certain input parameters. For example, if varying the treatment effect of an intervention, does the ICER remain above or below a certain willingness-to-pay threshold? It may be that small changes in an input parameter alter the conclusions and should be documented in the dissemination of the uncertainty analysis.

Two-way sensitivity analyses extend the one-way sensitivity analysis by varying two parameters simultaneously and assessing the impact on the results. For example, a decision maker may want to understand how both changes in price and effectiveness would impact the ICER. This may be presented in a table or figure format. Finally, probabilistic sensitivity analyses vary multiple input parameters simultaneously to assess the impact on the results. Probabilistic sensitivity analyses are presented in detail in Chapter 4.3.

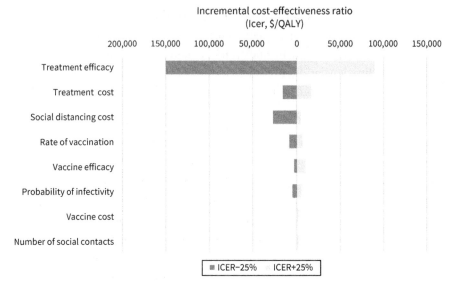

Fig. 3.5.2 Example tornado diagram of one-way sensitivity analyses for vaccine coverage for patients at-risk of COVID-19.

Source: Padula, Malaviya, Reid, Tierce, and Alexander (2020).

3.5.4.4 Data sources and distributions for parameter uncertainty

As discussed in Chapter 3.3, there are a variety of methods to incorporate uncertainty in input parameters. However, selecting the best available evidence in the literature can often involve subjective assessments of prior study designs. Input parameters ideally will include a point estimate and uncertainty around that estimate such as a 95% confidence interval. Input parameters ideally should be from the most recent and least biased sources of information. Many researchers employ a parameterized distribution of values as an input to a model (Briggs et al., 2006). Choosing a distribution can be useful for setting up a probabilistic analysis or even specifying the range of plausible values for one- and two-way sensitivity analyses.

3.5.5 Interpreting the incremental cost-effectiveness ratio

3.5.5.1 Identifying the single most cost-effective strategy

After calculating the ICER, we can use the sign of both the cost and benefit estimates as well as visual plots to help inform the most cost-effective strategy.

When comparing two strategies, there are four possibilities in terms of incremental cost and benefit on the CEA plane (Fig. 3.5.1):

- NE (upper-right) quadrant of the CEA plane: + incremental cost and + incremental benefit.
- SW (lower-left) quadrant of the CEA plane: – incremental cost and – incremental benefit.
- SE (lower-right) quadrant of the CEA plane: – incremental cost and + incremental benefit.
- NW (upper-left) quadrant of the CEA plane: + incremental cost and –incremental benefit.

While interpretation of ICERs requires a reference to the CEA plane, other measures of economic value may be useful for identifying a ranking of the most and least cost-effectiveness strategies when more than two strategies exist.

3.5.5.2 Ranking strategies from most to least cost-effective

While ICERs are often used to identify the single most cost-effective strategy, NHB or NMB may be more useful in cases with multiple treatments or interventions (Paulden, 2020; Stinnett & Mullahy, 1998). Some of the limitations of ICERs when identifying a ranking of cost-effectiveness strategies include leaving no "cost-effective" strategies after ruling out dominance and extended dominance as discussed earlier and the inability to identify the most cost-effective strategies when reviewing higher or lower ICERs (Paulden, 2020).

However, both NHB and NMB require that a willingness-to-pay threshold is specified. NHB and NMB are similar estimates of economic value but NHB is defined in units of health whereas NMB is defined in monetary units. The NHB has two main components: (1) the health benefit for patients who receive the treatment in question; and (2) the health loss experienced by other patients given the new treatment in question is covered, leaving fewer resources for health gains in other areas. To calculate NHB we first take the incremental gains in effectiveness (e.g., QALYs) less the ratio of incremental costs to the willingness-to-pay threshold (see Equation 3.1.6 in Chapter 3.1).

A positive NHB implies that overall population health would be increased if the new treatment were covered while a negative NHB implies the health benefits of the new treatment are not enough to outweigh the health losses that would arise from not funding other treatments. NMB uses a similar approach, however, the calculation results in a monetary value. NMB is calculated by multiplying the incremental health benefit by the willingness-to-pay threshold minus the incremental cost (see Equation 3.1.5 in Chapter 3.1).

A positive NMB indicates the treatment in question is cost-effective or the cost to derive the benefit is less than the maximum a decision maker is willing to pay for the benefit. NHB and NMB overcome some of the challenges in ICER interpretation because of the simplicity of the measure: the greater the NHB and NMB for a particular treatment, the more cost-effective that treatment is. This intuitive interpretation assists researchers and decision makers with identifying the most cost-effective strategies when two or more treatments are in question.

3.5.6 Limitations of economic evaluation methods for vaccine distribution

ICERs are defined by their use of a common denominator to measure change in effectiveness or change in utility. When the denominator measure is the QALY, it is widely considered to reflect incremental utility gain, as a metric comprising quality and quantity of life. This may be reported as the output of a cost–utility analysis, and is also accepted to be a type of CEA. This and other utility metrics, such as DALYs, are introduced in Chapter 4.2. Despite their wide use grounded in the economic concepts of utility and welfare economics, there are numerous concerns related to the use of QALYs (Nord, Daniels, & Kamlet, 2009) as discussed in Chapter 3.4.

Despite these chief concerns, the advantages of comparability among studies in the same therapeutic area and also across therapeutic areas facilitates resource allocation. Economic evaluation, and cost–utility analysis in particular, recognized the QALY as a preferred measure for clinical effectiveness. The US Panel on Cost-effectiveness in Health and Medicine concluded that QALYs are appropriate effectiveness measures by expressing health status as a function of physical and mental components that impact survival and life expectancy (Sanders et al., 2016). On the other hand, the Patient-Centered Outcomes Research Institute statutes explicitly prohibit any research "that discounts the value of a life because of an individual's disability," which implicates the QALY (Padula & McQueen, 2019; US Department of Health and Human Services, 2010). Thus, the use of ICER measures over recent decades has been supported with newly emerging measures to enhance, supplement, or replace these measures. There are numerous current efforts to improve on or replace QALYs to better reflect individual preferences and address many of the equity concerns.

There are ethical concerns around the use of QALYs and how they are used in decision-making(Ashcroft, 2005; Schneider, 2022). It is important to consider how individuals with worse-off baseline health can also gain health benefit as measured through the QALY, and therefore value, as a result of intervention than others with mild conditions. This raises another area of concern related to equity issues with CET. This threshold estimates what a user of healthcare services may be prepared to pay for a health benefit, assuming that there are competing demands for those resources. In the healthcare setting, the willingness-to-pay threshold is commonly used in cost-effective analyses to compare the resources consumed for each additional QALY gained for the intervention, against a predetermined willingness-to-pay threshold. The concern is that when there is spending above threshold, resources are taken away from one group to spend on another. This becomes an equity issue as health for one group is improved relative to another group. Equity distribution using a threshold is often not balanced and there are arguments that more should be spent on children, for example, or other groups who have been disadvantaged in the past to increase their health to the level of health of others. Critics of the specific threshold amounts may question whether thresholds represent opportunity costs. As of 2020, the UK's NICE uses a willingness-to-pay threshold of £20,000–£30,000 (0.70 and 1.04 times GDP, respectively) per QALY gained and it is used to make recommendations for the purchase of new technologies to the national health system based on their cost-effectiveness. In the US, the use of a willingness-to-pay threshold varies, depending on the payer. The US-based Institute for Clinical and Economic Review carries out CEAs and uses a CET of $50,000–$175,000 per QALY gained, using a higher threshold in some cases, such as for rare disease (Institute for Clinical and Economic Review, 2019).

Distributional CEA (Cookson et al., 2021) has been developed and applied to reflect the distribution of health outcomes across populations, and extended CEA has sought to incorporate concerns about financial risk protection to certain groups or individuals (Verguet et al., 2016). The key objectives of distributional CEA were described by Asaria, Griffin, and Cookson (2016) as improving total population health and reducing unfair health inequality by modeling and evaluating social distributions of health associated with different interventions. There have been examples of distributional CEA in LMICs for public health strategies such as an analysis of rotavirus vaccination in Ethiopia by Dawkins, Mirelman, Asaria, Johansson, and Cookson (2018). Griffin, Walker, and Sculpher (2020) analyzed the impact of air pollution reduction strategies from multiple perspectives using the quality-adjusted life expectancy framework.

3.5.7 Reporting quality of analysis with examples

Numerous tools are available to aid in the conduct or quality assessment of CEAs. On the one hand, guidance is useful when undertaking an analysis, to ensure that the appropriate inputs are used and that important components for a perspective are complete. On the other hand, when a decision maker is relying on published literature to make conclusions about value, it is useful to have a rubric for assessing the quality of a published study to evaluate whether the findings are reliable. When undertaking systematic reviews, it is useful for reviewers of economic evaluations to assess quality in a consistent and comprehensive manner (Watts & Li, 2019). For these reasons, it is useful to become familiar with several notable tools for assessing and reporting the quality of economic evaluation described in the following sections.

3.5.7.1 Components of a cost-effectiveness analysis report

The quality and reporting of CEA results is critical for decision makers to be able to compare results across studies and generalize results from one jurisdiction to another. Reporting guidelines are useful because they provide a standard set of results that CEA end-users should expect to see in a published CEA (Watts & Li, 2019). Additionally, the inputs and assumptions used for the analysis should be consistently reported across studies so that one can ascertain the methodological approach for the study. This also allows for comparability of results stemming from studies conducted with a similar methodological approach. Like all scientific papers, reports of CEAs should contain introduction, methods, results, and discussion sections, with specific components of the methods and results that are specific to CEA. For example, methods should specifically state the study perspective, time horizon, discount rate, and other key assumptions (Husereau et al., 2013). The results section should specifically state how uncertainty was characterized alongside the main results of incremental costs and effects.

3.5.7.2 Biases, limitations, and conflicts of interest

As described in previous chapters, model inputs rely on evidence synthesis. For each model parameter, there may be one or more published studies providing evidence for the input. These underlying studies are subject to bias depending on their rigor and this may lead to bias in the model inputs and resulting cost-effectiveness estimates. These data source considerations should be reported alongside the CEA methods.

Model-based CEAs are typically subject to limitations about the availability of reliable model inputs. For example, CEA models typically estimate cost-effectiveness over a longer horizon or larger population than has been studied in clinical trials. There are potential limitations to the assumptions used to produce the estimates, that the drug effects persist over that timeframe and similarly in populations beyond those studied in trials.

Sources of funding for CEA studies or conflicts of interest of study authors may exist and should be reported. Both the Consolidated Health Economic Evaluation Reporting Standards (CHEERS) and Quality of Health Economic Studies (QHES) checklists (described below) include items about study funding or conflict of interest.

3.5.7.3 Reference case and impact inventory

The comparability of methods used for CEA is facilitated by use of a "reference case" to list out a consistent set of methodological choices that will guide an analysis. One commonly used reference case example is the one proposed by the US Public Health Service Panel on Cost-Effectiveness in Health and Medicine and later updated in 2016 (Gold, Siegel, Russell, & Weinstein, 1996; Neumann, Ganiats, Russell, Sanders, & Siegel, 2016). Other reference case sources include NICE in the UK and the International Decision Support Initiative. A vaccine-specific reference case is provided in Chapter 4.4.

The impact inventory is a tool for analysts to comprehensively summarize the impacts of the intervention under consideration from both the healthcare sector and societal perspectives. All analyses conducted from the reference case should start with this inventory to ensure inclusion of all consequences that could affect the ICER. The impact inventory serves to identify consequences of interventions among formal and informal healthcare sectors (e.g., health outcomes, medical costs, and indirect medical and non-medical costs) as well as non-healthcare sectors (e.g., lost productivity, future consumption unrelated to health, and impacts on social services, criminal justice, education, and housing systems, among others). The inventory might also highlight impacts that are not typically considered in CEAs but important to include elsewhere in the evaluation.

3.5.7.4 CHEERS checklist

The CHEERS statement, published in 2013, includes a 24-item checklist and recommendations on minimum standards for CEA reporting (Husereau et al., 2022). At the time of publication, a panel of experts had convened to discuss proposed updates and revisions to the original CHEERS guidelines. The format of this checklist is particularly useful for peer reviewers, as well as researchers aiming to identify or extract study components for systematic reviews. The checklist recommendations are subdivided into six sections: (1) title and abstract, (2) introduction, (3) methods, (4) results, (5) discussion, and (6) other. There are specific recommendations for model-based evaluations versus trial-based evaluations. These address attributes of model-based evaluations such as model structure, inputs, and uncertainty. The CHEERS statement also addresses whether studies report sources of funding and potential conflicts of interest.

3.5.7.5 QHES assessment instrument

The QHES instrument was developed in 2003 to support quality assessment of cost-effectiveness studies (Ofman et al., 2003). This 16-question checklist assigns points for completion of the elements, resulting in a total score out of 100 points. The questions assign variable point values, implying increased importance and complexity of certain study attributes, such as analytic variables/inputs, cost methods, model components, and conclusions/recommendations (8 points each) versus smaller or less complex study attributes, such as subgroup specification (1 point), funding (3 points), and perspective (4 points).

References

Asaria, M., Griffin, S., & Cookson, R. (2016). Distributional cost-effectiveness analysis: A tutorial. *Medical Decision Making, 36*(1), 8–19. doi: 10.1177/0272989X15583266

Ashcroft, R. E. (2005). Quality of life as the basis of health care resource allocation: A philosopher's perspective on QALYs. *Virtual Mentor, 7*(2).

Bärnighausen, T., Bloom, D. E., Cafiero-Fonseca, E. T., & O'Brien, J. C. (2014). Valuing vaccination. *Proceedings of the National Academy of Sciences of the United States of America, 111*(34), 12313–12319. doi:10.1073/pnas.1400475111

Berkley, S. (2014). Improving access to vaccines through tiered pricing. *Lancet, 383*(9936), 2265–2267. doi:10.1016/s0140-6736(13)62424-1

Bertram, M. Y., Lauer, J. A., De Joncheere, K., Edejer, T., Hutubessy, R., Kieny, M.-P., & Hill, S. R. (2016). Cost-effectiveness thresholds: Pros and cons. *Bulletin of the World Health Organization, 94*(12), 925–930. doi:10.2471/BLT.15.164418

Briggs, A., Sculpher, M., & Claxton, K. (2006). *Decision modelling for health economic evaluation*. Oxford: Oxford University Press.

Briggs, A., Weinstein, M. C., Fenwick, E. A., Karnon, J., Sculpher, M. J., & Paltiel, A. D. (2012). Model parameter estimation and uncertainty analysis: A report of the ISPOR-SMDM Modeling Good Research Practices Task Force Working Group-6. *Medical Decision Making, 32*(5), 722–732. doi:10.1177/0272989x12458348

Chalkidou, K., Kettler, H., Ramakrishnan, G., Silverman, R., & Towse, A. (2020). *Leave no one behind: Using a benefit-based advance market commitment to incentivise development and global supply of COVID-19 vaccines*. Center for Global Development. https://www.cgdev. org/publication/leave-no-one-behind-using-benefit-based-advance-market-commitment-covid-vaccine

Chi, Y. L., Blecher, M., Chalkidou, K., Culyer, A., Claxton, K., Edoka, I., . . . Winch, A. (2020). What next after GDP-based cost-effectiveness thresholds? *Gates Open Research, 4*, 176. doi:10.12688/gatesopenres.13201.1

Claxton, K., Martin, S., Soares, M., Rice, N., Spackman, E., Hinde, S., . . . Sculpher, M. (2015). Methods for the estimation of the National Institute for Health and Care Excellence cost-effectiveness threshold. *Health Technology Assessment, 19*(14), 1–503, v–vi. doi:10.3310/hta19140

Clements, K. M., Chancellor, J., Nichol, K., DeLong, K., & Thompson, D. (2011). Cost-effectiveness of a recommendation of universal mass vaccination for seasonal influenza in the United States. *Value in Health, 14*(6), 800–811. doi:10.1016/j.jval.2011.03.005

Cookson, R., Griffin, S., Norheim, O. F., & Culyer, A. J. (2021). *Distributional cost-effectiveness analysis: Quantifying health equity impacts and trade-offs*. Oxford, UK: Oxford University Press.

Dawkins, B. R., Mirelman, A. J., Asaria, M., Johansson, K. A., & Cookson, R. A. (2018). Distributional cost-effectiveness analysis in low- and middle-income countries: illustrative example of rotavirus vaccination in Ethiopia. *Health Policy and Planning, 33*(3), 456–463. doi:10.1093/heapol/czx175

Edoka, I., Kohli-Lynch, C. N., Fraser, H., Hofman, K., Tempia, S., McMorrow, M., . . . Cohen, C. (2021). A cost-effectiveness analysis of South Africa's seasonal influenza vaccination programme. *Vaccine, 39*(2), 412–422. doi:10.1016/j.vaccine.2020.11.028

Edoka, I., & Stacey, N. K. (2020). Estimating a cost-effectiveness threshold for health care decision-making in South Africa. *Health Policy and Planning, 35*(5), 546–555. doi:10.1093/heapol/czz152

Farmer, P. (2015, February 3). Who lives and who dies: Paul Farmer on the iniquities of health-care funding. *London Review of Books, 37*(3). https://www.lrb.co.uk/the-paper/v37/n03/paul-farmer/who-lives-and-who-dies

Fesenfeld, M., Hutubessy, R., & Jit, M. (2013). Cost-effectiveness of human papillomavirus vaccination in low and middle income countries: A systematic review. *Vaccine, 31*(37), 3786–3804. doi:10.1016/j.vaccine.2013.06.060

Glassman, A., Cañón, O., & Silverman, R. (2016). How to get cost-effectiveness analysis right? The case of vaccine economics in Latin America. *Value Health, 19*(8), 913–920. doi:10.1016/j.jval.2016.04.014

Gold, M. R., Siegel, J., Russell, L., & Weinstein, M. (1996). *Cost-effectiveness in health and medicine.* New York, NY: Oxford University Press.

Gray, A. M., Clarke, P. M., Wolstenholme, J., & Wordsworth, S. (2011). *Applied methods of cost-effectiveness analysis in healthcare* (Vol. 3). Oxford: Oxford University Press.

Griffin, S., Walker, S., & Sculpher, M. (2020). Distributional cost effectiveness analysis of West Yorkshire low emission zone policies. *Health Economics, 29*(5), 567–579. doi:doi.org/10.1002/hec.4003

Hendriks, J., Hutubessy, R. C. W., Grohmann, G., Torelli, G., Friede, M., & Kieny, M. P. (2018). Quadrivalent influenza vaccines in low and middle income countries: Cost-effectiveness, affordability and availability. *Vaccine, 36*(28), 3993–3997. doi:10.1016/j.vaccine.2018.05.099

Husereau, D., Drummond, M., Augustovski, F., de Bekker-Grob, E., Briggs, A. H., Carswell, C., . . . Staniszewska, S. (2022). Consolidated Health Economic Evaluation Reporting Standards (CHEERS) 2022 Explanation and Elaboration: A Report of the ISPOR CHEERS II Good Practices Task Force. *Value Health, 25*(1), 10–31. doi:10.1016/j.jval.2021.10.008. Erratum in: Value Health. 2022 Jun;25(6):1060. PMID: 35031088.

Husereau, D., Drummond, M., Petrou, S., Carswell, C., Moher, D., Greenberg, D., . . . Loder, E. (2013). Consolidated Health Economic Evaluation Reporting Standards (CHEERS) statement. *Value in Health, 16*(2), e1–e5. doi:10.1016/j.jval.2013.02.010

Hutubessy, R., Chisholm, D., & Edejer, T. T. (2003). Generalized cost-effectiveness analysis for national-level priority-setting in the health sector. *Cost Effectiveness and Resource Allocation, 1*(1), 8. doi:10.1186/1478-7547-1-8

Institute for Clinical and Economic Review. (2019). *Value assessment framework 2020.* https://icer.org/our-approach/methods-process/value-assessment-framework/

Jauregui, B., Janusz, C. B., Clark, A. D., Sinha, A., Garcia, A. G., Resch, S., . . . Andrus, J. K. (2015). ProVac Global Initiative: A vision shaped by ten years of supporting evidence-based policy decisions. *Vaccine, 33*(1), A21–A27. doi:10.1016/j.vaccine.2014.12.080

Jit, M., Newall, A. T., & Beutels, P. (2013). Key issues for estimating the impact and cost-effectiveness of seasonal influenza vaccination strategies. *Human Vaccines & Immunotherapeutics, 9*(4), 834–840. doi:10.4161/hv.23637

Krubiner, C., & Faden, R. (2017). A matter of morality: Embedding ethics and equity in the health benefits policy. In A. Glassman, U. Giedon, & P. C. Smith (Eds.), *What's in, what's out? Designing benefits for universal health coverage* (pp. 290–326). Washington, DC: Center for Global Development.

Leech, A. A., Kim, D. D., Cohen, J. T., & Neumann, P. J. (2018). Use and misuse of cost-effectiveness analysis thresholds in low- and middle-income countries: Trends in cost-per-DALY studies. *Value in Health, 21*(7), 759–761. doi:10.1016/j.jval.2017.12.016

Loganathan, T., Ng, C. W., Lee, W. S., Hutubessy, R., Verguet, S., & Jit, M. (2018). Thresholds for decision-making: Informing the cost-effectiveness and affordability of rotavirus vaccines in Malaysia. *Health Policy and Planning, 33*(2), 204–214. doi:10.1093/heapol/czx166

Lomas, J., Martin, S., & Claxton, K. (2019). Estimating the marginal productivity of the English National Health Service from 2003 to 2012. *Value in Health, 22*(9), 995–1002. doi:10.1016/j.jval.2019.04.1926

Meyer, R. (2013, November 6). "The Biggest Fraud Ever Perpetrated on the World?" How a Twitter diatribe turned into an article in one of the world's most prestigious journals. *The Atlantic.* https://www.theatlantic.com/technology/archive/2013/11/is-economics-the-biggest-fraud-ever-perpetrated-on-the-world/281211/

Neumann, P., Ganiats, T., Russell, L., Sanders, G., & Siegel, J. (2016). *Cost-effectiveness in Health and Medicine.* New York, NY: Oxford University Press.

Nimdet, K., & Ngorsuraches, S. (2015). Willingness to pay per quality-adjusted life year for life-saving treatments in Thailand. *BMJ Open, 5*(10), e008123. doi:10.1136/bmjopen-2015-008123

Nord, E., Daniels, N., & Kamlet, M. (2009). QALYs: some challenges. *Value in Health*, *12*(1), S10–S15. doi:10.1111/j.1524-4733.2009.00516.x

Norheim, O. F., Baltussen, R., Johri, M., Chisholm, D., Nord, E., Brock, D., . . . Wikler, D. (2014). Guidance on priority setting in health care (GPS-Health): The inclusion of equity criteria not captured by cost-effectiveness analysis. *Cost Effectiveness and Resource Allocation*, *12*, 18. doi:10.1186/1478-7547-12-18

O'Mahony, J. F., & Paulden, M. (2019). The Joint Committee on Vaccination and Immunisation's advice on extending human papillomavirus vaccination to boys: Were cost-effectiveness analysis guidelines bent to achieve a politically acceptable decision? *Value in Health*, *22*(11), 1227–1230. doi:10.1016/j.jval.2019.07.010

Ochalek, J., Lomas, J., & Claxton, K. (2018). Estimating health opportunity costs in low-income and middle-income countries: A novel approach and evidence from cross-country data. *BMJ Global Health*, *3*(6), e000964. doi:10.1136/bmjgh-2018-000964

Ofman, J. J., Sullivan, S. D., Neumann, P. J., Chiou, C.-F., Henning, J. M., Wade, S. W., & Hay, J. W. (2003). Examining the value and quality of health economic analyses: Implications of Utilizing the QHES. *Journal of Managed Care Pharmacy*, *9*(1), 53–61. doi:10.18553/jmcp.2003.9.1.53

Padula, W. V., Malaviya, S., Reid, N., Tierce, J., & Alexander, C. (2020). Economic value of treatment and vaccine to address the COVID-19 pandemic: A U.S. cost-effectiveness and budget impact analysis. *Journal of Medical Economics*, *24*(1), 1060–1069. https://doi.org/10.1080/13696998.2021.1965732

Padula, W. V., & McQueen, R. B. (2019). Expanding the role of the Patient-Centered Outcomes Research Institute: Reauthorization and facilitating value assessments. *Applied Health Economics and Health Policy*, *17*(6), 757–759. doi:10.1007/s40258-019-00525-z

Paulden, M. (2020). Calculating and interpreting ICERs and net benefit. *PharmacoEconomics*, *38*(8), 785–807. doi:10.1007/s40273-020-00914-6

Principi, N., Camilloni, B., & Esposito, S. (2018). Influenza immunization policies: Which could be the main reasons for differences among countries? *Human Vaccines & Immunotherapeutics*, *14*(3), 684–692. doi:10.1080/21645515.2017.1405188

Revill, P., Walker, S. M., Madan, J., Ciaranello, A., Mwase, T., Gibb, D. M., . . . Sculpher, M. J. (2014). *Using cost-effectiveness thresholds to determine value for money in low-and middle-income country healthcare systems: Are current international norms fit for purpose?* Centre for Health Economics, University of York. http://eprints.whiterose.ac.uk/136186/

Rumbold, B., Baker, R., Ferraz, O., Hawkes, S., Krubiner, C., Littlejohns, P., . . . Hunt, P. (2017). Universal health coverage, priority setting, and the human right to health. *Lancet*, *390*(10095), 712–714. doi:10.1016/s0140-6736(17)30931-5

Sanders, G. D., Neumann, P. J., Basu, A., Brock, D. W., Feeny, D., Krahn, M., . . . Ganiats, T. G. (2016). Recommendations for conduct, methodological practices, and reporting of cost-effectiveness analyses: Second Panel on Cost-Effectiveness in Health and Medicine. *JAMA*, *316*(10), 1093–1103. doi:10.1001/jama.2016.12195

Schneider, P. (2022). The QALY is ableist: On the unethical implications of health states worse than dead. *Quality of Life Research*, *31*(5), 1545–1552. doi:10.1007/s11136-021-03052-4. Epub 2021 Dec 9. PMID: 34882282; PMCID: PMC9023412.

Schwarzer, R., Rochau, U., Saverno, K., Jahn, B., Bornschein, B., Muehlberger, N., . . . Siebert, U. (2015). Systematic overview of cost-effectiveness thresholds in ten countries across four continents. *Journal of Comparative Effectiveness Research*, *4*(5), 485–504. doi:10.2217/cer.15.38

Stinnett, A. A., & Mullahy, J. (1998). Net health benefits: A new framework for the analysis of uncertainty in cost-effectiveness analysis. *Medical Decision Making*, *18*(2 Suppl), S68–S80. doi:10.1177/0272989x98018002s09

Stinnett, A. A., & Paltiel, A. D. (1996). Mathematical programming for the efficient allocation of health care resources. *Journal of Health Economics, 15*(5), 641–653. doi:10.1016/s0167-6296(96)00493-6

Teerawattananon, Y., & Tritasavit, N. (2015). A learning experience from price negotiations for vaccines. *Vaccine, 33*(1), A11–A12. doi:10.1016/j.vaccine.2014.12.050

Teerawattananon, Y., Tritasavit, N., Suchonwanich, N., & Kingkaew, P. (2014). The use of economic evaluation for guiding the pharmaceutical reimbursement list in Thailand. *Zeitschrift fur Evidenz, Fortbildung und Qualitat im Gesundheitswesen, 108*(7), 397–404. doi:10.1016/j.zefq.2014.06.017

Thavorncharoensap, M., Teerawattananon, Y., Natanant, S., Kulpeng, W., Yothasamut, J., & Werayingyong, P. (2013). Estimating the willingness to pay for a quality-adjusted life year in Thailand: Does the context of health gain matter? *ClinicoEconomics and Outcomes Research: CEOR, 5*, 29–36. doi:10.2147/CEOR.S38062

US Department of Health and Human Services. (2010). *Patient Protection and Affordable Care Act.* U.S. Government Publishing Office. https://www.congress.gov/111/plaws/publ148/PLAW-111publ148.pdf

Vallejo-Torres, L., García-Lorenzo, B., & Serrano-Aguilar, P. (2018). Estimating a cost-effectiveness threshold for the Spanish NHS. *Health Economics, 27*(4), 746–761. doi:10.1002/hec.3633

Vanness, D. J., Lomas, J., & Ahn, H. (2021). A health opportunity cost threshold for cost-effectiveness analysis in the United States. *Annals of Internal Medicine, 174*(1), 25–32. doi:10.7326/m20-1392

Verguet, S., Kim, J. J., & Jamison, D. T. (2016). Extended cost-effectiveness analysis for health policy assessment: A tutorial. *PharmacoEconomics, 34*(9), 913–923. doi:10.1007/s40273-016-0414-z

Watts, R. D., & Li, I. W. (2019). Use of checklists in reviews of health economic evaluations, 2010 to 2018. *Value in Health, 22*(3), 377–382. doi:10.1016/j.jval.2018.10.006

Woods, B., Revill, P., Sculpher, M., & Claxton, K. (2016). Country-level cost-effectiveness thresholds: Initial estimates and the need for further research. *Value in Health, 19*(8), 929–935. doi:10.1016/j.jval.2016.02.017

World Health Organization. (2014a). *Making fair choices on the path to universal health coverage.* https://www.who.int/publications/i/item/9789241507158

World Health Organization. (2016). *Guidance on the economic evaluation of influenza vaccination.* https://apps.who.int/iris/bitstream/handle/10665/250086/WHO-IVB-16.05-eng.pdf

World Health Organization. (2020c). *Seasonal influenza vaccines: An overview for decision makers.* https://apps.who.int/iris/bitstream/handle/10665/336951/9789240010154-eng.pdf

3.6

Budget impact analysis and return on investment

Elizabeth Watts

3.6.1 Budget impact analysis

Economic evaluations for investment cases may be enhanced by performing a budget impact analysis (BIA), which demonstrates affordability independent of a vaccine's cost-effectiveness. While a vaccine may be cost-effective, the scale of the program may have an outsize impact on the country's (or insurer's) budget relative to other health spending (Bilinski et al., 2017). A well-conducted BIA can inform budgeting and planning for vaccine decision-making.

BIA defines who pays for the difference in cost for the vaccine program compared to the status quo and frames the cost relative to how much is spent on other health interventions. BIA is not the total cost of the program, which is influenced by the size of the target population and vaccine uptake (or coverage), but the cost per person paying for the vaccine. Thus, BIA is typically performed from the payer's perspective (Sullivan et al., 2014). For publicly funded programs, the number of payers is the number of taxpayers. For private insurance schemes, the number of payers is the number of insurance plan members.

The budget impact is calculated from the difference in cost for the vaccine program compared to the status quo or alternative intervention. Additionally, future cost savings that may accrue from preventing the disease may be subtracted from the cost if those savings would accrue to the payer (Sullivan et al., 2014).

BIA strictly refers to costs of a program and can be extrapolated using the numerator of the incremental cost-effectiveness ratio from a cost-effectiveness analysis (CEA). Building off of a CEA that estimates the

Elizabeth Watts, *Budget impact analysis and return on investment* In: *Handbook of Applied Health Economics in Vaccines.*
Edited by: David Bishai, Logan Brenzel and William V. Padula, Oxford University Press. © Oxford University Press 2023.
DOI: 10.1093/oso/9780192896087.003.0019

difference in cost per vaccinated individual, the total difference in cost can be estimated by multiplying the per-person cost difference by the target population for the vaccine. Budget impact is then estimated by dividing the total cost by the number of individuals who pay either taxes or premiums into the health system or insurance scheme that will cover the cost of the vaccine. If the government or insurance scheme will only pay for a portion of the vaccine cost, this should be reflected in the BIA.

Since BIA is calculated from the payer's perspective, the time horizon should reflect the budgeting period (1–3 years), rather than the lifetime of the vaccine effect, as typically presented in a CEA (Sullivan et al., 2014). Analyses covering a long time horizon have high uncertainty, which may be subject to changing technology or changes in the target population (Sullivan et al., 2014). Changes in technology may include the development of more effective vaccines, or changes in formulation. Likewise, the target population may change due to demographic factors or changes in recommendations for the vaccine delivery. Lastly, costs in BIA should not be discounted because they will reflect the cost in the respective year of payment (Sullivan et al., 2014).

Consider a case of hepatitis B vaccine where adding the vaccine would cost an additional US $34,685.21 per patient with an at-risk population of 10,000 over 50 years (the estimated life expectancy of individuals without infection) over the current standard of treatment. If the vaccine program will be fully funded through a private insurance scheme with 100,000 members, the budget impact would be calculated by dividing the total cost by the number of insurance program members. The resulting budget impact would be that members would pay an additional $3,468.52 over the impact period of 50 years. In annual terms, the cost would be $69.37 per member per year, or $5.78 per member per month. This case is considered further in Chapter 3.7.

From the numerator of the incremental cost-effectiveness ratio, the estimated per-patient program cost is $34,685.21:

$$\frac{\$34,685.21}{10,000 \text{ at} - \text{risk individuals}}$$

Given there are 100,000 members, divide the total program cost to compute the per-member cost:

$$\frac{\$346,852,080}{100,000 \text{ members}} = \$3,469.52 \text{ per member}$$

Divide the lifetime cost per payer by the number of years:

$$\frac{\$3,469.52}{50\,\text{years}} = \$69.37\,\text{per member per year}$$

This cost can be further contextualized by comparing the budget impact of the vaccine program to the total annual payments per member. For example, if the plan members contribute $1,800 per year to the insurance scheme, the additional cost for the vaccine program would represent a 3.9% increase in the cost of the insurance program to add the hepatitis B vaccine. Alternatively, the cost could be compared to the expenditure for existing vaccines covered by the insurance plan.

Budget impact shows the additional cost for decision makers by presenting the relative additional cost of the vaccine compared to what is already being spent on health or other vaccines. It allows decision makers to assess whether introducing a cost-effective vaccine will be affordable.

3.6.2 Return on investment analysis

Return on investment (ROI) analysis is a useful presentation format for decision makers and donors considering investment in immunization programs. In contrast to CEA which compares the health impact of vaccine programs to the costs, ROI compares benefits to costs in monetary terms. ROI is the ratio of net benefits (benefits minus costs) to costs. It is sometimes presented as the number of years required for the health system to break even and recoup costs.

Costs of vaccine programs include costs of vaccines (vaccine doses, syringes, and safety boxes), the cost of delivering vaccines (cold chain and healthcare labor costs), as well as social mobilization efforts. Vaccine costs may be adjusted by applying a buffer stock rate and wastage rate. When conducting ROI as an extension of CEA, the costs included for the ROI analysis should align with the assumptions used in the CEA.

Economic benefits of immunization should be clearly defined and presented in monetary terms, not quality-adjusted life years or disability-adjusted life years. Benefits may be calculated using several different methods. A conservative approach is the cost-of-illness approach, which examines averted costs of vaccine-preventable diseases, such as costs of treatment, household out-of-pocket expenditure (transportation costs), and productivity loss (caregiver missed work or productivity loss due to disability or death). If calculating ROI from the payer perspective, economic benefits should only include cost savings for the government or healthcare sector. A broader approach may include additional cost savings to households, such as transportation costs and lost wages due to caregiver absenteeism.

Other approaches for estimating economic benefits of vaccines include the value of statistical life approach or value of statistical life-year approach (Robinson et al., 2019), which reflect the average willingness to pay to reduce risk of death for individuals in a population. Given the number of ways to estimate economic benefits of vaccines and the impact these different perspectives have on results (Ozawa et al., 2016; Sim, Watts, Constenla, Brenzel, & Patenaude, 2020), it is prudent to present results using multiple approaches and to clearly describe the methodology (Sim, Jit, Constenla, Peters, & Hutubessy, 2019).

An important consideration when comparing economic benefits and costs of vaccine programs is that benefits may accrue years after the initial investment and implementation of vaccine programs. When estimating the ROI, benefits should be discounted to the year of initial investment or the year of vaccination. Typically, economists apply a 3% discount rate, but alternative discount rates (between 0% and 5%) should be explored in case they have a large impact on the result.

ROI is computed by dividing net benefits by costs.

Equation 3.6.1. ROI:

$$ROI = \frac{Benefits - Costs}{Costs} \times 100\%$$

As shown in Equation 3.6.1, if the ROI is positive, the benefits exceed costs. An ROI of 50% means that for every dollar invested, there is a 50% return or $1.5 in benefits ($0.5 in net benefits). An ROI of 2000% means that for every dollar invested, $21 in benefits ($20 in net benefits) are generated. An alternative calculation is the benefit–cost ratio (BCR), which divides benefits by costs. If the BCR is greater than 1, benefits exceed costs.

ROI may also be presented as the number of years needed to recoup costs after the initial investment. However, it is important to remember that ROI is the average net benefit per dollar invested and is not adjusted for changes in benefits or costs over time (Padula, Lee, & Pronovost, 2017). To calculate the time to recoup costs, the time horizon considered is divided by the ROI. For example, if assessing a vaccine program with an ROI of 2.0 over 10 years, costs would be recouped after only 5 years (Padula et al., 2017).

The above example of hepatitis B vaccine can also be applied to an ROI analysis. We saw earlier that the vaccine program cost for 10,000 at-risk individuals would be $346,852,080. Let's assume we estimated that the vaccine would generate a present value of $450,000,000 in economic benefits in this population. The ROI would be calculated as follows:

First subtract the costs from the benefits to calculate net benefits:

$$Net\,benefits = \$450,000,000 - \$346,852,080$$

Then divide net benefits by costs and multiply by 100%:

$$ROI = \frac{\$103,147,920}{\$346,852,080} \times 100\%$$

$$ROI = 29.7\%$$

Implementing the hepatitis B vaccine in this population would yield a return of 30 cents per dollar invested, on average. Because the ROI is greater than 0, the benefits of implementing the vaccine exceed the costs. Likewise, the BCR (calculated by dividing benefits by costs) of 1.3 shows that benefits of this vaccine exceed costs because they are greater than 1.

Researchers should be mindful of which parameters are most influential over the results and which parameters have the greatest uncertainty and perform sensitivity analysis to reflect the uncertainty. One-way sensitivity analysis may also be used to demonstrate which variables have the largest impact on the results. Multivariate sensitivity will show overall uncertainty for all parameters included in sensitivity analysis.

When presenting ROI to decision makers, net benefits should be presented alongside the ROI, as net benefits demonstrate scale of benefits which is not inferable from the ROI or BCR. Decision-makers may be inclined to compare the ROI for the vaccine to other health or non-health investments. In this case, it is best to clearly state the methods used to estimate the ROI. Depending on the approach used to estimate the economic benefits, ROI may be comparable to benefits and costs of alternative investments, not only in the health sector, but also in education, infrastructure, and other competing priorities. Recent studies on the ROI of vaccines showed that vaccines against ten pathogens would return $20 in benefits for each dollar invested using a cost-of-illness approach and $52 in benefits using a value of statistical life approach in 94 low- and middle-income countries (Sim et al., 2020). Other health interventions, including nutrition supplementation and tuberculosis

Table 3.6.1 Select return on investment estimates of public health interventions

Intervention	Country or region	ROI	Approach for estimating economic benefits
HIV testing (Hutchinson et al., 2012)	US	1.95	Cost of illness averted
Supervised injection facilities (Andresen & Boyd, 2010)	Canada	3.6	Cost of illness averted
Syringe exchange (Nguyen, Weir, Des Jarlais, Pinkerton, & Holtgrave, 2014)	US	7.6	Cost of illness averted
Vaccines against ten pathogens (Sim et al., 2020)	LMICs	19.8	Cost of illness averted
Tuberculosis prevention (Stop TB Partnership, 2019)	LMICs	44	Value of statistical life
Childhood nutrition (Horton & Hoddinott, 2014)	LMICs	44	Value of statistical life
Vaccines against ten pathogens (Sim et al., 2020)	LMICs	52.2	Value of statistical life

LMICs, low- and middle-income countries.

prevention, have also been evaluated using a value of statistical life approach (Table 3.6.1) and reflect high returns. ROIs that estimate economic benefits by estimating averted costs typically have lower ROIs than if a broader approach was taken, which may be a more appropriate approach depending on the target audience for the analysis. A systematic review of published ROI analyses focused on public health interventions estimated a median ROI of 14.3 across investments in public health interventions (Masters, Anwar, Collins, Cookson, & Capewell, 2017).

References

Andresen, M., & Boyd, N. (2010). A cost-benefit and cost-effectiveness analysis of Vancouver's supervised injection facility. *International Journal of Drug Policy, 21*(1), 70–76. doi:10.1016/j.drugpo.2009.03.004

Bilinski, A., Neumann, P., Cohen, J., Thorat, T., McDaniel, K., & Salomon, J. A. (2017). When cost-effective interventions are unaffordable: Integrating cost-effectiveness and budget impact in priority setting for global health programs. *PLOS Medicine, 14*(10), e1002397. doi:10.1371/journal.pmed.1002397

Horton, S., & Hoddinott, J. (2014). *Benefits and costs of the food and nutrition targets for the post-2015 development agenda.* Copenhagen Consensus Center. https://www.ign.org/document.cfm?page_id=142003378

Hutchinson, A. B., Farnham, P. G., Duffy, N., Woliski, R., Sansom, S., Dooley, S., . . . Mermin, J. (2012). Return on public health investment: CDC's expanded HIV testing initiative. *Journal of Acquired Immunodeficiency Syndrome, 59*(3), 281–286. doi:10.1097/QAI.0b013e31823e5bee

Masters, R., Anwar, E., Collins, B., Cookson, R., & Capewell, S. (2017). Return on investment of public health interventions: A systematic review. *Journal of Epidemiology and Community Health, 71*(8), 827–834. doi:10.1136/jech-2016-208141

Nguyen, T., Weir, B. W., Des Jarlais, D. C., Pinkerton, S. D., & Holtgrave, D. R. (2014). Syringe exchange in the United States: A national level economic evaluation of hypothetical increases in investment. *AIDS and Behavior, 18*, 2144–2155. doi:10.1007/s10461-014-0789-9

Ozawa, S., Clark, S., Portnoy, A., Grewal, S., Brenzel, L., & Walker, D. G. (2016). Return on investment from childhood immunization in low- and middle-income countries, 2011–20. *Health Affairs, 35*(2), 199–207. doi:10.1377/hlthaff.2015.1086

Padula, W. V., Lee, K. K. H., & Pronovost, P. J. (2017). Using economic evaluation to illustrate value of care for improving patient safety and quality: Choosing the right method. *Journal of Patient Safety, 17*(6), e568–e574. doi:10.1097/PTS.0000000000000410

Robinson, L. A., Hammitt, J. K., Cecchini, M., Chalkidou, K., Claxton, K., Cropper, M., . . . Wong, B. (2019). *Reference case guidelines for benefit-cost analysis in global health and development.* Bill & Melinda Gates Foundation. https://cdn1.sph.harvard.edu/wp-content/uploads/sites/2447/2019/05/BCA-Guidelines-May-2019.pdf

Sim, S. Y., Jit, M., Constenla, D., Peters, D. H., & Hutubessy, R. (2019). A scoping review of investment cases for vaccines and immunization programs. *Value in Health, 22*(8), 942–952. doi:10.1016/j.jval.2019.04.002

Sim, S. Y., Watts, E., Constenla, D., Brenzel, L., & Patenaude, B. N. (2020). Return on investment from immunization against 10 pathogens in 94 low-and middle-income countries, 2011–30. *Health Affairs, 39*(8), 1343–1353. doi:10.1377/hlthaff.2020.00103

Stop TB Partnership. (2019). *The paradigm shift 2018–2022.* Geneva: Stop TB Partnership.

Sullivan, S. D., Mauskopf, J. A., Augustovski, F., Jaime Caro, J., Lee, K. M., Minchin, M., . . . Shau, W.-Y. (2014). Budget impact analysis—principles of good practice: Report of the ISPOR 2012 Budget Impact Analysis Good Practice II Task Force. *Value in Health, 17*(1), 5–14. doi:10.1016/j.jval.2013.08.2291

3.7

Introduction to decision tree modeling

William V. Padula

Decision tree modeling is a difficult task that requires attention to the clinical pathway in addition to the key outcomes. There is no one way to make a decision tree. It may be best to know that all decision trees have three major components:

- A decision node—where comparators are pitched against one another.
- Chance nodes—points where clinical outcomes are weighted by the probabilities of their potential.
- Terminal nodes—clinical endpoints where costs and effectiveness measures accumulate.

Costs and effectiveness measures are weighted by the probability of clinical outcomes that occur at each chance node.

For vaccine outcomes, it may be best to start with a standardized model structure such as the classic Susceptible–Infected–Recovered (SIR) model since such a practice has clinical validity and allows you to forgo complicated model development and focus on parameter estimation.

To understand decision tree modeling, a case study can help introduce the principles. Therefore, we provide the following case study of the hepatitis B vaccine to walk through the exercise. More examples of vaccine economic models that produce both health and economic benefits of vaccines can be found through the Vaccine Impact Modeling Consortium (VIMC; http://www.vaccineimpact.org).

William V. Padula, *Introduction to decision tree modeling* In: *Handbook of Applied Health Economics in Vaccines*.
Edited by: David Bishai, Logan Brenzel and William V. Padula, Oxford University Press. © Oxford University Press 2023.
DOI: 10.1093/oso/9780192896087.003.0020

3.7.1 Case study of hepatitis B vaccine

Hepatitis B is a concerning and debilitating infectious disease worldwide that can be transmitted through blood, sexual contact, or from mother to child at birth. If infected, a patient can have short-term (acute) or long-term (chronic) consequences related to the disease, including costs for continuous healthcare. Fortunately, there is a vaccine on the market for hepatitis B virus to protect people in high-risk areas from infection.

The vaccine is considered highly valuable to people who are high risk based on behavioral activity or local prevalence of disease. However, there is situationally equipoise about the value of hepatitis B vaccination for primary prevention in the general population. Questions about value have much to do with the impact that herd immunity can have on entire populations. Value also varies by whether people are low risk either because they are located in areas where prevalence of hepatitis B virus is low, or because their own behavior would minimize exposure to the infection.

The case of hepatitis B vaccine provides a useful exercise for conducting cost-effectiveness analysis and budget impact analysis from multiple perspectives. As it turns out, depending on the perspective (e.g., healthcare sector, payer, patient), the value may vary substantially. This exercise uses a straightforward decision tree in order to calculate the cost-effectiveness and budget impact from each of these perspectives.

3.7.1.1 Conceptual framework

To begin this exercise, open the Microsoft Excel worksheet entitled "Hep B Part A" and start on the worksheet tab [DECISION MODEL]. Additional content on (Hep B Part A) is available online, 10.1093/oso/ 9780192896087.012.0001. You will note the structure of the model (Fig. 3.7.1). Some important information about the model design should be noted here:

- *Study design.* The model uses the classic epidemiological framework referred to as SIR in order to perform cost-effectiveness analysis and budget impact analysis.
- *Model structure.* This model is exclusively a decision tree; Markov model approaches are covered in Chapter 4.2.
- *Perspective.* The model uses information in order to make judgments about value from three perspectives—healthcare sector, payer, and patient.

HepB_CEA-Tree_PartA

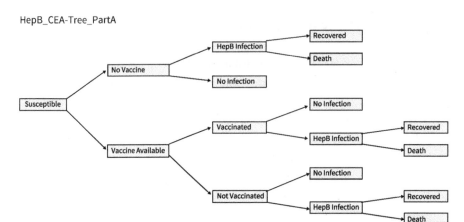

Fig. 3.7.1 Example hepatitis B vaccine decision tree for conducting economic evaluation.

- *Comparators.* The model compares instances for either "Vaccine Available" or "No Vaccine."
- *Time horizon.* This model provides data on outcomes for individuals through 50 years. Patients who become infected with hepatitis B virus may not have the same degree of survival or life expectancy on average.
- *Endpoints.* The SIR model provides classic endpoints including No Infection, Recovered, and Death. These endpoints impact a number of key measures important to economic evaluation, including costs and health utility.
- *Main outcome measures.* This model is built with the goal of being able to conduct economic evaluation in order to derive information about the incremental cost-effectiveness ratio (ICER) and budget impact in terms of per member per month.

3.7.1.2 Decision model

The SIR framework assumes that not all patients are infected at baseline, and that some individuals who become infected can recover after an acute phase, which is consistent with the timeline of hepatitis B virus. In addition, a vaccine can protect many individuals from contracting hepatitis B virus, so that they remain in a long-term susceptible state. The following paragraphs describe the model in greater detail.

During their life course, patients start in the Susceptible (S) state. For communities where a vaccine is not available, individuals' experiences are simulated in the upper arm of the model which refers to the "No Vaccine" comparator. At any given node, individual outcomes are weighted by the probability of these outcomes as noted by population prevalence measures. Many individuals who do not receive a vaccine will go directly to the terminal node entitled "No Infection." At this endpoint, there are no costs incurred for a vaccine or healthcare costs related to hepatitis B virus. Alternatively, a patient can advance to "HepB Infection" if they contract the virus, which is the infected (I) state of the SIR model. This rate of infection as reflected in this decision tree is small but non-zero. Patients who are infected with hepatitis B virus then advance to the two terminal nodes of this branch, "Recovered" (R) or "Death."

The alternative comparator arm of the model "Vaccine Available" reflects scenarios where a vaccine exists but may not be accessible or necessary for all individuals in the population. Whatever the reason may be, a proportion of individuals are "Vaccinated." Once vaccinated, we can safely assume that most individuals in the model are protected from infection, and the same sub-tree presents as in the "No Vaccine" arm. These options including "No Infection" or "HepB Infection," which proceeds onto "Recovered" and "Death." The other component of the "Vaccine Available" comparator includes an option for "Not Vaccinated" due to issues based on access or lack of need for the vaccine, perhaps due to herd immunity or other measures. After "Vaccine Available," the same nodes for infection present as in the other endpoints of the decision tree. When decision trees have similar sub-trees past major decision nodes, this is referred to as model symmetry.

3.7.1.3 Parameter estimation

Under the [PARAMETERS] worksheet of the exercise, you are presented with information about critical data points needed to perform economic evaluation in this decision model. Key parameters include information about probabilities of outcomes, effect modifiers with the presence of a vaccine, and cost-sharing proportions between key stakeholder in the model. There are also a number of measures of costs for vaccine and provider administration, as well as hepatitis B treatment. Finally, there are data about health utility in units of disability-adjusted life years (DALYs) and survival. The values for these data are currently left out of the model, so the empty cells in column B are highlighted *red*. You will have to extract these data from the forthcoming passages to put into the model to perform calculations and interpret results. As you put these data into the cells in column B, the highlighted color of the cells will change to *yellow*.

3.7.2 Part A: data extraction

Open up the file "Hep B Part A" if you have not already, and navigate to the [PARAMETERS] tab. The following information is critical to the economic evaluation of the hepatitis B vaccine. Most of these data are translated from the case study of hepatitis B vaccination in adults according to Hoerger et al. (2013). As data are presented, you should input this information into the appropriate cell.

I. Probabilities:
    A. Hepatitis B occurs in the population at an incidence rate of 1%.
    B. The probability of recovery from hepatitis B is 5% if infected.
    C. The probability of receiving a vaccine for hepatitis B, if available, is 85%.
    D. The probability of risk reduction for hepatitis B infection with a vaccine is 95%, suggesting that this vaccine is highly efficacious.
    E. The vaccine provides herd immunity to those in the population who remain unvaccinated, which reduces risk of infection by a probability of 75%.
    F. A payer (i.e., health insurance) will cover 90% of the cost of the vaccine's price.
    G. A payer will cover 80% of the cost of vaccine administration, by which a provider (e.g., physician, nurse, pharmacist, or public health worker) injects the vaccine into an individual.
    H. If a patient is infected with hepatitis B virus, they are responsible for 25% of all diagnostic and treatment costs for the duration of care.
II. Costs:
    A. The cost of the vaccine is US $28.00 per patient.
    B. The cost of vaccine administration is US $14.42 per patient.
    C. The cost of a provider to diagnose hepatitis B virus in an individual is US $250.00.
    D. The annual cost to manage and treat hepatitis B virus is US $1,824.00.
III. Health utility and survival:
    A. Patients diagnosed with hepatitis B who die with the virus lose 0.050 DALYs, and have an average life expectancy of 5 years.
    B. Patients diagnosed with hepatitis B who recover from the virus lost 0.025 DALYs, and have an average life expectancy of 20 years.
    C. Patients who are not infected have a population average disutility 0.010 DALYs, and have an average life expectancy of 50 years.

As you transcribe these data into the appropriate cell, you will notice that the cells in column B turn from *red* to *yellow*. You'll also notice that data are translated into probabilities for [DECISION MODEL]. It is important to note here that the probabilities in the model are comprehensive of all population health outcomes at each node. Given that the decision nodes are dichotomous (i.e., two outcomes per node), you only need one probability per node to calculate the outcomes. All nodes should add up to 100%, so knowing one of the two nodes allows you to calculate the difference for the alternative node. For example, click on cell F7 under No Vaccine ⇨ No Infection. This cell does not specify its own probability, but is calculated by subtracting the probability of hepatitis B infection (i.e., hepatitis B incidence) from 100%. The probabilities of Death and Not Vaccinated in the model are also remainders from known parameters.

In addition, not all information about probabilities in the model are translated directly translated into a probability. The probabilities of risk reduction for hepatitis B infection due to the presence of a vaccine or herd immunity are not actually probability of decision nodes, but effect modifiers. For example, click on cell H12 and you will see that the rate of hepatitis B infection is multiplied by the difference of the vaccine risk-reduction from 100%. The same type of calculation for herd immunity is presented in cell H18 since the presence of herd immunity protects unvaccinated people from hepatitis B infection. However, vaccination does not impact the rates of death or recovery if a patient does become infected.

3.7.3 Part B: exploring cost-effectiveness analysis

If you feel that you have correctly input all parameters into the model in Part A, then you can continue with the current working model. Otherwise, we recommend opening the second iteration of the model "Hep B Part B" to continue following along this exercise. ⬤ Additional content on (Hep B Part B) is available online, 10.1093/oso/9780192896087.012.0001.

Health state probabilities are calculated in real-time in [DECISION MODEL] as data are populated under [PARAMETERS]. These probabilities provide critical data that act as weights on costs, health utilities and survival for economic evaluation. At this point, we recommend that you click through some of the probabilities below health states on [DECISION MODEL] in order to understand where the probabilities come from in [PARAMETERS] and how they are calculated.

The probability weights from the model endpoints are presented in the [C-E ANALYSIS] tab under column B. These probabilities are calculated as the product of node probabilities for a specific pathway. For instance, the endpoint probability of "No Vaccine ⇨ HepB Infection ⇨ Recovered" is determined by the probabilities of hepatitis B infection multiplied by recovery $(0.01 \times 0.05 = 0.0005)$.

Once probabilities and outcomes are calculated, there should be a value in column B associated with each pathway. As a rule, these probabilities should add up to 100% for all health states in a decision tree arm. You can build a check into the model to confirm this by summing up all probabilities in each arm and ensure that they add up to 1.0. This is illustrated in column C for each arm of the model.

For this part of the exercise, try building in the check yourself using the "SUM()" function in excel. Do this in the following steps:

1. Sum probabilities for No Vaccine:
    a. Place the cursor over cell C9 which should be a *red*, blank cell.
    b. Enter the following formula to calculate the total probabilities of the No Vaccine Arm: =SUM(B4:B8)
    c. Then click; the color of the cell should change to *yellow*.
2. Sum probabilities for Vaccine Available:
    a. Place the cursor over cell C21 which should be a *red*, blank cell.
    b. Enter the following formula to calculate the total probabilities of the No Vaccine Arm: =SUM(B10:B20)
    c. Then click; the color of the cell should change to *yellow*.

If the probabilities do not total 1.0 in cells C9 and C21, then you have may an error in the way that you put probabilities into the model.

Columns D through K have to do with cost outcomes. These are broken down into several categories of fixed and variable costs that offer some time-dependency to the model's function. These costs are also broken down by perspective, since some costs are pertinent only to the payer or patient perspective. We can safely assume that the summation of payer and patient costs represent healthcare sector costs as well.

In columns D and E are fixed costs to payers and patients. These fixed costs are the costs that only would come up once related to vaccination or hepatitis B management during the course of a patient's lifetime. For patients with hepatitis B infection, we assume that the cost of diagnosis is a one-time fixed cost upfront to establish that the patient is infected. Thus, all individuals who are infected have this cost applied to them, regardless of whether they are in the Vaccine Available or No Vaccine arms of the model. The other fixed costs are that of the Vaccine and Vaccine Administration. These costs are only applied to patients in the Vaccine Available arm of the model who receive the vaccine. The costs are broken down into payer and patient proportions based on the information you would have put into the [PARAMETERS] to ensure that costs are distributed between both perspectives. While payers pay for the majority of these costs, patients (or their guardians) are responsible for an "out-of-pocket" portion of costs to ensure responsible utilization of these services by individuals in the community, and could be interpreted as a typical co-pay.

In columns F and G are annual, or variable, costs incurred by patients who become infected with hepatitis B, either with or without a vaccination. We assume that patients who are infected incur an average annual cost of hepatitis B treatment and management no matter what, which again is broken down into payer and patient components.

The total costs to each perspective appear in columns H and I, which are a summation of the one-time fixed cost, and the annual costs from each perspective multiplied by the assumed duration of survival for a model subgroup. For instance, in the pathway No Vaccine ⇨ No Infection, there are US $0.00 since there is neither a cost for vaccination nor treatment from any perspective. In another instance, a patient in No Vaccine ⇨ HepB Infection ⇨ Recovered, the total cost is calculated by multiplying the annual cost of hepatitis B treatment by the average life expectancy with hepatitis B infection (recovered), added to the one-time cost of hepatitis B diagnosis. Whereas the alternate pathway, No Vaccine ⇨ HepB Infection ⇨ Death, is calculated in the same fashion, but the cost of treatment is multiplied by an specified life expectancy for hepatitis B infection until death. In a final instance, we should point out that costs in the Vaccine Available arm include the fixed cost of the Vaccine and its administration distributed to payers and patients if the model specifies that the pathway included that the individual was Vaccinated.

Columns J and K provide important information about costs in the process of developing an economic model, which is to weight costs to each perspective by the probability of outcome (column B). While costs for hepatitis B treatment or vaccination can seem high, their weight in the model only matters to the extent of the probability of an outcome. Thus, weighted costs in columns J and K are calculated simply by multiplying the total costs to patients and payers by the corresponding probability of outcomes in the same row. Note that a single probability of outcome is applied to all perspectives. It is unusual that you would have different probabilities of outcomes for different perspectives when building a simple model such as this decision tree.

Next, we provide important information about health utility and survival. This model analyzes information about patient health utility in units of DALYs. However, DALYs, as interpreted for an economic model, do not provide direct data for results. DALYs provide information about the disability accumulated with a disease, but we want to understand the utility, or gain of health status and function as a result of avoiding infectious disease with a vaccine. Therefore, it is important here to convert DALYs to "DALYs Averted" so that we can express utility on a scale of 0.0 (total disability) to 1.0 (no disability). Thus, column L calculated DALYs averted by subtracting the reported DALYs for a particular endpoint health state from 1.0.

Column M provides the corresponding life expectancy with each health state. In column N, these weighted life expectancies are calculated by multiplying life expectancy (column M) and probability of outcome (column B). In column O, Total DALYs Averted can be illustrated from multiplying DALYs Averted (column L) by Life Expectancy (column M). In the final column P, critical information about weighted health utility in units of DALYs averted is expressed by multiplying Total DALYs Averted (column O) by Probability of Outcome (column B). This information is used in the forthcoming cost-effectiveness analysis calculation.

3.7.4 Part C: determining the incremental cost-effectiveness ratio

If you feel that you have correctly input all parameters into the model in Part B, then you can continue with the current working model. Otherwise, we recommend opening the third iteration of the model "Hep B Part C" to continue following along this exercise. ☰ Additional content on (Hep B Part C) is available online, 10.1093/oso/9780192896087.012.0001.

You now have a working model where all information is available in order to make determinations about the cost-effectiveness of hepatitis B vaccine from different perspectives. Go to the [C-E RESULTS] tab to perform these calculations. You will note that many of the cells on this tab are currently blank and *red*. You will need to reference data from other tabs in the model to complete the calculations.

Select cell C4, which is the payer cost of No Vaccine. This is the sum of all weighted payer costs on the [C-E ANALYSIS] tab. Using the "SUM()" command, enter a formula in C4 that references the three weighted payer costs in column J of the [C-E ANALYSIS] tab and adds them up in total. (Hint: the formula should appear in the same syntax as Part B, Step 1b.)

Continue these steps of adding up costs from the payer and patient perspectives on the [C-E RESULTS] tab by filling in cells C5, D4, and D5. You will need to use the same "SUM()" command to reference values in columns J and K on the [C-E ANALYSIS] tab. Note that for the vaccine comparator (values in row 5), there are 6 cells that you must reference in columns J and K on the [C-E ANALYSIS] tab.

Once you have costs from each perspective, you can calculate the total costs from the healthcare sector perspective for the two alternatives. Place formulas in cells B4 and B5 that add up the costs from payer and patient perspectives in each arm of the model for corresponding rows (i.e., rows 4 and 5).

Now you are ready to total up the DALYs averted for each arm of the study in rows 8 and 9. Because DALYs averted is a universal measure of health utility, we assume here that it does not vary by perspective (that is, the same amount of DALYs averted is observed to the patient, payer, and the healthcare sector).

Select cell D8, which is the patient DALYs averted of No Vaccine. This is the sum of all weighted DALYs averted on the [C-E Analysis] tab. Using the "SUM()" command, enter a formula in D8 that references the three weighted DALYs averted in column P of the [C-E Analysis] tab and adds them up in total. (Hint: the formula should appear in the same syntax as Part B, Step 1b.)

Continue these steps of adding up DALYs averted from the payer, patient, and healthcare sector perspectives on the [C-E RESULTS] tab by filling in cells D9, B8, B9, C8, and C9. You will need to use the same "SUM()" command to reference values in column P on the [C-E ANALYSIS] tab. Note that for the vaccine comparator (values in row 9), there are 6 cells that you must reference in column P on the [C-E ANALYSIS] tab.

You'll notice that as you input the total costs and DALYs averted from each perspective, the model will automatically calculate differences in costs and effectiveness between perspectives. This information is what you need to calculate the ICERs for each perspective in row 12.

For the ICER calculation, start with the total ICER calculation first from the healthcare sector perspective. Create a formula in cell B12 that divides the value in cell B6 by the value in cell B10. (Hint: make sure to use the "=" sign at the beginning of your formula.)

For the formulas in cells C12 and D12, you can copy/paste the formula from cell B12, and excel will automatically update the column reference points for you.

You should now be able to see the ICER values and observe the cost-effectiveness determination (cells B15:D17) at different willingness-to-pay thresholds. How do the ICERs vary by perspective? Which option is cost effective from which perspective at US $50,000/DALY averted versus US $150,000/DALY averted?

3.7.5 Part D: exploring budget impact analysis

If you feel that you have correctly input all parameters into the model in Part C, then you can continue with the current working model. Otherwise, we recommend opening the fourth iteration of the model "Hep B Part D" to continue following along this exercise. ☰ Additional content on (Hep B Part D) is available online, 10.1093/oso/9780192896087.012.0001.

You now have a working model where all information is available in order to make determinations about cost-effectiveness. The next step is to calculate budget impact. To start, go to the [BUDGET IMPACT] tab. There are two blank cells, B3 and B4, which you will need the following data to populate:

- Assume that you are working with a health insurance payer that covers health plans for 100,000 people. Use this information in B3.
- Assume that 10% of your population would benefit from immediate intervention with the hepatitis B vaccine. Input the 10% value in cell B4.

The remaining values in column B for the budget impact analysis should automatically populate. What you will now see is how the payer cost difference for vaccine in [C-E RESULTS] cell C6 plays into the budget impact analysis. The total cost of the vaccine program does not present a burden to the 10,000 recipients of the vaccine, but rather the 100,000 individuals who participate in a risk pool who can help pay for it. Since the benefits of the vaccine are modeled over a total time horizon of up to 50 years for the cohort specified, this time plays out in dividing up total budget impact by year, and then by month. The final budget impact value, represented as per-member per-year or per-member per-month (cell B10) estimates are important measures to many payers (both state and commercial payers) since they operate on revenues from monthly premiums or annual tax collections.

3.7.6 Part E: interpreting budget impact

If you feel that you have correctly input all parameters into the model in Part D, then you can continue with the current working model. Otherwise, we recommend opening the final iteration of the model "Hep B Part E" to continue following along this exercise. ☰ Additional content on (Hep B Part E) is available online, 10.1093/oso/9780192896087.012.0001.

Does the per-member per-month budget impact seem like a reasonable investment of a payer's risk pool? Does this budget impact compare to other classic examples of vaccine interventions in terms of affordability for a payer to commit to? How does the budget impact compare to the cost-effectiveness of the hepatitis B vaccine at certain willingness-to-pay thresholds?

Reference

Hoerger, T. J., Schillie, S., Wittenborn, J. S., Bradley, C. L., Zhou, F., Byrd, K., & Murphy, T. V. (2013). Cost-effectiveness of hepatitis B vaccination in adults with diagnosed diabetes. *Diabetes Care, 36*(1), 63–69. doi:10.2337/dc12-0759

4

ADVANCED METHODS IN
ECONOMIC EVALUATION

Edited by William V. Padula, Emmanuel F. Drabo, and Ijeoma Edoka

4.0

Section introduction: advanced methods in economic evaluation

Emmanuel F. Drabo and William V. Padula

Economic evaluation has emerged in health as the science of assessing value, to inform the efficient use of scarce healthcare resources. To meet the objective, it is critical that the information generated by economic evaluation studies be as accurate as possible. This implies that both the structure of the model and data quality meet higher standards than one might find in a simple model with limited parameter inputs. Both data quality and model structure will be explored in greater detail in this section. The World Health Organization also provides a valuable resource for additional tips on modeling complex systems of vaccine delivery (World Health Organization: Immunization Vaccines and Biologicals, 2019).

4.0.1 Rationale for advanced models

Health economic evaluation models are computer-based simulation models which focus on the population-level impacts of diseases and disease mitigation strategies can help overcome these challenges to the evaluation of policies by combining the best available data (e.g., epidemic, clinical, economic) from multiple sources, to permit comparisons of the current and future epidemiological, clinical, and economic impacts of multiple alternative disease-related interventions or strategies, and for different population subgroups.

Ideally, decisions would be guided by evidence from randomized controlled trials. However, randomized controlled trials are not always possible to conduct, and may be impractical for providing economic-specific evidence (e.g., costs and probabilities of some long-term outcomes). For example, as there may be multiple strategies to assess, and given that strategies may vary in "intensity" of implementation or may combine multiple interventions, it is impractical and costly to compare them in a single randomized controlled

Emmanuel F. Drabo and William V. Padula, *Section introduction: advanced methods in economic evaluation* In: *Handbook of Applied Health Economics in Vaccines*. Edited by: David Bishai, Logan Brenzel and William V. Padula, Oxford University Press.
© Oxford University Press 2023. DOI: 10.1093/oso/9780192896087.003.0021

trial. In these cases, modeling techniques such as decision trees can be useful. However, to account for the long-term consequences of various decisions, more complex models are needed. These models can be used to extrapolate results from the observed clinical evidence over a short time frame to a longer time frame, randomized controlled trials are often conducted over a relatively short period of time (Sonnenberg & Beck, 1993).

4.0.2 Model structure

Health economic evaluation models can estimate the distribution of the population or a cohort of individuals targeted or affected by a given vaccination strategy in various health states (e.g., healthy, sick, or dead), at any given point in time. In addition, they quantify how health itself is affected by alternative strategies. By moving from simple decision trees to a more complex and all-encompassing model approach, such as Markov models, economic analysis can begin to better reflect the actual sequelae of infectious diseases. Markov models can also more accurately capture the impact on health that a vaccine could potentially have over time, given that Markov models encapsulate many elements of time dependency.

4.0.3 Material covered

This section draws on a wide range of methods and applications developed specifically for advanced economic modeling in vaccine economics to offer a synopsis of current and emerging methods of modeling approaches for health economic evaluation. The section is organized into four chapters which walk the reader through these advanced vaccine economic modeling techniques and their applications with concrete examples and exercises, starting with simpler Markov models, and moving progressively towards more complex modeling approaches such as transmission models.

Chapter 4.1 introduces the reader to Markov modeling using an applied exercise with a hepatitis B vaccination decision problem.

Chapter 4.2 introduces the reader to static and dynamic modeling such as disease transmission models, with examples from both high- and low-income settings. Readers will become familiar with when to use each type of model.

Chapter 4.3 focuses on probabilistic sensitivity analysis and value of information.

Chapter 4.4 provides a reference case for vaccine economic evaluation using a novel coronavirus disease 2019 (COVID-19) vaccine program Markov model.

References

Sonnenberg, F. A., & Beck, J. R. (1993). Markov models in medical decision making: A practical guide. *Medical Decision Making, 13*(4), 322–338. doi:10.1177/0272989X9301300409

World Health Organization: Immunization Vaccines and Biologicals. (2019). *WHO guide for standardization of economic evaluations of immunization programmes.* https://www.who.int/immunization/documents/who_ivb_19.10/en/

4.1

Introduction to Markov modeling

Emmanuel F. Drabo and William V. Padula

To assess vaccination strategies more accurately in terms of their cost-effectiveness and to help guide public health decisions-making, it is critical to account for both the short- and long-term consequences of each available strategy. As randomized controlled trials may be impractical to assess long-term outcomes, models are needed to extrapolate results from the observed clinical evidence over both short- to long-term time frames (Sonnenberg & Beck, 1993).

Economic models examining time-dependent outcomes are constructed to estimate the distribution of the population or a cohort of individuals targeted or affected by a vaccination strategy in various health states (e.g., healthy, sick, or dead). In addition, models quantify how health itself is affected by alternative strategies—both in terms of intermediate changes in health status, as well as health endpoints. The economic and health consequences associated with a chosen strategy are measured as costs (e.g., direct medical care or drug costs) and health outcomes (e.g., life years, quality of life), respectively, and assigned to each health status, to estimate the expected cost and effectiveness of that strategy.

Chapter 3.7 introduced the decision tree model for vaccine economics, a simplified type of modeling approach for extrapolating the long-term outcomes of a vaccination strategy. While decision trees are useful for modeling instantaneous or one-time probabilistic events, they are limited in capturing the effects of the duration of the time spent in each health state. This chapter introduces the reader to Markov decision-analytic models, which are a widely used modeling approach in economic evaluation (Drummond, Sculpher, Claxton, Stoddart, & Torrance, 2015b).

In 1906, Andrey Markov introduced the Markov assumption, *that all following states are independent of all past states.* Markov models depict transitioning fluidly between health states based on prior probabilities of assumed outcomes. However, Markov models with dynamic features still allow a modeler to partition events so that patients with certain features are limited in terms of what can happen next. For instance, a person cannot develop pneumonia without first contracting influenza, but a person with influenza could

Emmanuel F. Drabo and William V. Padula, *Introduction to Markov modeling* In: *Handbook of Applied Health Economics in Vaccines*. Edited by: David Bishai, Logan Brenzel and William V. Padula, Oxford University Press. © Oxford University Press 2023.
DOI: 10.1093/oso/9780192896087.003.0022

have a probability of transitioning to a state of pneumonia based on our understanding of prior probabilities. More about this will be explained later throughout this chapter and additional considerations and data are presented in Appendix 4 and "SVIRD". ⊟ Additional content on (SVIRD) is available online, 10.1093/oso/9780192896087.012.0001.

4.1.1 Definition of a Markov model

Markov models can represent disease processes that evolve over time. These models can be designed to keep track of the costs and health-related quality of life (HRQoL) changes of spending time in a particular health status, by representing health status as a series of finite, discrete health states. Changes in health status over time are captured through transition probabilities between health states. This process of transitioning between states can then be modelled as finite-state Markov chains with the corresponding state transition probabilities. These models are particularly useful in the context of decision problems involving risk that continues and potentially changes over time, when the timing of events is important to outcomes, and when events occur more than once (Sonnenberg & Beck, 1993).

Markov models are well suited for the value assessment of vaccination strategies, as they can capture disease transmission patterns and disease recurrence, and estimate long-term costs and health outcomes (e.g., life years gained, quality-adjusted life years (QALYs)) associated with alternative vaccination strategies. It would be straightforward to sum up the total time spent in each health state and multiply this by the appropriate HRQoL factors and costs per unit time for each health state to derive the total intervention health effects and costs for transitioning between states.

Markov modeling provides a more convenient way of modeling the economic and health outcomes associated with vaccination decisions. The Markov modeling approach achieves this by modeling the process of transitioning between states as finite-state Markov chains and the corresponding state transition probabilities.

The foundational elements of a Markov model are *health states*. A health state, s, can correspond to an illness status (e.g., healthy versus sick), a particular disease stage, the presence of treatment, the receipt of a vaccine, some other disease-related status (e.g., circumcision status, screening status, etc.), or death. These health states must be *mutually exclusive* and *exhaustive*. Two states are said to be mutually exclusive if the same individual cannot be in both simultaneously, at any given point in time. The state set is said to be exhaustive if it includes all possible states relevant to the disease process. The other necessary element of a Markov model is the *transition* of individuals in a cohort between health states, according to their risk of contracting a disease or developing a condition, the natural progression of the disease or its underlying biological or behavioral factors, or due to the presence of a health intervention such as vaccination or treatment. For this reason, Markov models are sometimes referred to as *transition models*.

Each transition between any two health states (s, s') has a *transition probability*, $T(s, s')$. Although Markov models often have far more than two states, the basic concepts can be presented by considering just two states. The transition probabilities between any two states can be described by a square two-dimensional *transition probability matrix, T*:

$$T =$$

	S	S'
S	$T(s,s)$	$T(s,s')$
S'	$T(s',s)$	$T(s',s')$

The rows of the transition matrix represent the current state (s) of a given individual in the cohort or population, and the columns represent the transition state (s). Each cell (s, s') of the transition matrix represents the transition probability $T(s, s')$ between a current state s and a transition state s'. The value of each transition probability ranges between 0.0 and 1.0. Each row of the state transition matrix must also sum to 1, as the states are mutually exclusive, and one must be in a state. Transitions occur over a period, called a *cycle*. At any cycle t, the probability of being in (i.e., transitioning to) a given state s' is the product of the probability of being in state s at the start of the model, and the probability of transitioning to state s'. This can be more generally denoted by the following formula:

$$S \times T^t$$

where S is a vector of the probabilities of being in each state s at the start of the model, and T^t is the product of multiplying t state transition matrices. It should be noted here that it is possible for the person to remain in the current state, in which case $s = s'$. Finally, each health state can have a *cost* and *benefit* associated to it. These costs and benefits are called *rewards* or *payoffs*, $R(s)$.

In Markov chains, it is possible to have a state, s', from which individuals cannot move out once they enter. If such a state exists, it is called an *absorbing* state, and the Markov chain is referred to as an *absorbing Markov chain*. Any non-absorbing state in an absorbing Markov chain is called *transient*. When $S \times T^t = S$, we say that the system is at a stationary (or steady) state. For a more in-depth treatment of the use of Markov models in health economic evaluation, the reader should refer to prior work by Beck and Pauker (1983), Sonnenberg and Beck (1993), and Briggs and Sculpher (1998).

4.1.2 Steps in developing a Markov model

The development of transparent and policy-relevant Markov models for economic evaluation of vaccines involves the following critical steps. First, one must clearly define the states and allowable transitions that govern the disease and decision process, as well as how a vaccine may or may not alter the pathway of disease progression for some, if not all, individuals in the population being modeled.

Second, the analyst must select an appropriate cycle length. When thinking about the patient's journey, we must consider the duration and frequency of stay in each state, and the associated costs and outcomes of each state. The cycle length, that is, the minimum time people spend in a state, is a convenient way to measure duration of stay. The timescale of a Markov model depends on the biology and economics of the events. If infectious diseases are progressing in important ways on a daily basis, the time should be days; if they are progressing over months, the time cycle should be months, and so on. Cycle lengths could be as brief as on the scale of hours or days, or as long as months or years, if not more depending on the situation.

Related to cycle length is the time horizon, which was discussed with respect to decision trees in Chapter 3.7. This is the amount of time that an infectious disease or vaccine-related immunity may be relevant. Thus, time horizons can also be as brief as days, months, or years, but rarely exceed the duration of immunity offered by a vaccine, or a patient's life expectancy. For a study of an influenza vaccine, a 12-month time horizon is relevant since most flu shots are only indicated for that time period. However, other vaccines such as yellow fever and polio are considered to confer immunity ranging closer to a patient's full life expectancy.

Third, a set of transition probabilities between states must be specified to construct the state transition matrix.

Fourth, a cost and health outcome (e.g., natural unit, utility) must be assigned to each health state.

Fifth, the initial set-up of the population across the various health states must be determined.

Sixth, methods of evaluation of the alternative strategies, such as cost-effectiveness analysis, must be predefined.

Finally, a perspective should be well defined at the time that the model is being conceived so that the model accurately reflects health outcomes with respect to costs and clinical benefits being accrued that matter to the perspective. As discussed in the previous chapter, perspectives can range from patient, to provider, to health system, to payer, to government, to society, or some combination of these examples.

4.1.3 Example of a Markov model: hepatitis B vaccination transitions

To illustrate these concepts, consider the hepatitis B vaccination decision problem in the example in Chapter 3.7, adapted from Hoerger et al. (2013). The original study by Hoerger et al. (2013) found that with a 10% uptake rate, hepatitis B vaccination among all US adults with diagnosed diabetes would lead to 528,047 people vaccinated which could prevent 4,271 acute and 256 chronic hepatitis B infections, at an incremental healthcare cost of $91.4 million. The intervention was estimated to generate 1,218 QALYs, thus translating into a cost-effectiveness ratio of $75.094 per QALY gained.

Our adaption of Hoerger et al.'s Markov model of the hepatitis B vaccination decision problem includes five health states: Susceptible (S, i.e., uninfected, but at risk of infection), Vaccinated (V), Infected (I), Recovered (R), and Dead (D). Models of this type are referred to in the epidemiological modeling literature as SVIRD models. This model can be depicted using an *influence* or *state transition diagram*, to show the transitions of individuals between health states (Fig. 4.1.1).

Looking at Fig. 4.1.1, we can notice that the five health states, represented by the ovals, are mutually exclusive, that is, individuals can only be Susceptible, Vaccinated, Infected, Recovered, or Dead within the model. For example, if people are in the Susceptible state, they can become infected and transition to the Infected state, become vaccinated and transition to the Vaccinated state, die of natural cause and transition to the Death state, or remain Susceptible. Similarly, Vaccinated individuals can receive protection from the vaccine and remain in the Vaccinated state, lose protection from the vaccine (if the vaccine

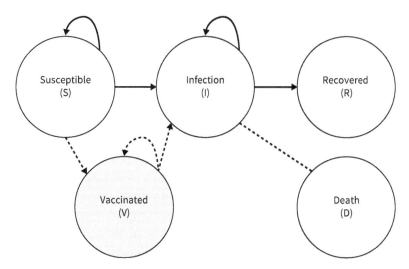

Fig. 4.1.1 State transition diagram of the hepatitis B vaccine Markov model. The states of the model are represented by the circles; the transitions between health states are represented by the arrows.

is imperfect, or when the immunity from the vaccine wanes) and become infected, thus transitioning into the Infected state, or die of other causes and transition to the Dead state.

Once in the Infected state, individuals can recover from the infection and move to the Recovered state, die of other causes or from hepatitis B complication and transition to the Dead state, or remain Infected. Those who recover are assumed to gain lifetime immunity and remain in the Recovered state or die of other causes and transition to the Dead state. Once people are in the Dead state, they cannot move from that state to any other state; hence, the Dead state is an *absorbing* state, and all other states are non-absorbing *transient* states. The directed arrows that connect the ovals (health states) represent the directions of the transitions between states. Each of these arrows is associated with a state transition probability, $T(s, s')$. It is also worthwhile noticing that in this model, individuals cannot return to their initial state once they leave it. Equally noteworthy is the observation that it is possible to remain in the same health state after a cycle.

4.1.4 Parameterization of Markov models

To best inform decision-making, it is critical that the Markov models incorporate the best available evidence on the process that is being modeled, and the interventions that are being evaluated (Briggs & Sculpher, 1998). To achieve this, the input parameters for the model typically incorporate a wide range of information from various sources, such as estimated vaccine efficacy from clinical trials, disease evolution from epidemiological cohorts, quality-of-life values or disability weights from population-level studies, transition probabilities from life tables, and so on. The implementation of the Markov model should also be sufficiently flexible to accommodate these various sources of data. As done with decision models, transition probabilities for Markov models are derived from clinical trials, observational data, meta-analyses, expert panels, surveys, and other relevant sources of evidence. Chapter 3.3 provides more details on how to identify, appraise, synthesize, and transform data from disparate sources to inform decision-analytic models.

We draw from the reported clinical, epidemiological, and economic input parameters in the Hoerger et al. (2013) study to parameterize the model. To illustrate, we have summarized in Table 4.1.1 the transition probabilities (matrix) associated with this Markov model for the no-vaccination (status quo) policy, for a cohort of diabetics aged 20 years.

These transition matrices should be read from left to right. Each cell represents the probability of transitioning from a state s to another state s'. For example, the probability of transitioning from the Susceptible state (S) to the Infected state (I) is 0.70. For the actual input data used to calculate the entries of the transition matrix depicted in Table 4.1.1, the reader should refer to Table 4.1.2 and the "Parameters" tab of the Excel file for the model.

As observed earlier, the probabilities in each row of the transition matrices add up to 1. When developing a Markov model, one should always check that this fundamental property holds. The constraint that the sum of the transition probabilities from one state to all other states must sum up to 1 captures the notion that we must always account for all transitions in each cycle, and the idea that probabilities are exhaustive and mutually exclusive. As noted earlier,

Table 4.1.1 Illustrative state transition probabilities for the vaccination scenario

	S	V	I	R	D	Check
Susceptible (S)	0.198	0.100	0.700	0.000	0.002	1.000
Vaccinated (V)	0.000	0.998	0.000045	0.000	0.002	1.000
Infected (I)	0.000	0.000	0.129	0.865	0.006	1.000
Recovered (R)	0.000	0.000	0.000	0.998	0.002	1.000
Deaths (D)	0.000	0.000	0.000	0.000	1.000	1.000

it is worthwhile noticing that the Dead state is a final (absorbing) state, so that the probability of remaining in the Dead state is 1. Entries of the transition matrix with values of 0 reflect the fact that such transitions are not permitted. For example, given that individuals cannot transition from the Infected state to the Susceptible state, the transition probability from I to S is 0. The transition matrix therefore must agree with the transition diagram.

4.1.5 Adding cost and benefits

We will first conduct a cost analysis using the Markov model we have introduced. In their study, Hoerger et al. (2013) reported the costs associated with healthcare utilization, as well as the health outcomes in different health states. We use these cost estimates to conduct the cost analysis of the vaccination and no-vaccination interventions in our illustrative example. Our cost data include vaccination costs (e.g., cost-share of the vaccine covered by a payer, vaccine price, etc.), the costs of hepatitis B diagnosis, the costs of treating acute hepatitis B infection, as well as the costs of treating chronic hepatitis B. These costs are summarized in Table 4.1.2. The costs summarized in the table are costs per cycle and per person. It is worthwhile noticing that while costs increase with worse states, costs in the worst state (Dead state) are 0. We also draw from these estimates to calculate the health outcomes associated with each health state.

4.1.6 Simulating the transitions of a cohort and conducting a cost-effectiveness analysis

With these data, we can calculate the expected costs and expected health outcomes of each vaccination strategy.

In our example, we simulated the transitions of a representative cohort of 1,000 diabetic patients aged 20 years, in each type of vaccination intervention (vaccination versus no-vaccination policies) over 59 years, with each cycle corresponding to 1 year. The 59-year time horizon is used because the average life expectancy of uninfected individuals (Susceptible and Vaccinated) in the cohort is approximately 59 years. Hence, the analysis is effectively a *lifetime horizon*.

At each cycle of the simulation, individuals age, and some die (e.g., 1,868 out of 1 million individuals in the first cycle under the first strategy). We can

Table 4.1.2 Model input parameter and values

Parameter	Value	Source
Probabilities		
Acute hepatitis B transmission probabilities		
Rate of asymptomatic infections (acute)	0.700	Hoerger et al. (2013)
Hospitalization rate	0.380	Hoerger et al. (2013)
Share of hospitalizations that are fulminant cases	0.040	Hoerger et al. (2013)
Probability of progression from acute to chronic hepatitis, weighted	0.053	Calculation
Probability of death during an acute infection	0.003	Calculation
Probability of recovery from an acute infection	0.942	Calculation
Chronic hepatitis B transmission probabilities		
Prevalence of chronic hepatitis B	0.082	Schillie, Xing, Murphy, & Hu (2012)
Average annual mortality rate among persons with chronic hepatitis B	0.036	Calculated from the chronic hepatitis B Markov model of Hoerger et al. (2013)
Vaccination probabilities		
Probability of accepting the vaccine	0.100	Assumption (Hoerger et al., 2013)
Awareness of hepatitis B infection		
Proportion of chronic hepatitis B aware of infection	0.339	Kim, Billah, Lieu, & Weinstein (2006)
Proportion of acute hepatitis B aware of infection	0.345	
Costs	US $	
Acute hepatitis B costs		
Annual cost to treat a hepatitis B infection	1,744.00	Calculation
Test for antibody to hepatitis B-core antigen (anti-HBc)	15.00	Kim et al. (2006)
Cost of chronic hepatitis B diagnosis (serologic testing for hepatitis B surface antigen (HBsAg))	20.00	Assumption
Out-of-pocket cost-share for hepatitis B diagnosis to patient	0.25	Assumption
Out-of-pocket cost-share for hepatitis B infection treatment to patient	0.25	Assumption
Vaccination costs		
Cost of vaccine	28.00	Centers for Disease Control and Prevention (2011); Hoerger et al. (2013)
Cost of vaccine administration	14.42	Hoerger et al. (2013); Miriti et al. (2008)
Cost-share of vaccine covered by payer	0.90	Assumption
Cost-share of vaccine administration by payer	0.80	Assumption

Table 4.1.2 Continued

Parameter	Value	Source
Utilities: quality-adjusted life years	QALYs	
EQ-5D health utility score		
Diabetes (EQ-5D)	0.751	Hoerger et al. (2013); Sullivan & Ghushchyan (2006)
HRQoL utility weights		
Susceptible	1.000	Assumption
Vaccinated	1.000	Assumption
Infected	0.992	Calculated from the input parameters and Markov model of Hoerger et al. (2013)
Recovered	1.000	Assumption
Discount rates		
Discount rate	0.030	Assumption

therefore use this information to calculate the *life years* in each cycle. In the first cycle, under the No Vaccination strategy, 1,868 people died in the cohort, but 998,132 were alive, and accumulated 998,132 life years. Similarly, in the second cycle, 996,263 people were alive, and accumulated 996,263 years of life. We can repeat these calculations and derive the accumulated years of life associated with each cycle. At the end of the 59 cycles, we sum all the years of life over the 59 cycles to obtain the total life years. We can also use this information to produce the *survival curve*. The area under the survival curve represents the total years of life accumulated under the strategy.

Now, we need to calculate the total costs associated with each strategy. To do this, we need estimates of the annual costs of spending a year in each health state, as well as estimates of the expected total number of individuals in each state at each cycle. We must also calculate and add both the fixed and variable costs associated with each strategy, such as hepatitis B diagnosis costs, and vaccination costs.

In our simplified example, we only track the direct vaccination program and medical costs. We assume that the there are no additional medical costs associated with spending time in the Susceptible, Vaccinated, Recovered, and Death states. Hence, only the Infected state produces direct medical costs. However, at each cycle, newly vaccinated individuals will incur program costs in the form of vaccination. Similarly, a fraction of infected individuals will incur hepatitis B diagnosis costs. Of course, from a societal perspective, more cost components should be included; for example, we should be accounting for productivity loss from mortality, or from morbidity. Nevertheless, these complexities are omitted here for ease of exposition of the model.

In our model, the Infected state consists of both individuals with an acute infection, and those with a chronic infection. There are even more nuances, as shown in the Hoerger et al. (2013) study. Again, for simplicity, we aggregated these substates into acute and chronic infections. The annual expected cost of spending a year in the Infected state was estimated to be $1,744 (see Appendix 5 for derivations). The calculation of the total costs simply requires multiplying the annual expected costs of spending time in each state with the expected prevalence of individuals in each state during each period. We must also add the total expected program costs during each period. For example, for this cohort, 100,000 new individuals were vaccinated during the first cycle, accumulating $4,118,447 in program costs.

Now that we have the total life years and total costs over the time horizon for any given strategy (vaccination versus no vaccination), we can accumulate these total annual life years and costs over all periods to derive the cumulative life years and costs. For this cohort, 48,848,055 total undiscounted life years are accumulated under a no-vaccination strategy, compared to 48,848,808 total undiscounted life years accumulated under the vaccination strategy. Hence, the total number of life years gained under a vaccination strategy, relative to the no-vaccination strategy, is 753 life years. Similarly, the total costs accumulated under the no-vaccination strategy was $63,272,588 compared with $66,470,281 under the vaccination strategy. Hence, the incremental costs of the vaccination strategy, relative to no vaccination, is $3,197,693. With the calculated incremental costs and life year gains, we can calculate the incremental cost-effectiveness ratio (ICER) associated with the vaccination strategy, relative to no vaccination; this ICER estimate is $4,247 per life year gained. If a decision maker was willing to pay this price per life year gained, vaccination would be good value for money. Notice that neither the costs nor life years are discounted yet.

Adjusting for quality (i.e., preferences) is relatively straightforward in Markov models. Since each health state has a preference weight, that is, HRQoL weight, associated with it, we can multiply these weights by the utility score for the diabetic population, and the average time spent in each state during each cycle. The relative effectiveness of vaccination compared to no vaccination would then be the difference in the accumulated QALYs produced by the two strategies. In our example, the HRQoL weights associated with the Susceptible, Vaccinated, and Recovered states are 1.00 for each state. The corresponding weights for the Infected and Death states are 0.992 (see Appendix 5 for weighting and derivations), and 0.00, respectively. Notice that the HRQoL weights for the Infected state are high here; this is because the vast majority of infection cases are acute infections which resolve. The EuroQol five-dimensional (EQ-5D) utility score for diabetes patients is 0.751 (Hoerger et al., 2013; Sullivan & Ghushchyan, 2006). Deriving the QALYs associated with each intervention only required calculating the QALYs at each cycle and accumulating them over the observation period. The QALY associated with any given health state at any given cycle is calculated by multiplying the utility score for the population of interest (diabetes patients) with the total number of individuals in that health state, the duration of time spent in the state, and the HRQoL utility weight associated with the state. The total QALYs for the cycle is simply calculated by aggregating the state-level QALYs across all health states. For example, under the Vaccination strategy, the total QALYs associated with the uninfected (Susceptible, Vaccinated, and Recovered) states during the first cycle is 748,914 QALYs (0.751 × 1 year × [1.00 × 897,222 Susceptible + 1.00 × 100,000 Vaccinated + 1.00 × 0 Recovered). For the Infected state, a total of 678 QALYs (0.751 × 1 year × [0.992 × 910 Infected]) are produced during the first cycle. The number of QALYs produced by the Death state is 0. The total number of QALYs produced during the cycle, across all states, is therefore 749,591 QALYs. We can then do these calculations for each cycle of the model and trace the total QALYs associated with each. A total of 36,685,366 QALYs are accumulated over the observation period and across all health states, under the Vaccination strategy, compared to 36,684,672 QALYs under the No Vaccination strategy, thus resulting in 694 incremental QALYs gained under the Vaccination strategy. This suggests an ICER of $4,605 per QALY gained.

We can also add life years and calculate the disability-adjusted life years, as we have done with the decision tree model presented in Chapter 3.7. We will not expand on these calculations here, for brevity.

Discounting is also easy to do in Markov models; one simply needs to calculate the present values of the cycle-level costs and benefits associated with each strategy, and aggregate over the total number of cycles. In our example, we assume an annual discount rate of 3% for both costs and utilities. The discounted total costs, life years, and QALYs after the first cycle are $1,544,799, 969,060 life years, and 727,759 QALYs, respectively, under the Vaccination strategy. The cumulative discounted costs, life years, and QALYs over the entire simulation period are $49,254,863, 24,674,647 life years, and 18,530,600 QALYs, respectively, for the Vaccination strategy. For the No Vaccination strategy, the corresponding estimates are $38,448,013, 24,674,257 life years, and 18,530,235 QALYs, respectively. Together, these estimates suggest that on a discounted basis, the ICER for the Vaccination strategy, when compared to the No Vaccination strategy is $27,733 per life year gained and $29,635 per QALY gained.

It is worthwhile noting that the usual exercise of adjusting inputs (e.g., translating all costs into a single year's value) must be conducted, although we have not discussed it here.

4.1.7 Half-cycle correction

It should be noted that in the approach described above to calculate the life years accumulated in each cycle, we have implicitly assumed that those who die died at the start of the cycle. However, they could have died at any point during the cycle, thus we should take this into account to avoid underestimating costs and benefits. Specifically, since people die during each cycle and have spent some time alive during the cycle in which they died, it seems reasonable that we should credit this time alive (as well as its associated costs) to the strategy. This assumption is less of an issue if it is applied to all strategies being evaluated, and when the cycle length is short.

A reasonable and less biased approach would be to assume that people die in the middle of the cycle. This is a result of assuming that individuals die, uniformly, during the cycle. In other words, we would assume that over each cycle, death follows a uniform distribution, that is, the probability of death is the same every time during the cycle. This assumption is known as the *half-cycle correction*. It consists of adding half the time to those who died during the cycle. We have illustrated it in our Excel example.

4.1.8 Markov models as "trees"

In Chapter 3.7, we introduced the decision tree modeling approach for examining this problem. For recurrent events, however, the decision tree approach is not suitable. While it is possible to construct a recursive decision tree with one tree per cycle, it would be too complicated to do so as one would rapidly run into the "bushy" tree problem. By this, we mean that a decision tree with many independent nodes representing state transitions and time-dependent outcomes over long time horizons may be overly complex to construct.

Fortunately, the same problem can be represented as a Markovian chain process to help address much more complex questions such as vaccination against influenza.

Influenza provides a helpful example for this purpose because on an annual basis, a flu shot offers the patient immunity from the infection for 12 months. However, after 12 months, the immunity wanes and the vaccination process should be started all over again. If looking at the value of an influenza immunization program beyond 12 months, then a Markov model certainly provides simplicity in its *Susceptible, Infected, Recovered,* and/or *Vaccinated* structure as compared with trees branching out for recurrent years of vaccination.

4.1.9 Memoryless property of Markov cohort models

Markov models of the type described above assume that transitions to a state are independent of the past or the duration an individual has been in a state. In other words, there is no "memory" of the past. This is known as the *memoryless property* or *Markov assumption.*

The memoryless property is a limitation of Markov models as in many situations the duration of stay in a health state influences the chances of outcomes. For example, most individuals with hepatitis C virus are known to have delayed onset of symptoms. One could mitigate this limitation by adding additional transition states (e.g., asymptomatic, acute symptoms, chronic symptoms, liver transplantation, etc.), and making transition probabilities conditional on past events.

As we have assumed in our hepatitis B vaccination example, we allowed for different probabilities of death by order of liver transplantation.

References

Beck, J. R., & Pauker, S. G. (1983). The Markov process in medical prognosis. *Medical Decision Making, 3*(4), 419–458. doi:10.1177/0272989X8300300403

Briggs, A., & Sculpher, M. (1998). An introduction to Markov modelling for economic evaluation. *PharmacoEconomics, 13*(4), 397–409. doi:10.2165/00019053-199813040-00003

Centers for Disease Control and Prevention. (2011). *CDC vaccine price list: Adult vaccine price list.* http://www.cdc.gov/vaccines/programs/vfc/cdc-vac-price-list.htm

Drummond, M., Sculpher, M., Claxton, K., Stoddart, G. L., & Torrance, G. W. (2015). *Methods for the economic evaluation of health care programmes* (4th ed.). Oxford: Oxford University Press.

Hoerger, T. J., Schillie, S., Wittenborn, J. S., Bradley, C. L., Zhou, F., Byrd, K., & Murphy, T. V. (2013). Cost-effectiveness of hepatitis B vaccination in adults with diagnosed diabetes. *Diabetes Care, 36*(1), 63–69. doi:10.2337/dc12-0759

Kim, S. Y., Billah, K., Lieu, T. A., & Weinstein, M. C. (2006). Cost effectiveness of hepatitis B vaccination at HIV counseling and testing sites. *American Journal of Preventive Medicine, 30*(6), 498–506. doi:10.1016/j.amepre.2006.01.017

Miriti, M. K. K., Billah, K., Weinbaum, C., Subiadur, J., Zimmerman, R., Murray, P.,... Buffington, J. (2008). Economic benefits of hepatitis B vaccination at sexually transmitted disease clinics in the U.S. *Public Health Reports (Washington, D.C.: 1974), 123*(4), 504–513. doi:10.1177/003335490812300412

Schillie, S. F., Xing, J., Murphy, T. V., & Hu, D. J. (2012). Prevalence of hepatitis B virus infection among persons with diagnosed diabetes mellitus in the United States, 1999–2010. *Journal of Viral Hepatitis, 19*(9), 674–676. doi:10.1111/j.1365-2893.2012.01616.x

Sonnenberg, F. A., & Beck, J. R. (1993). Markov models in medical decision making: A practical guide. *Medical Decision Making, 13*(4), 322–338. doi:10.1177/0272989X9301300409

Sullivan, P. W., & Ghushchyan, V. (2006). Preference-based EQ-5D index scores for chronic conditions in the United States. *Medical Decision Making, 26*(4), 410–420. doi:10.1177/0272989x06290495

4.2

Static and dynamic modeling

Ann Levin and Colleen Burgess

In order to calculate the costs and health utilities associated with the implementation of various vaccine programs, we must first have a grasp of the epidemiological impacts of these strategies. To do this, we must be able to predict the morbidity and mortality associated with the given infectious disease, as well as any variations in these outcomes resulting from vaccination and other interventions. This involves the utilization of epidemiological modeling techniques. This chapter presents a discussion of static and dynamic modeling of infectious diseases and the advantages and disadvantages of using the two approaches. Researchers employ this type of modeling for estimating the impact of vaccination on morbidity and mortality for economic evaluations.

4.2.1 When is a static model appropriate? When is a dynamic model needed?

There are two approaches to modeling the impact of infectious diseases on morbidity and mortality: static and dynamic. A static model assumes that the force of infection is constant or changes only as a function of age and other individual characteristics. Static models estimate the direct effect of vaccination on vaccinated individuals—that is, the reduction in morbidity and mortality—and are affected by the incidence and prevalence of the disease and efficacy of the vaccine. Static models can generate outcomes quickly and fairly simply and can often be constructed using easily accessible software programs such as Microsoft Excel or Google Sheets. The mathematics involved in static models tend to be relatively straightforward, such as applying an infection rate to a population to calculate the expected number of disease cases over a short period of time. These types of models can obscure significant epidemiological interactions, however, such as the geographic

Ann Levin and Colleen Burgess, *Static and dynamic modeling* In: *Handbook of Applied Health Economics in Vaccines*. Edited by: David Bishai, Logan Brenzel and William V. Padula, Oxford University Press. © Oxford University Press 2023. DOI: 10.1093/oso/9780192896087.003.0023 heterogeneity of vaccinated populations, or the threshold for herd immunity required to drive an outbreak to extinction.

A dynamic model, on the other hand, captures both direct and indirect effects of vaccination on vaccinated and unvaccinated individuals, including herd immunity.

In contrast with static models, a dynamic disease transmission model assumes that the force of infection can vary throughout the course of time and as a function of population interactions, often in nonlinear ways. To simulate transmission, dynamic models take into account data on the contact patterns of individuals, the distribution of the infection in the population, and the transmissibility of the infection (Kim & Goldie, 2008). If the protective effect of vaccination is sufficiently high and enough individuals are vaccinated, the herd immunity threshold can be reached. This threshold is "the proportion of a population that needs to be immune in order to halt the spread of a communicable disease" (Nymark, Sharma, Miller, Enemark, & Griffiths, 2017). That is, if enough individuals are vaccinated, others are less likely to be infected since fewer persons around them are susceptible to the disease. Some diseases are highly transmissible, such as measles, and most of the population need to be immune to the disease to achieve herd immunity. Other diseases such as polio and *Haemophilus influenza* type b are not as transmissible and have a lower threshold (Nymark et al., 2017).

Dynamic models are preferable for modeling the impact of a vaccine when considerations of herd immunity are likely to be important. Best practice guidelines on economic evaluation of vaccines recommend dynamic models when "the rate at which susceptible individual acquire infection is reduced due to vaccination or when it is not possible to obtain a conservative estimate with a static model" (Nymark et al., 2017). Static models can be used as a conservative estimate when indirect effects are not expected to be influential, the disease is not infectious (e.g., cancer), and there is no human-to-human transmission (e.g., rabies, tetanus, Japanese encephalitis) (World Health Organization: Immunization Vaccines and Biologicals, 2019). See Fig. 4.2.1 for a flowchart for deciding whether to use static or dynamic models.

4.2.2 Disease transmission modeling

In this section, different types of static and dynamic models are described (Table 4.2.1).

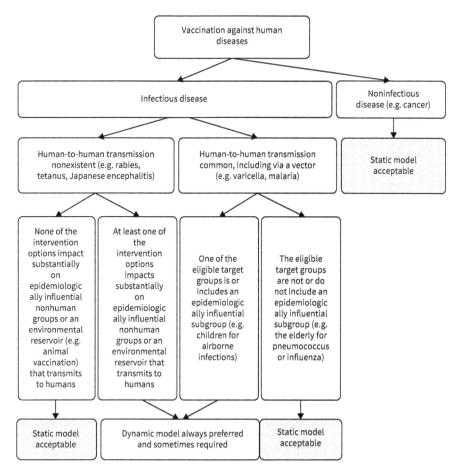

Fig. 4.2.1 Flow chart on when to use static and dynamic models.

Source: Reproduced from *WHO guide for standardization of economic evaluations of immunization programmes*, WHO, Copyright (2019).

4.2.2.1 Deterministic models

The transition from one disease state to the next is governed by rates or probabilities, depending on the type of model. A deterministic model assumes that there is no randomness to the way the disease behaves in the population, and that the system can be fully described by a set of mathematical equations and parameters. A deterministic model for the simple Susceptible–Infected–Recovered–Vaccinated (SIRV) system can be represented by a system of ordinary differential equations:

Table 4.2.1 Classification of mathematical model types used in health economic evaluation

	Static	Dynamic
Deterministic		

Aggregate level (compartmental/ cohort)	1. Deterministic aggregate-level static model
	  1.1 Decision trees
	  1.2 State-transition models (e.g., Markov model)
	  1.3 Hybrid models (e.g., a decision tree embedded with Markov models)
		2. Deterministic aggregate-level (compartmental) dynamic model
		  2.1 Discrete difference equations model (discrete time)
		  2.2 Ordinary differential equation (ODE) model (continuous time)
		  2.3 Partial differential equation (PDE) model (continuous time)
		  2.4 Other types of models that allow for interaction

Individual level	Uncommon	Uncommon
Stochastic (probabilistic)		
Aggregate level (compartmental/ cohort)	3. Stochastic aggregate-level static model, e.g., Monte Carlo simulation (sampling of outcomes) of a decision tree or a state-transition model	4. Stochastic aggregate-level dynamic model, e.g., individual sampling of compartmental dynamic model

Individual level	5. Static microsimulation model (e.g., Monte Carlo microsimulation of a decision tree or a state-transition model)	6. Dynamic microsimulation model
		  6.1 Monte Carlo simulation of a Markov model with interaction
		  6.2 Discrete-event simulation model
		  6.3 Agent-based model

Equation 4.2.1. Deterministic model:

$$\frac{dS}{dt} = -\beta SI - \rho S$$

$$\frac{dI}{dt} = -\beta SI - \gamma I$$

$$\frac{dR}{dt} = \gamma I$$

$$\frac{dV}{dt} = \rho S$$

The transition from susceptible to infected is governed by the disease transmission rate β and the number or proportion of infected people in the population, I. Individuals can also leave the susceptible population via vaccination, at a rate ρ which is governed by vaccination coverage and vaccine effectiveness. Once infected, an individual recovers at the rate γ, which is generally driven by the duration of the infectious period for the disease. In a deterministic model, the rates β, ρ and γ are constants or functional forms which can be defined clearly in mathematical terms.

A deterministic model assumes the system is fully describable by a defined set of equations and parameters, and thus every time the deterministic model is run it will always generate the same result. In contrast, a stochastic model assumes the presence of randomness which could affect a single parameter or multiple components within the system. The presence of uncertainty surrounding transitions between disease states can be represented by defining rate parameters as random values or probability distributions around a mean, as opposed to a constant value or smooth mathematical function. Such stochasticity can represent random events such as an influx of immigrants, the arrival of an infected tourist, the unexpected loss of vaccine efficacy due to a breakdown in the cold chain, or even a mutation in the virus. Because of this randomness, a stochastic model will generate a different result each time the model is run. Therefore, when utilized, stochastic models must be run for many iterations—in the order of hundreds or thousands—in order to explore the range of possible results. This will result in the clustering of model outcomes, and central estimates and ranges for epidemiological outputs such as cases and deaths can then be fed into economic calculations to determine the resulting spread of costs and health utilities.

While some deterministic models are solvable, in many cases, the mathematics behind transmission models are complex enough that it is impossible to solve the equations for an explicit solution.

4.2.2.2 SIRV model

From a disease perspective, a population can be divided into subgroups based on disease states—those who are susceptible to disease (S); those who are currently infected and able to transmit the disease to others (I); and those who have already been infected, have since recovered, and presumably now possess some level of immunity to re-infection (R). Taken together, this defines what is called an "SIR" model—Susceptible–Infected–Recovered (Fig. 4.2.2). The structure of the SIR model parallels the progression of a disease outbreak as the population flows from one group into the next.

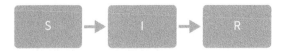

Fig. 4.2.2 Susceptible–Infected–Recovered (SIR) model.

Susceptibles become infected via disease transmission, and infected individuals recover from illness. The basic SIR model can be modified in a myriad of ways—the inclusion of an "incubating" phase, adding both acute and chronic stages of infection, or incorporating disease-related mortality, along with the inclusion of age structure, geographic variation, and so on.

Including vaccination in the model introduces a new subgroup: those who have been vaccinated against the disease and possess partial or full protection against infection, which may or may not wane over time (V). Now we have the "SIRV" model (Fig. 4.2.3).

In the SIRV model, individuals leave the susceptible population either by infection or by vaccination, and once in the vaccinated category, they no longer participate in disease transmission within the population (depending on vaccine efficacy, the potential for breakthrough infections, etc.). The inclusion of the vaccinated subgroup (in the simplest implementation) has the direct effect of reducing the size of the susceptible subgroup—which subsequently reduces the future size of the infected class.

The deterministic SIRV differential equation model is continuous—that is, transitions occur smoothly over time.

4.2.2.3 Contact matrices

For all of the transmission model structures described above, the functional form of the disease transmission rate β is highly dependent upon the disease being modeled. However, for all direct transmission diseases (i.e., diseases which do not require a vector or fomite for transmission) β will depend on

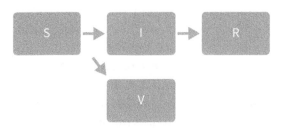

Fig. 4.2.3 Susceptible–Infected–Recovered–Vaccinated (SIRV) model.

effective interactions between susceptible and infected individuals. The definition of an effective interaction varies by disease—for bloodborne pathogens this implies direct contact with the blood or blood products of an infected person; for sexually transmitted diseases this requires sexual contact between susceptible and infected partners; and for respiratory viruses this includes close proximity contacts that result in the inhalation of respiratory secretions from an infectious individual. The effectiveness of the interaction can depend on the attack rate of the disease, the duration of exposure, the infectious dose, and many other factors including the implementation of disease interventions.

Contacts within populations are often driven by social or demographic factors, including age structure, family structure, work status or job function, socioeconomic status, and so on. Quantification of these interactions can be incorporated into disease transmission models to add realism to transmission functions and reflect non-vaccination contact-related interventions such as personal protective equipment, school closures, social distancing, and quarantine.

Mathematically, this quantification often takes the form of a contact matrix. A contact matrix is a pairwise quantitative description of the number of contacts per unit time between individuals in any two subpopulations. One of the most utilized age-structured contact matrix systems in epidemiological modeling is the set of POLYMOD matrices which provide estimates for the number of unique contacts per day between different age groups in eight different European countries, based on daily contact diaries (Mossong et al., 2008). This was later expanded to 152 countries by mathematical methods (Prem, Cook, & Jit, 2017). Contact matrices based upon other population subdivisions can be based on any number of other structures, such as the number of patients a healthcare worker interacts with daily, or the average ridership of public transportation systems.

4.2.2.4 Stochastic models

A stochastic model simulates the world by assuming that events occur randomly rather than assuming that events occur in a prespecified manner as in the case of deterministic models (Kim & Goldie, 2008). While adding complexity, a stochastic model provides a more comprehensive evaluation of the impact of variability and uncertainty. These types of models can be used when modeling an infectious disease outbreak in a small population because these are affected by chance and infectious agents are transmitted with different transmission probabilities (Kim & Goldie, 2008).

Stochastic models can be simulated numerically on a computer using programming languages such as R or software applications such as Matlab or Mathematica, for example, to generate morbidity and mortality results which can be used to calculate costs, quality-adjusted life years, disability-adjusted life years, incremental cost-effectiveness ratios, and other health utility outcomes. When disease transmission models are simulated on a computer, however, it is often more straightforward to work with variables in discrete time, working with incremental time units of a single day, week, month, and so on, based on the dynamics of the disease. This changes the interpretation of the parameters in the SIRV model, which now takes the following form:

Equation 4.2.2. Stochastic model:

$$S_{t+1} = -\beta S_t I_t - \rho S_t$$

$$I_{t+1} = \beta S_t I_t - \gamma I_t$$

$$R_{t+1} = \gamma I_t$$

$$V_{t+1} = \rho S_t$$

4.2.2.5 Dynamic stochastic microsimulation

A microsimulation is an individual-based model "in which individual instantiations of a system—such as a patient's lifetime or the course of an epidemic—are generated using a random process to 'draw' from probability distributions a large number of times, in order to examine the central tendency and possibly the distribution of outcomes" (Weinstein, 2006). Some examples of dynamic stochastic microsimulations are:

- Monte Carlo simulations of a Markov model.
- Discrete-event simulation models.
- Agent-based models.

4.2.2.6 Discrete event simulation

Discrete event simulations assume that events occur at a discrete time interval, known as time steps, rather than at any time on a continuum as in a

continuous model. While a continuous model may provide more accurate results, the computational burden is large and such models are sometimes not
solvable. Thus, modelers often prefer to approximate continuous solutions
with discrete models. The time steps used often affect the model's results and
thus it is important to choose the interval carefully.

4.2.2.7 Agent-based models

The agent-based model is a type of dynamic microsimulation model and is
a class of model for simulating the actions and interactions of autonomous
agents with their own behavioral rules.

4.2.3 Data requirements for validation

It has been said that "all models are wrong, but some are useful" (Box, 1976).
However, if we are trying to provide scientific policy guidance such as an investment case for the introduction of a new vaccine, or a detailed comparison between vaccination strategies, it is critical to minimize the degree to
which our model is "wrong," and simultaneously maximize its "usefulness."
We want our infectious disease transmission model to be as close to reality as
possible—that is, the model must be validated against real-world data. Model
validation can employ a variety of different statistical techniques to compare
model-generated outputs to real data sets. The output generated by the models
described above includes cases (and possibly deaths) associated with the transmission of a given infectious disease within a specific setting. Thus, we need to
acquire location-specific case-count, disease incidence, or seroprevalence data
sets to use as our comparator in the model validation process. This can be historical reported disease cases, if the disease is reportable, and accounting for
potential underreporting, specific to that population. This level of data spec-
ificity can be difficult to find though. In the case in which population-specific
real-world data cannot be found, it may be appropriate to use another population or location, for which quality data is available, as a proxy—based on simi-
larity between the two populations in terms of demographic, social, economic,
and political characteristics, along with comparable structure of the respective
health systems.

The quality of data sets used for model validation is very important, as is
understanding the original source of the data and any manipulations that

have been made to it. If, for example, mortality was counted differently for populations under 80 years old than for those above 80 in the data set, this could prohibit any one-to-one comparison with model outputs unless similar age-specific transformation is applied to model-generated outcomes as well.

4.2.4 Examples of static and dynamic modeling for vaccination models

An example of static modeling is Atherly, Lewis, Tate, Parashar, and Rheingans' (2012) study that used a decision-analytic model to project the health outcomes and direct costs of introducing the rotavirus vaccination in GAVI-eligible countries during 2011–2030 (Atherly, Lewis, Tate, Parashar, & Rheingans, 2012). To estimate health outcomes, they used national estimates of rotavirus medical visits and deaths. They applied regional-specific vaccine efficacy rates to low- and lower-middle income countries as well as pooled random effects for countries with high child mortality rates (under-five mortality rates >30/1,000) to project cases averted. Scenario analyses were also conducted for variables with uncertainty and indirect effects (assuming herd immunity).

In another static modeling study, Sander et al. (2010) conducted a cost–utility analysis of the universal influenza immunization program in Canada. They used multivariate regression models to project influenza infections, controlling for age, sex, province, influenza surveillance, and temporal trends. They then estimated the reduction in infection rates with vaccination. They used this information to calculate quality-adjusted life years lost from influenza.

Two studies that use dynamic modeling are Khan et al.'s (2018) study on the introduction of an oral cholera vaccine in Dhaka, Bangladesh, and Burger, Sy, Nygård, Kristiansen, and Kim's (2015) study on the cost-effectiveness of a delayed catch-up program using the 4-valent human papillomavirus vaccine in Norway. Khan et al. estimated the impact of different vaccination targeting strategies in Dhaka, Bangladesh, with an SIR model of cholera transmission that simulates how a person can be infected by another individual or from the environment (Khan et al., 2018). Burger et al. used a model that simulates sexual mixing and HPV transmission among females and males to project which females will acquire an HPV-16 or -18 infection, the two types that cause 70% of cervical cancers (Burger et al., 2015). They also used a microsimulation model of cervical carcinogenesis to capture cervical cancer outcomes associated with all HPV types and screening strategies.

References

Atherly, D. E., Lewis, K. D., Tate, J., Parashar, U. D., & Rheingans, R. D. (2012). Projected health and economic impact of rotavirus vaccination in GAVI-eligible countries: 2011–2030. *Vaccine, 30*(Suppl 1), A7–A14. doi:10.1016/j.vaccine.2011.12.096

Box, G. E. P. (1976). Science and statistics. *Journal of the American Statistical Association, 71*(356), 791–799. doi:10.1080/01621459.1976.10480949

Burger, E. A., Sy, S., Nygård, M., Kristiansen, I. S., & Kim, J. J. (2015). Too late to vaccinate? The incremental benefits and cost-effectiveness of a delayed catch-up program using the 4-valent human papillomavirus vaccine in Norway. *Journal of Infectious Diseases, 211*(2), 206–215. doi:10.1093/infdis/jiu413

Khan, A. I., Levin, A., Chao, D. L., DeRoeck, D., Dimitrov, D. T., Khan, J. A. M.,... Qadri, F. (2018). The impact and cost-effectiveness of controlling cholera through the use of oral cholera vaccines in urban Bangladesh: A disease modeling and economic analysis. *PLOS Neglected Tropical Diseases, 12*(10), e0006652. doi:10.1371/journal.pntd.0006652

Kim, S. Y., & Goldie, S. J. (2008). Cost-effectiveness analyses of vaccination programmes: A focused review of modelling approaches. *PharmacoEconomics, 26*(3), 191–215. doi:10.2165/00019053-200826030-00004

Mossong, J., Hens, N., Jit, M., Beutels, P., Auranen, K., Mikolajczyk, R.,... Edmunds, W. J. (2008). Social contacts and mixing patterns relevant to the spread of infectious diseases. *PLOS Medicine, 5*(3), e74. doi:10.1371/journal.pmed.0050074

Nymark, L. S., Sharma, T., Miller, A., Enemark, U., & Griffiths, U. K. (2017). Inclusion of the value of herd immunity in economic evaluations of vaccines. A systematic review of methods used. *Vaccine, 35*(49 Pt B), 6828–6841. doi:10.1016/j.vaccine.2017.10.024

Prem, K., Cook, A. R., & Jit, M. (2017). Projecting social contact matrices in 152 countries using contact surveys and demographic data. *PLOS Computational Biology, 13*(9), e1005697. doi:10.1371/journal.pcbi.1005697

Sander, B., Kwong, J. C., Bauch, C. T., Maetzel, A., McGeer, A., Raboud, J. M., & Krahn, M. (2010). Economic appraisal of Ontario's Universal Influenza Immunization Program: A cost-utility analysis. *PLoS Medicine, 7*(4), e1000256. doi:10.1371/journal.pmed.1000256

Weinstein, M. C. (2006). Recent developments in decision-analytic modelling for economic evaluation. *PharmacoEconomics, 24*(11), 1043–1053. doi:10.2165/00019053-200624110-00002

World Health Organization: Immunization Vaccines and Biologicals. (2019). *WHO guide for standardization of economic evaluations of immunization programmes.* https://apps.who.int/iris/bitstream/handle/10665/329389/WHO-IVB-19.10-eng.pdf

4.3

Probabilistic sensitivity analysis and value of information analysis

Ciaran N. Kohli-Lynch

All research findings are subject to uncertainty. We never know the true efficacy of a vaccine, but rather a range of likely values based on observations from clinical trial and population health data. Uncertainty arises in clinical studies because data measurement and sampling are never perfect, leading to potential biases in study results. A variety of statistical methods have been developed to define reasonable "confidence intervals" for study results—or the potential variability around an expected value (e.g., the mean treatment effect of a vaccine). Like other areas of research, uncertainty exists in decision-analytic modelling. Three types of uncertainty are important to consider:

- Methodological uncertainty.
- Structural uncertainty.
- Parametric uncertainty.

This chapter reviews the impact of uncertainty on economic modeling. It focuses mainly on parametric uncertainty, given the impact that such uncertainty can have on estimates of vaccine value.

Parametric uncertainty refers to uncertainty around the inputs for a decision model. Decision-analytic modelling often involves synthesizing data from multiple studies. Inevitably, uncertainty in these input data propagates into modelling results. Probabilistic sensitivity analysis (PSA) quantifies the impact of parametric uncertainty on model outputs.

As discussed in Chapter 3.5, we can explore the impact of parametric uncertainty through deterministic sensitivity analysis. The Second Panel on Cost-Effectiveness in Health and Medicine notes that PSA is a more thorough approach for quantifying the uncertainty inherent in decision modelling

Ciaran N. Kohli-Lynch, *Probabilistic sensitivity analysis and value of information analysis* In: *Handbook of Applied Health Economics in Vaccines*. Edited by: David Bishai, Logan Brenzel and William V. Padula, Oxford University Press. © Oxford University Press 2023. DOI: 10.1093/oso/9780192896087.003.0024

(Sanders et al., 2016). It involves modelling parameter values as distributions rather than point estimates and running a model multiple times with input values stochastically sampled from these distributions. Value of information analysis produces actionable decisions based on the results of PSA. It quantifies the costs and benefits of investing in further research to reduce uncertainty in a decision.

4.3.1 Uncertainty in economic evaluation

Uncertainty in decision-analytic modelling can broadly be separated into three categories: methodological, structural, and parametric uncertainty (Bojke, Claxton, Sculpher, & Palmer, 2009; Briggs, 2000). These types of uncertainty arise through different processes and must be addressed differentially.

4.3.1.1 Methodological uncertainty

Methodological uncertainty refers to the fact that different analytic approaches may be adopted in a modelling study. Uncertainty in some model parameters does not arise due to imprecise data, but rather because of disagreement in the optimal approach needed to address a research question. This handbook has explored key analytic considerations when conducting an economic evaluation of a vaccination program. These include study perspective, inclusion of unrelated disease (or "background") costs, and the metric used to value health benefit (e.g., quality-adjusted life years (QALYs), disability-adjusted life years (DALYs) averted).

The aim of a healthcare decision maker is to choose which treatments to implement, given multiple options and a limited budget. Hence, decision modelling studies are most informative when they adhere to a common methodological approach that enables comparisons between multiple different interventions. Consistency in analytic approaches can be achieved by adopting a "reference case" of core analytic methodology (International Decision Support Initiative, 2017; National Institute for Health and Clinical Excellence, 2013; Sanders et al., 2016). Optimally, each decision maker would define their own reference case. Researchers can explore the impact and appropriateness of reference case criteria in sensitivity analyses.

4.3.1.2 Structural uncertainty

Structural uncertainty pertains to decisions made by researchers when constructing a decision model. These include the type of model employed (e.g., decision tree, Markov model, dynamic transmission model), the way transition probabilities are defined (e.g., fixed versus time-dependent probabilities), and the health states included in a model (e.g., health outcomes and clinical endpoints).

Cost-effectiveness analysis is often a complex process laden with assumptions. There is a constant trade-off between research time, computing efficiency, and model accuracy. Two researchers asked to analyze the same question with the same input data will likely produce different models. Neither model is likely to comprehensively track all patient outcomes, but they may capture the outcomes of greatest interest, economic impact, or epidemiologic burden.

The solutions for dealing with structural uncertainty are demanding. The Second Panel on Cost-Effectiveness in Health and Medicine proposes that structural uncertainty can be reduced by tasking multiple research teams with model development and averaging outcomes across different models (Sanders et al., 2016). This is clearly a resource-intensive process and determining weights to apply to different models is difficult. It is sometimes possible to "parameterize" sources of structural uncertainty. Imagine there is uncertainty regarding whether a health state should be included in a Markov model. This health state could be included conditional on a probability which aligns with the researchers' prior beliefs that it is an important part of the disease pathway.

4.3.1.3 Parametric uncertainty

Parametric uncertainty relates to uncertainty in the input parameters for a model. Estimates of parameters will inevitably be imprecise. Costs, health state valuations, and probabilities are all sources of parametric uncertainty. Any value which is estimated through observational or experimental means, such as a cohort study or clinical trial, can be described as a *random variable*. Because these variables are estimated through partly random processes, like the process of recruiting a generalizable cohort, there is inherent uncertainty in their true value.

Model inputs are often derived from published literature (see Chapter 3.3). Greenhalgh (1997) provides a hierarchy for the reliability, validity, and generalizability of published data. In descending order, Greenhalgh's hierarchy includes:

- Systematic reviews and meta-analyses of randomized controlled trials.
- Randomized controlled trials with definitive results.
- Randomized controlled trials with non-definitive results.
- Cohort studies.
- Case–control studies.
- Cross-sectional surveys.
- Case reports.

In research areas with little quantitative data, expert opinion may be included at the end of this list (Leal, Wordsworth, Legood, & Blair, 2007). Deriving model inputs from any of these methods will introduce parametric uncertainty into the decision modelling process.

Published studies often present a point estimate, or expected value for the value of a parameter, alongside a confidence interval (CI). The point estimate of random variable X can be referred to as its expected value, $E[X]$. In a sample of random variables, the arithmetic mean, often represented by $\bar{x}$, is an unbiased estimator of $E[X]$. The CI represents a plausible range for the true value of the parameter. It describes uncertainty in the point estimate and is a function of the variance of a random variable. The sample variance, s^2, is an unbiased estimator of the population variance, σ^2.

Clinical research cannot establish the true value of a parameter due to "sampling" and "non-sampling" errors. Sampling errors exist because most clinical research elicits information from a subset of the total population of interest. A randomized controlled trial for a new vaccine will only recruit a small proportion of the potential patient population. It is therefore impossible to establish what the exact treatment effect would be in the overall population. Non-sampling errors arise due to imperfectly conducted research. Survey answers may be misunderstood, data collection may be incomplete, anthropomorphic variables may be incorrectly measured, and data may be incorrectly processed.

The CI indicates the likely range for the value of a parameter. For example, a meta-analysis by Cochrane synthesized results from randomized controlled trials of vaccination against human papillomaviruses in young women to prevent cervical precancer (Arbyn, Xu, Simoens, & Martin-Hirsch, 2018). They found that the relative risk of precancer for young women receiving the human papillomavirus vaccine versus placebo was 0.05 with a 95% CI of 0.03–0.10.

With 95% confidence, they state that the true relative risk in the studied population lies between 0.03 and 0.10. Using the point estimate as a parameter in a decision modelling study would disregard this acknowledged uncertainty.

Parametric uncertainty should not be confused with subgroup-level variability. The former refers to uncertainty in the true value of a parameter for a population. The latter refers to real differences in parameters that exist between patient subgroups (Kohli-Lynch & Briggs, 2019). When there is reason to believe that parameters vary based on identifiable patient characteristics (e.g., age, sex, presence of biomarker), decision analysis should be conducted separately for each subgroup (Sculpher, 2008).

4.3.2 Probabilistic sensitivity analysis

It is important to reflect parametric uncertainty in decision modelling studies. Failing to address this uncertainty will bias cost-effectiveness estimates. Additionally, quantifying uncertainty allows researchers to assess the benefits of obtaining more information regarding model inputs. A standard approach for dealing with uncertainty in decision modelling studies is to conduct PSA.

4.3.2.1 Basic concept

PSA involves running a decision model multiple times. Each run of the model can be referred to as an *iteration*. Key parameters are not included in the model as unitary values when conducting a PSA. Instead, parameters are included as draws from probability distributions. Probability distributions are functions that assign probabilities to the range of possible values that the variable can assume, based on the likelihood that they are the true value. For example, the probability distribution for a fair coin toss would be a function that assigns a probability of 0.5 to outcome "heads" and a probability of 0.5 to outcome "tails." The standard normal distribution, shown in Fig. 4.3.1, is another probability distribution. It has a mean value of 0 and a standard deviation of 1, with dispersion around the mean described by a mathematical formula. Similar distributions, often with a different mean and standard deviation, are commonly used to describe biomedical phenomena.

Using a probability distribution rather than a point estimate to represent a model parameter acknowledges the fact that there is uncertainty surrounding the true value of the parameter. Every time the model is run in a

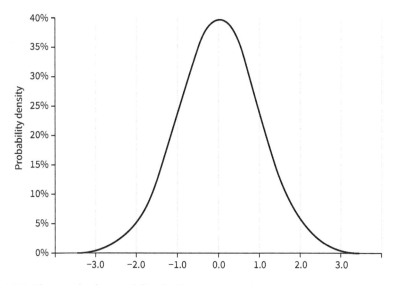

Fig. 4.3.1 The standard normal distribution.

PSA, a different set of parametric inputs are probabilistically sampled from their respective distributions. The process of running the model repeatedly with probabilistically sampled inputs is called "Monte Carlo simulation." At the end of each run, model outcomes (e.g., QALYs, DALYs averted, costs) are recorded. Mean cost-effectiveness is then calculated by averaging across all recorded outcomes. The multiple estimates produced during a PSA enable estimation of confidence intervals for model outputs.

Consider the model shown in Fig. 4.3.2, adapted from a cost-effectiveness analysis of the seasonal influenza vaccine in South Africa (Edoka et al., 2021). This decision tree model estimates the cost-effectiveness of vaccinating elderly individuals. There is considerable uncertainty in many of the parameters that determine the cost-effectiveness of the vaccination program. Unvaccinated elderly individuals have a 3.2% (95% CI 1.4–5.6%) probability of developing seasonal influenza, a 4.4% (95% CI 1.8–7.8%) probability of dying if they contract the disease, and incur a loss of 0.031 QALYs (95% CI 0.025–0.037 QALYs) if they develop severe influenza. A vaccine is available with 58% (95% CI 34–73%) effectiveness.

Deterministic analysis refers to running a decision model with point estimate inputs. When we evaluate the seasonal influenza model deterministically, we estimate that the vaccination program would produce 294 QALYs at a cost of around $615,000 (USD in 2018). This leads to an incremental cost-effectiveness ratio (ICER) of around $2,090/QALY and is displayed on

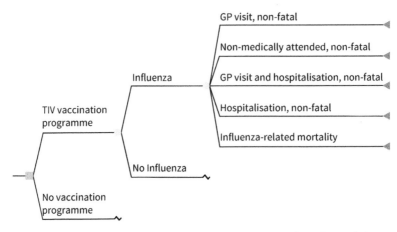

Fig. 4.3.2 Decision tree model, seasonal influenza vaccination for elderly adults in South Africa. TIV, trivalent inactivated influenza vaccine.

Source: Reprinted from *Vaccine*, *39*(2), Edoka, I., Kohli-Lynch, C. N., Fraser, H., Hofman, K., Tempia, S., McMorrow, M.,... Cohen, C., A cost-effectiveness analysis of South Africa's seasonal influenza vaccination programme, 412–422, (2021), with permission from Elsevier.

the cost-effectiveness plane with a black cross (Fig. 4.3). South Africa's cost-effectiveness threshold should be $3,040/QALY according to recent research (Edoka & Stacey, 2020). This threshold is shown on the cost-effectiveness plane. As the deterministic estimate of cost-effectiveness lies below the threshold, it should be implemented based on this result.

We could also run the seasonal influenza model probabilistically. The cloud of red spots on Fig. 4.3.3 shows the results of 1,000 PSA iterations. In each iteration, input parameters for the model were pulled from respective probability distributions and led to varying estimates for the cost-effectiveness of the vaccine. Using PSA, uncertainty in the model inputs has been propagated into the model outputs and we gain a greater understanding of the uncertainty inherent in the decision-making process. Additionally, the average cost-effectiveness across the 1,000 PSA iterations will vary, albeit marginally, from the deterministic outcome of the model.

While there is no objective means of determining how many iterations are required to produce accurate estimates with a PSA, it is common to run a model several thousand times. Ultimately, the number of iterations chosen should reduce any uncertainty that arises simply due to the Monte Carlo simulation (Hatswell, Bullement, Briggs, Paulden, & Stevenson, 2018). There should be "model convergence" whereby PSAs with the same number of iterations produce similar mean outputs.

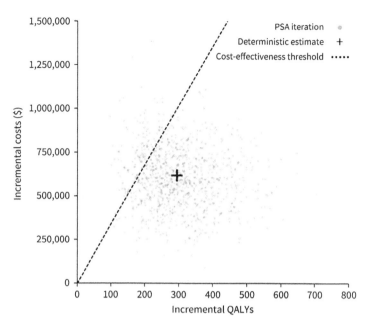

Fig. 4.3.3 Cost-effectiveness scatter plot with deterministic and probabilistic results.

4.3.2.2 Purpose of probabilistic sensitivity analysis

Most clinical research relies on statistical tests to validate findings. While these tests vary, researchers typically strive to prove that their findings have a type-1 error rate of 5% or lower (i.e., p-value <0.05), meaning they have 95% confidence that the null hypothesis of a study can be rejected. In most clinical studies, the null hypothesis states that some new treatment is equally as effective as a comparator. If an effect is observed with a p-value less than 0.05, there is strong evidence of a difference in effect between the treatment and comparator. Confidence intervals and p-values can be derived for cost-effectiveness estimates in decision modelling studies through PSA.

One use of a PSA is to determine whether we can reject the null hypothesis that two treatment options are equally cost-effective. Regulatory bodies often require that manufacturers of novel healthcare products prove that a treatment is efficacious before approving it for widespread use. Healthcare payers may be similarly loath to fund an intervention if they are not confident that it is more cost-effective than established comparators.

Claxton (1999) argues that arbitrary hurdles like the statistical tests described above should be avoided when deciding whether to implement a healthcare intervention. If a healthcare decision maker must choose between a new intervention and standard care, they should implement the intervention which is most cost-effective according to a central cost-effectiveness estimate, regardless of uncertainty. It is pure historical happenstance that determines which option from a set of competing interventions is currently considered standard care. While some decisions will inevitably be incorrect, the net effect of this approach will be that net benefit in the population is maximized.

The Arrow–Lind principle states that, under certain circumstances, the cost of investing in social programs with some uncertainty in outcome tends to 0 as the population becomes very large (Arrow & Lind, 1970). This supports the idea that healthcare decision makers should base decisions on central estimates when evaluating investment opportunities when the risk of an incorrect decision is spread over a large population.

If a central estimate of cost-effectiveness is sufficient to inform healthcare decision-making, regardless of its confidence interval, it is worth considering the necessity and relevance of PSA. Expected cost-effectiveness results derived from deterministic analysis are often biased. Conducting a PSA helps correct this bias and produce an accurate estimate of cost-effectiveness. Beyond improving model accuracy, PSA also provides information regarding uncertainty in the estimates produced by a decision model. This information can be used to elicit the probability of making an incorrect decision based on model results and estimate the value of reducing uncertainty in the decision.

Consider the results shown in Fig. 4.3.3. The central estimate for the ICER is below the cost-effectiveness threshold. Based on this result, the treatment should be implemented. However, 21% of PSA simulations are above the threshold. Accordingly, there is a 21% chance that a decision based on the central estimate will be incorrect and the vaccine will not be cost-effective for elderly individuals in South Africa. Further research to reduce this uncertainty may be desirable.

4.3.2.3 Expected cost-effectiveness

When we evaluate a decision model, we are interested in its *expected value*. All decision models are essentially functions; that is, they are mathematical operators that accept a range of inputs which they combine to estimate outputs (e.g., health and cost outcomes). To calculate the expected value of a function,

$g(x)$, we must evaluate the function at each possible value of input variable, x. Next, we weight each outcome by the likelihood that it is the true parameter value and sum across all potential inputs.

The process of calculating the expected value of a function with continuous inputs can be presented mathematically as follows: $E[g(X)] = \int g(x)p(x)dx$. The function $p(x)$ is a probability distribution, outlining all the possible values that the random variable x may assume and the likelihood that they are the true parameter value. A random variable x is described as *discrete* when it has countable number of possible values. The expected value of a function of a discrete random variable can be estimated as $E[g(x)] = \sum_x p(x)g(x)$. More generally, the expected value of function $g(X)$ of any random variable x can be expressed as $E_x[g(X)]$.

For most decision models, evaluating $E_x[g(X)]$ is very difficult. Even simple models represent long, complicated functions with multiple interacting parameters. We can estimate the expected outcome of a model by running a PSA. This imitates the process described in the calculations above. We assess the output of the model at a range of input values which are sampled from probability distributions. The distributions are chosen to ensure that likely values are sampled more frequently than unlikely values. As we increase the number of PSA runs and average over observed outcomes, our cost-effectiveness estimate tends towards the expected value of the model.

Depending on the complexity of a decision model, we may be able to use non-probabilistic methods to obtain an unbiased estimate for the expected value of the model. The scale and complexity of decision models vary greatly, from simple decision trees to complex microsimulation and discrete event simulation models and beyond. The least complicated decision models, including some worksheet-based models and decision trees, are "linear in their input variables." This means that the model can be expressed as a series of terms added together. An example of a simple linear function is $g(X) = mX + c$, where X is a random variable with expected value $E[X]$ and m and c are constant. A common proof in mathematics shows that the expected value of a linear function is equal to the value of the function evaluated at the expected value of its parameters. Mathematically, $E_x[g(X)] = g(E[x])$. For our purposes, this means that some simple decision models can be run deterministically without biasing results. Running a PSA adds no additional information regarding the expected cost-effectiveness of an intervention in this scenario.

Most decision-analytic models are nonlinear in their input variables. They cannot be expressed as a simple linear function. Rather, they represent complicated, multivariate functions where parameters combine multiplicatively and in power relations. Even the simplest Markov models quickly become nonlinear as transition probabilities must be cross-multiplied and combined as powers to estimate outcomes. Unlike linear models, the expected value of a linear function is not equal to the value of the function evaluated at the expected value of its parameters. Mathematically, $E_x[g(X)] \neq g(E[x])$. Hence, plugging point estimates for parameters into a nonlinear decision model produces biased estimates. It is important to recognize that running a nonlinear model deterministically is unlikely to cause large biases in model results; $E_x[g(X)]$ rarely differs greatly from $g(E[x])$. Nonetheless, using probabilistic methods is mathematically more accurate.

4.3.2.4 Making models probabilistic

Conducting a PSA involves running a model several times with different input parameters. Values for parameters are chosen by sampling from probability distributions. Suitable distributions for parameters should be defined with consideration for the point estimate of the parameter, its variance, and logical constraints on the values that it can take.

Many types of probability distributions exist. Key among these is the normal distribution, shown in Fig. 4.3.1. Values for this distribution are distributed symmetrically around the population mean and decrease in frequency as they move away from the mean. While other distributions share these characteristics, the normal distribution is important as it describes a wide range of natural phenomena. Indeed, according to the *central limit theorem*, the normal distribution describes the sampling distribution of the mean of any set of random variables with a sufficient sample size. In practice, few parameters are derived from large enough samples to justify using the normal distribution to describe their distribution in a PSA.

Often logical data constraints make it preferable to employ alternatives to the normal distribution in PSA. Fig. 4.3.4 displays an illustrative histogram of influenza vaccine costs observed in a fictional South African costing study with 1,000 observations. Similar data were used to inform this parameter in the seasonal influenza vaccine model. Most vaccines cost less than $5.00, but some payers spent significantly more per dose. Such price variation is common in multi-payer markets where large insurers can negotiate discounts from listed prices when buying products in bulk. The observed

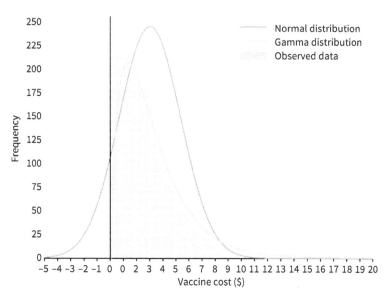

Fig. 4.3.4 Influenza vaccine cost, normal distribution, and gamma distribution.

vaccine cost data are *skewed*, meaning they are not symmetrically distributed around the mean. If we use descriptive statistics from this dataset to produce a normal distribution, it will not provide an accurate model for the skewed data.

A normal distribution is depicted by the red curve on Fig. 4.3.4. It was constructed using the mean ($3.00) and standard error ($2.34) from the vaccine cost data and is scaled to estimate the frequency of different costs expected in a cohort of 1,000 observations. This distribution assigns non-negative likelihood to negative costs. Negative unit vaccine costs are impossible; no benevolent manufacturer is paying insurers to provide the seasonal influenza vaccine in South Africa. We must find an alternative distribution to describe this parameter. The alternative distribution would preferably maintain the observed mean and variance from the data but must not allow sampling of negative unit costs.

While many distributions can be employed to describe uncertainty in a random variable, the choice of distribution for a parameter in a decision model is often straightforward. The core parameters in most decision models relate to costs, utilities, probabilities, and treatment effect sizes. Each of these parameter types is well described by a limited number of common distributions. Appendix 6 includes a detailed description of some candidate distributions for different types of parameters. In addition, it describes how distributions can be operationalized when conducting PSA in Microsoft Excel.

4.3.2.5 Interpreting probabilistic sensitivity analysis results

Once a PSA has been conducted, there are several ways to report its results. These include reporting expected values derived from simulations, reporting uncertainty intervals for estimates, and visually presenting results in scatter plots and cost-effectiveness acceptability curves.

4.3.2.5.1 Expected outcomes and confidence intervals

Results from a PSA can be used to compute the expected value of a model. Effectively, this involves averaging over all model outcomes recorded in the PSA. As discussed in Chapter 2.3, computing the expected value of the model through PSA produces an unbiased estimate of model outcomes. In the seasonal influenza example, the 95% CI for QALYs gained from vaccination in elderly individuals was 140–525. The 95% CI for costs was $282,000–$939,000.

Net monetary benefit (NMB) is a more useful measure than the ICER for representing uncertainty in cost-effectiveness estimates. ICERs are not continuously defined. If no change in outcome is observed, the denominator is 0 and the ICER is undefined. In addition, two ICERs may have very different interpretations. Negative ICERs can represent cost-saving or dominated treatment strategies. Finally, when analyzing multiple treatment strategies, the relative ranking of strategies may vary in ICER calculations. NMB has the benefit of being linear and continuously defined. Additionally, when comparing the NMB of multiple treatment strategies, the option with the highest value is always the most cost-effective.

4.3.2.5.2 Cost-effectiveness scatter plots

Cost-effectiveness scatter plots are a visual means of presenting the results from a PSA. These are cost-effectiveness planes with the outcomes of all PSA iterations presented together. It is common to present all results incremental to a standard comparator, which is represented at the origin of the figure. Fig. 4.3.3 shows the cost-effectiveness scatter plot for the seasonal influenza vaccine example.

When two interventions are being considered, we can directly calculate the probability that an intervention is cost-effective through observation of the cost-effectiveness scatter plot. First, we plot a cost-effectiveness threshold on a scatter plot of incremental costs and incremental QALYs for an intervention versus a comparator. Next, we count the number of PSA iterations that lie below the cost-effectiveness threshold. In Fig. 4.3, 81% of PSA iterations produced cost-effectiveness estimates below a threshold of $3,040/QALY. We can infer that the treatment has an 81% probability of being cost-effective. While the process is slightly more complicated for multiple treatment options, the general process is the same. In this situation, using NMB to represent cost-effectiveness simplifies the calculation.

There is typically some relationship between costs and effects in a decision modelling study. For example, if a treatment successfully prevents disease-related events it may also reduce costs associated with these events. This means that we cannot infer the uncertainty in cost-effectiveness directly from the confidence intervals for costs and effects. Instead, we need to represent the joint density of costs and effects. Visually, uncertainty in cost-effectiveness can be represented with confidence ellipses around points on a cost-effectiveness scatter plot, fitted using a system of equations that account for potential correlations between costs and effects (Briggs, O'Brien, & Blackhouse, 2002; Nixon, Wonderling, & Grieve, 2010).

4.3.2.5.3 Cost-effectiveness acceptability curves

Suppose that the cost-effectiveness threshold in Fig. 4.3.3 was increased to $5,000/QALY. More PSA iterations would now fall below the threshold on the cost-effectiveness scatter plot. Our estimated probability of the treatment being cost-effectiveness would increase. Intuitively, this makes sense: the more a decision maker is willing to pay for an increase in health, the likelier a novel treatment which improves health will be cost-effective.

It is often informative to show the likelihood that a treatment is cost-effective over a range of different cost-effectiveness thresholds. We can count the number of PSA iterations for a treatment that are cost-effective at a range of different thresholds and present these graphically. This graph is called a *cost-effectiveness acceptability curve*. Fig. 4.3.5 shows the cost-effectiveness acceptability curve for vaccinating elderly individuals in South Africa against seasonal influenza. A threshold of $3,040/QALY is represented on the cost-effectiveness acceptability curve by a dashed line. As noted previously, vaccinating this population has an 81% probability of being cost-effective at this threshold.

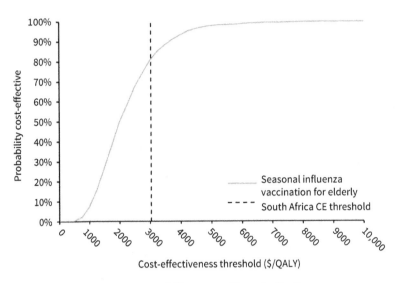

Fig. 4.3.5 Cost-effectiveness acceptability curve. CE, cost-effectiveness.

4.3.3 Value of information analysis

The results from a PSA can be used to estimate the value of further re-search. There will always be some uncertainty surrounding decisions to implement new health technologies. Reducing this uncertainty lowers the likelihood that a decision maker will implement a treatment that is not cost-effective or reject one that is cost-effective. Value of information analysis quantifies the gains in expected health benefit associated with re-duced uncertainty.

Three measures are fundamental in value of information analysis. These are expected value of perfect information (EVPI), expected value of perfect parameter information (EVPPI), and expected value of sample information (EVSI). This section will describe each of these measures and how they can be used to inform healthcare decision-making.

As a motivating example, consider a football team that needs to score more goals and decides to recruit a new striker. They have two potential signings on their shortlist. Club statisticians use data from previous seasons to estimate how many goals each striker will score in the upcoming season. Some uncer-tainty will surround each of these estimates, driven by variables which can be studied (e.g., age, fitness, form). If the club recruited a clairvoyant manager, they could spend their money on the player who will definitely score the most goals.[1] There may be some benefit in resolving uncertainty in one specific parameter. For example, perfect information regarding each player's future injury risk would be beneficial. Finally, even without perfect information, collecting additional information on each player's fitness would be useful as it would ultimately reduce uncertainty in expected goals scored. These three options align with the concepts of EVPI, EVPPI, and EVSI, respectively.

4.3.3.1 Expected value of perfect information

The EVPI refers to the amount of money a decision maker would pay for all uncertainty in a decision to be resolved. A clairvoyant decision maker will always make correct implementation decisions. Hence, they avoid any losses associated with incorrect decision-making.

When choosing which of multiple mutually exclusive treatments to implement, a decision maker must consider the expected cost-effectiveness of these treatments. With current, imperfect information, it is possible that an incorrect decision will be made. This would occur if the most cost-effective treatment was not implemented. A decision maker with perfect information will always implement the most cost-effective treatment.

When assessing multiple interventions, there is uncertainty around model parameters. A set of different eventualities exists. Each combination of model parameters reflects a different eventuality. Only one of these eventualities is the true state of the world. Depending on the eventuality modelled, the relative cost-effectiveness of the interventions will vary. In each eventuality, only one intervention will be optimal. A decision maker with perfect information knows which eventuality will occur and will always choose to implement the optimal treatment strategy for this situation. A decision maker with imperfect information will choose to implement the treatment with the highest expected cost-effectiveness, weighted by the probability of each eventuality occurring.

The mathematical procedure for estimating EVPI is outlined in Appendix 6. It involves probabilistically running a model multiple times and simulating the decisions that would be made by decision makers with current and perfect information.

---

[1] Such a clairvoyant manager has not been on the job market since Martin O'Neill managed the Celtic football team in Glasgow, Scotland, from 2000 to 2005 taking the team to win 75% of its games.

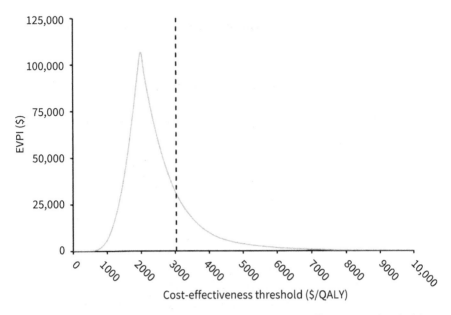

Fig. 4.3.6 Expected value of perfect information versus cost-effectiveness threshold.

Fig. 4.3.6 shows the EVPI for the South African seasonal influenza vaccine program at different cost-effectiveness thresholds. A threshold of \$3,040/QALY is represented by a dashed line. The EVPI is near 0 when the threshold is near 0 because there is strong certainty that the vaccination program will generate incremental costs. At low thresholds, QALY gains are assigned little value and it is unlikely that an expensive new treatment will be cost-effective. Therefore, the expected NMB of not vaccinating, $E(NMB_{no\ vaccine})$, is greater than expected NMB of the vaccination program, $E(NMB_{vaccine})$. The decision maker with current information will reject the program and current information is adequate to support this decision.

We know that the vaccine likely produces health benefits and as the threshold increases, these benefits are assigned higher value. Hence, the probability that the vaccination program is cost-effective will increase as the threshold increases. While the threshold remains low (below \$2,090/QALY) but increases, the decision maker with current information will still choose not to implement the vaccination program. As the threshold grows, health gains are assigned more value and the possibility that this decision is incorrect grows. Accordingly, the value of obtaining more information grows.

An inflection point occurs at a threshold of \$2,090/QALY, the ICER associated with the vaccination program. At this threshold, $E(NMB_{vaccine})$ becomes larger than $E(NMB_{no\ vaccine})$ and the decision maker with current information will choose to implement the vaccination program. As the threshold increases beyond the inflection point, health benefits are assigned progressively greater value and the probability that implementing the vaccination program was cost-ineffective falls. Hence the possibility of an incorrect decision with current information declines alongside the value of additional research.

The EVPI can help determine whether a decision maker should fund additional research. Future research will reduce the gap between expected NMB with perfect information and expected NMB with current information. Spending more than EVPI on this research will lead to an expected net loss in population health. If EVPI is greater than the proposed cost of a study, then the research funds would be better spent elsewhere in the healthcare budget. We can therefore regard EVPI as an upper bound that a healthcare decision maker should spend on a research project regarding a treatment decision.

The EVPI associated with a healthcare decision does not imply a cost at which research should be pursued. It is necessary but not sufficient that further research costs less than the EVPI. For the seasonal influenza vaccine in South Africa, a decision maker may desire additional information on the cost-effectiveness of vaccinating elderly individuals. According to Fig. 4.3.6, the EVPI is approximately $31,000 at a cost-effectiveness threshold of $3,040/QALY. If the cost required to conduct a proposed trial is below this value, a decision maker cannot not rule out conducting the research. The sample size for a trial of that cost may be too small to plausibly change a treatment decision. Further information, namely the EVSI of the proposed study, is required before pursuing this study.

4.3.3.2 Expected value of perfect parameter information

Clinical research generally focuses on a small set of parameters rather than the entire uncertainty in a treatment decision. Randomized controlled trials of new vaccines generally examine the efficacy or effectiveness of a vaccine. Some studies focus on alternative parameters (e.g., costs, adverse events). Hence, research typically reduces uncertainty in a limited number of parameters. The EVPPI quantifies the expected value associated with removing one source of uncertainty from the decision-making calculus.

Conceptually, EVPPI is very similar to EVPI; it is equal to the difference between expected NMB with perfect parameter information and the expected

NMB with current information. The expected NMB with perfect parameter information is equal to the expected NMB for a decision maker with perfect information regarding some proper subset of the decision-making parameters. The mathematical formulation of EVPPI is presented in Appendix 6.

If there are multiple sources of uncertainty in a healthcare decision, calculating the EVPPI for various uncertain parameters may help guide future research. The parameter with the highest EVPPI is the parameter which would be most beneficial to have complete information on. Of course, it may be more costly to study some parameters than others.

As before, the EVPPI associated with a decision provides an upper bound to the resources that should be expended on future research. If a randomized controlled trial which assesses the effectiveness of a vaccine will cost less than the EVPPI, a decision maker should not necessarily fund this trial. Estimating EVSI would help to determine whether the research should be pursued.

4.3.3.3 Expected value of sample information

The EVPI and EVPPI associated with a decision estimate the maximum amount of money that should be spent on new research. Simply costing less than EVPI and EVPPI is not sufficient to justify funding a new study. Collecting additional information will not eliminate uncertainty in a decision but will increase the likelihood that the most cost-effective treatment strategy will be adopted. The EVSI estimates the value of pursuing a specific new research study, dependent on an expected reduction in uncertainty. This estimate can be used to determine how much money should be spent on a new study.

The EVSI represents the gain in NMB that a decision maker expects to achieve with new information. It is equal to the difference between the expected NMB with current information and the expected NMB with sample information. The process for calculating expected NMB with sample information is outlined in Appendix 6. It accounts for existing levels of uncertainty and the type of data being collected by a proposed study.

References

Arbyn, M., Xu, L., Simoens, C., & Martin-Hirsch, P. P. (2018). Prophylactic vaccination against human papillomaviruses to prevent cervical cancer and its precursors. *Cochrane Database of Systematic Reviews, 5*(5), CD009069. doi:10.1002/14651858.CD009069.pub3

Arrow, K., & Lind, R. C. (1970). Uncertainty and the evaluation of public investment decisions. *American Economic Review, 60*(3), 364–378. https://EconPapers.repec.org/RePEc:aea:aec rev:v:60:y:1970:i:3:p:364-78

Bojke, L., Claxton, K., Sculpher, M., & Palmer, S. (2009). Characterizing structural uncertainty in decision analytic models: A review and application of methods. *Value in Health, 12*(5), 739–749. doi:10.1111/j.1524-4733.2008.00502.x

Briggs, A. (2000). Handling uncertainty in cost-effectiveness models. *PharmacoEconomics, 17*(5), 479–500. doi:10.2165/00019053-200017050-00006

Briggs, A., O'Brien, B. J., & Blackhouse, G. (2002). Thinking outside the box: Recent advances in the analysis and presentation of uncertainty in cost-effectiveness studies. *Annual Review of Public Health, 23*, 377–401. doi:10.1146/annurev.publhealth.23.100901.140534

Claxton, K. (1999). The irrelevance of inference: A decision-making approach to the stochastic evaluation of health care technologies. *Journal of Health Economics, 18*(3), 341–364. doi:10.1016/s0167-6296(98)00039-3

Edoka, I., Kohli-Lynch, C. N., Fraser, H., Hofman, K., Tempia, S., McMorrow, M.,… Cohen, C. (2021). A cost-effectiveness analysis of South Africa's seasonal influenza vaccination programme. *Vaccine, 39*(2), 412–422. doi:10.1016/j.vaccine.2020.11.028

Edoka, I., & Stacey, N. K. (2020). Estimating a cost-effectiveness threshold for health care decision-making in South Africa. *Health Policy and Planning, 35*(5), 546–555. doi:10.1093/heapol/czz152

Greenhalgh, T. (1997). How to read a paper: Getting your bearings (deciding what the paper is about). *BMJ, 315*(7102), 243. doi:10.1136/bmj.315.7102.243

Hatswell, A. J., Bullement, A., Briggs, A., Paulden, M., & Stevenson, M. D. (2018). Probabilistic sensitivity analysis in cost-effectiveness models: Determining model convergence in cohort models. *PharmacoEconomics, 36*(12), 1421–1426. https://EconPapers.repec.org/RePEc:spr:pharme:v:36:y:2018:i:12:d:10.1007_s40273-018-0697-3

International Decision Support Initiative. (2017). *IDSI reference case for economic evaluation.* https://www.idsihealth.org/resource-items/idsi-reference-case-for-economic-evaluation

Kohli-Lynch, C. N., & Briggs, A. H. (2019). *Heterogeneity in cost-effectiveness analysis.* Oxford: Oxford University Press.

Leal, J., Wordsworth, S., Legood, R., & Blair, E. (2007). Eliciting expert opinion for economic models: An applied example. *Value in Health, 10*(3), 195–203. doi:10.1111/j.1524-4733.2007.00169.x

National Institute for Health and Clinical Excellence. (2013). *Guide to the methods of technology appraisal 2013.* https://www.nice.org.uk/process/pmg9/resources/guide-to-the-methods-of-technology-appraisal-2013-pdf-2007975843781

Nixon, R., Wonderling, D., & Grieve, R. (2010). Non-parametric methods for cost-effectiveness analysis: The central limit theorem and the bootstrap compared. *Health Economics, 19*, 316–333. doi:10.1002/hec.1477

Sanders, G. D., Neumann, P. J., Basu, A., Brock, D. W., Feeny, D., Krahn, M.,… Ganiats, T. G. (2016). Recommendations for conduct, methodological practices, and reporting of cost-effectiveness analyses: Second Panel on Cost-Effectiveness in Health and Medicine. *JAMA, 316*(10), 1093–1103. doi:10.1001/jama.2016.12195

Sculpher, M. (2008). Subgroups and heterogeneity in cost-effectiveness analysis. *PharmacoEconomics, 26*(9), 799–806. doi:10.2165/00019053-200826090-00009

4.4

Economic evaluation reference case with Markov model

William V. Padula, Shreena Malaviya, Natalie M. Reid, Jonothan Tierce, and G. Caleb Alexander

Sometimes the best way to understand the use of a classical infectious disease Markov model such as the *Susceptible–Exposed–Infected–Recovered* (SEIR) framework is to see it applied to an actual example.

This chapter draws material from an earlier technical report based on a model developed in the early phases of the coronavirus disease 2019 (COVID-19) outbreak in the US to better under the value of vaccines relative to treatments. The data in the model were calibrated to reach the date of September 22, 2020 when the US surpassed the grim milestone of 200,000 deaths from COVID-19. Although this infectious disease has had a prolonged and profound fatal impact on societies worldwide, these early epidemiologic data combined with our understanding of the economics of vaccines provide some valuable information on the opportunity costs avoided with the introduction of a vaccine.

This chapter illustrates some of the conceptual elements of a typical cost-effectiveness analysis of a vaccine being considered for adoption. The full technical report is available on SSRN as report number 358664 entitled, "Economic value of treatment and vaccine to address the COVID-19 pandemic: A U.S. cost-effectiveness and budget impact analysis."

4.4.1 Introduction

The severe acute respiratory syndrome coronavirus 2 (SARS-CoV-2) virus causing COVID-19 rapidly transmitted through nearly 200 countries, infected hundreds of millions of individuals, and resulted in millions of deaths since its onset in China in late 2019. While dozens of countries were heavily impacted,

William V. Padula, Shreena Malaviya, Natalie M. Reid, Jonothan Tierce, and G. Caleb Alexander, *Economic evaluation reference case with Markov model* In: *Handbook of Applied Health Economics in Vaccines*. Edited by: David Bishai, Logan Brenzel and William V. Padula, Oxford University Press. © Oxford University Press 2023. DOI: 10.1093/oso/9780192896087.003.0025 the US has experienced one of the highest levels of early-onset morbidity and mortality from the pandemic, with over 4 million individuals infected and over 200,000 succumbing from COVID-19 as of September 22, 2020 (Johns Hopkins Coronavirus Resource Center, 2020). Widely cited projections available in September 2020 suggested that circumstances would worsen before they improved (Institute for Health Metrics & Evaluation, 2020).

The magnitude of morbidity and mortality from the pandemic, as well as its economic impact and effect on all sectors of society, galvanized the scientific community and unleashed enormous activity devoted to identifying treatments that reduce viral replication or host response, as well as vaccines that ultimately diminish viral transmissibility. A review of World Health Organization and US clinical trial registries revealed over 300 clinical trials testing the therapeutic benefits of 92 drugs or plasma against COVID-19, including 64 in monotherapy and 28 different combinations (J. M. Sanders, Monogue, Jodlowski, & Cutrell, 2020) by late 2020. Vaccines to protect against COVID-19 infection (Park, 2020), were presumed an important tool in COVID-19 control.

Treatments and vaccines offer different value propositions. Treatments reduce the downstream disease burden on the health system and are only taken on an as-needed basis. Yet, they are only useful among those who become infected, they do not prevent the initial spread of infection, especially among asymptomatic carriers, and they typically require a provider's prescription.

Vaccines are valued differently. Vaccines should be given to as many who have access and are highly vulnerable. As the number of vaccinated people grows, non-vaccinated individuals benefit through herd immunity (Mauskopf et al., 2018). Vaccines have the benefit of preventing the downstream effects of disease, keeping societies more productive and worry free, and reducing the need for isolating social measures. However, vaccines are often not as efficiently targeted as treatments in the sense that they must be given to many individuals who never would have contracted the disease, leading to high upfront costs for governments and payers that invest in their coverage (Carvalho, Jit, Cox, Yoong, & Hutubessy, 2018).

Despite the catastrophic nature of the COVID-19 pandemic and the unprecedented scientific effort to address it, the relative value of a treatment or vaccine for COVID-19 had not been immediately characterized (Apuzzo & Kirkpatrick, 2020). We quantified this value using economic modelling based on rates of COVID-19 infection in the US as of September 22, 2020. This approach can be used to generate fundamental new knowledge regarding the economic value of vaccines for infectious disease outbreak with respect to commonly assumed alternatives (e.g., acute treatment, social distancing measures).

4.4.2 Methods

4.4.2.1 Study design

We developed a Markov model to evaluate the cost-effectiveness of disruptive strategies developed in response to the COVID-19 pandemic. We used the model to compare two innovative technologies, a treatment or vaccination, to current status quo for most communities in the US: doing nothing or social distancing. The model was designed using a SEIR structure, which has been used to construct a number of epidemiological and mathematical models for the spread of COVID-19 (Hou et al., 2020; Iwata & Miyakoshi, 2020; Wei et al., 2020).

In accordance with guidelines established by the Second Panel on Cost-Effectiveness in Health & Medicine, we used a US societal perspective to measure resource utilization, financial burden, and health effects (G. D. Sanders et al., 2016). The model's time horizon was 365 days with 1-day cycles. We used a discounting rate of 3% where applicable, and we adjusted all costs for inflation to represent 2020 US dollars, measuring effectiveness in units of quality-adjusted life years (QALYs).

We sought several findings from the model results. By applying the economic model to the roughly 330 million US residents according to the 2020 census, we were able to both calibrate model outcomes with current real-world data on disease outcomes as of September 22, 2020. We simulated the impact of COVID-19 and potential solutions on the US population in terms of total cost, number of infections, number of hospitalizations, and mortality. The model was also purposed to measure the incremental cost-effectiveness ratio (ICER) and budget impact. ICERs were interpreted at a willingness-to-pay threshold of $50,000/QALY.

4.4.2.2 Model structure

Our SEIR model simulated the transition of the US population through ten mutually exclusive health states (Fig. 4.4.1). All patients began in a

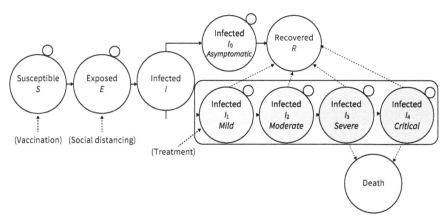

Fig. 4.4.1 Markov model of disease progression with coronavirus disease 2019 (COVID-19). Patients progressed through a modified "SEIR" process (Susceptible–Exposed–Infected–Recovered). The infection phases were staged from 0 through 4 in terms of increasing escalation, including use of critical care services. Patients who did not recover from COVID-19 died. Model alternatives to doing nothing included social distancing, treatment during the I_1 infected phase, or a vaccination to avoid entry into the susceptible phase.

susceptible (S) population. Over the course of time, patients would then become exposed (E) to COVID-19 infection. Upon exposure, a proportion of the population would become infected (I). We assumed five separate infected states (I_0–I_4) based on current information about COVID-19 (Cascella, Rajnik, Cuomo, Dulebohn, & Di Napoli, 2020; Shi et al., 2020). The states that did not require hospitalization included (I_0) asymptomatic, (I_1) uncomplicated or mild symptoms, and (I_2) moderate symptoms without signs of severe pneumonia. Patients who required hospitalization to manage symptoms were broken up into two states: (I_3) severe or (I_4) critical (Shi et al., 2020). Any patient who survived infection transitioned to recovered (R). Patients in I_3 or I_4 also risked death.

4.4.2.3 Mitigation strategies

We customized the comparator arms of the model to capture health state transitions as appropriate in reference to the base case. The treatment arm considered a therapy at the onset of mild symptoms during the I_1 phase to increase the probability of transition to R prior to any chance of escalation. In particular, we assumed an antiviral medication similar to zanamivir (brand name: Relenza; manufacturer: GlaxoSmithKline) in terms of list price, efficacy, and course of treatment for the base-case analysis (Monto et al., 2002). We also conducted uncertainty tests to evaluate scenarios where a hypothetical treatment differed from zanamivir (e.g., higher price, lower efficacy, etc.).

The vaccination arm separated a large proportion of the population out of the susceptible pool, contributing to an assumed herd immunity (Fine, Eames, & Heymann, 2011). In this scenario, we assumed that 60% of the population would be vaccinated, consistent with recommendations by Gavi, the Vaccine Alliance (Gavi, 2020e).

4.4.2.4 Model parameters
4.4.2.4.1 Costs
We applied micro-costing methods to a literature review to calculate the costs associated with each symptomatic infection state and prevention or treatment strategy (Table 4.4.1) (Xu, Grossetta Nardini, & Ruger, 2014). The model state costs were obtained from published literature. Individuals in health states S, E, I_0, and R were expected to have no additional costs. Infected patients were assessed the cost of a lost work day, based on methods recommended by the US Bureau of Labor Statistics. Cost of a lost work day was calculated from the US gross domestic product of $21 trillion distributed among 330 million individuals, averaging 261 work days each to represent an average of $243.81 per person per day (Bureau of Labor Statistics, 2008).

The societal costs of a new treatment or vaccine were assumed from the US list prices for similar technologies, zanamivir or the influenza vaccine, in accordance with World Health Organization methods guidance on costing (World Health Organization, 2015).

4.4.2.4.2 Probabilities
Most model probabilities were obtained from official reports of COVID-19 outcomes, which were current as of September 22, 2020, through these sources: the Johns Hopkins Coronavirus Resource Center (https://coronavirus.jhu.edu/, Baltimore, MD, USA); the US Centers for Disease Control and Prevention (https://www.cdc.gov/coronavirus/2019-ncov/, Atlanta, GA, USA); the World Health Organization (https://www.who.int/, Geneva, Switzerland); and the Institute for Health Metrics and Evaluation (https://covid19.healthdata.org/united-states-of-america, Seattle, WA, USA). In a small number of instances where data were not available through these sources,

Table 4.4.1 Model parameters based on infection statistics and assumptions as of September 22, 2020

Parameter	Expected value	Range for sensitivity analysis		Source
		Lower bound	Upper bound	
Infection population statistics				
US population (2020)	330 million			
Probability of social contact (b)	0.053			Yang et al. (2020)
Social contacts per person (c)	7.00	5.00	9.00	Eames, Tilston, Brooks Pollock, & Edmunds (2012)
Inverse average infectious period (γ)	0.14			Yang et al. (2020)
Transmission rate (β)	0.37			($b \times c$)
Basic reproduction number (R_0)	2.57	1.95	3.25	(β/γ)
Social contacts per person with social distancing	3.00			Assumed
Transition probabilities				
S to E	0.307	0.000	1.00	Yang et al. (2020)
E to I	0.005	0.004	0.006	Johns Hopkins Coronavirus Resource Center (2020); Yang et al. (2020)
I to I_0	0.250	−0.429	0.929	Whitehead (2020)
I_0 to $R^\star$	1.000			Assumed
I to $I_1^\star$	0.750			
I_1 to $I_2^\star$	0.191			
I_1 to R	0.809	0.000	1.000	Chinese Center for Disease Control and Prevention (2020)

(continued)

Table 4.4.1 Continued

Parameter	Expected value	Range for sensitivity analysis		Source
		Lower bound	Upper bound	
I_2 to I_3	0.314	0.000	10.000	Centers for Disease Control and Prevention (2020)
I_2 to R^*	0.686			
I_3 to I_4	0.115	0.000	0.531	Centers for Disease Control and Prevention (2020)
I_3 to R^*	0.859			
I_3 to death	0.026	0.000	0.084	Johns Hopkins Coronavirus Resource Center (2020); Centers for Disease Control and Prevention (2020)
I_4 to R^*	0.974			
I_4 to death	0.026	0.000	0.100	Johns Hopkins Coronavirus Resource Center (2020); Centers for Disease Control and Prevention (2020)
Effect modifiers of interventions				
Treatment efficacy	0.820	0.000	1.000	Monto et al. (2002)
Vaccine efficacy	0.900	0.000	1.000	Assumed
Proportion vaccinated	0.600	0.000	1.000	Gavi (2020)
S to E with social distancing	0.157	0.000	1.000	Anderson, Heesterbeek, Klinkenberg, & Hollingsworth (2020)
Risk reduction with social distancing	0.600	0.000	1.000	Anderson et al. (2020)
Risk reduction from herd immunity	0.500	0.000	1.000	Assumed

Daily costs (USD 2020)

I₁ costs

Sick day	$122.86	$92.15	$153.58	Bureau of Labor Statistics (2008)
Medications	$0.95	$0.71	$1.19	Drugs.com (2020a, 2020c)

I₂ costs

Sick day	$252.87	$189.65	$316.09	Bureau of Labor Statistics (2008)
Medications	$5.07	$3.80	$6.34	Drugs.com (2020a, 2020b)
Primary care visit and tests	$1,248.70	$936.53	$1,560.88	Castlight Health (2020)
Urgent care visit and tests	$1,553.38	$1,165.04	$1,941.73	Castlight Health (2020)
Emergency care visit and tests	$9,253.25	$6,939.94	$11,566.56	Castlight Health (2020)

I₃ and I₄ costs

Primary care visit, tests, and X-ray	$8,850.19	$6,637.64	$11,062.74	Castlight Health (2020)
Urgent care visit, tests, and X-ray	$9,143.51	$6,857.63	$11,429.39	Castlight Health (2020)
Emergency care visit, tests, and X-ray	$16,843.31	$12,632.48	$21,054.14	Castlight Health (2020)
Hospital bed (I_3)	$1,432.57	$1,074.43	$1,790.71	Rae, Claxton, Kurani, McDermott, & Cox (2020)
ICU bed (I_4)	$3,898.85	$2,924.14	$4,873.56	Rae et al. (2020)

Intervention costs

Treatment	$1,000.00	$750.00	$1,250.00	Assumed
Vaccine	$100.00	$75.00	$125.00	Assumed

(*continued*)

Table 4.4.1 Continued

Parameter	Expected value	Range for sensitivity analysis		Source
		Lower bound	Upper bound	
Utilities (QALYs)				
Utility of susceptible (S)	0.880	0.018	1.000	Khan, Muennig, Gardam, & Zivin, 2005; Sullivan & Ghushchyan (2006)
Utility of exposed (E)	0.880	0.018	1.000	Khan et al. (2005)
Utility of infected (I)	0.833	0.017	1.000	Khan et al. (2005)
Utility of asymptomatic (I_0)	0.833	0.017	1.000	Khan et al. (2005)
Utility of mild symptoms (I_1)	0.614	0.012	1.000	Yang et al. (2020)
Utility of moderate symptoms (I_2)	0.500	0.010	0.990	Khan et al. (2005)
Utility of severe symptoms (I_3)	0.250	0.005	0.495	Khan et al. (2005)
Utility of critical care (I_4)	0.050	0.001	0.099	Khan et al. (2005)
Utility of death	0.000			Anchor
Utility of recover (R)	0.880	0.018	1.000	Khan et al. (2005); Sullivan & Ghushchyan (2006)
Utility with vaccine	0.900	0.018	1.000	Khan et al. (2005); Lee et al. (2015); Sullivan & Ghushchyan (2006)

such as for historical outcomes of comparators based on influenza treatment and vaccination, we obtained model probabilities from the peer-reviewed systematic review and clinical trials literature.

4.4.2.4.3 Health utilities

We measured utilities in units of QALYs based on five-dimensional EuroQol (EQ-5D) index scores collected from the US Medical Expenditure Panel Survey (MEPS) (Shaw, Johnson, & Coons, 2005; Sullivan & Ghushchyan, 2006; Sullivan, Lawrence, & Ghushchyan, 2005). In general, QALYs range from 0.0 (death) to 1.0 (full health). We assumed the US population average was 0.88 QALYs (Sullivan & Ghushchyan, 2006). Patients infected and symptomatic had utilities that reflected less desirable health states. In the hypothetical state with the availability of a vaccine for COVID-19, we assumed a higher population average of 0.90 QALYs since utilities are a reflection of preferences, and individuals would likely have preferred the availability of vaccines to forgo the threat of an infectious disease (Lee et al., 2015).

4.4.2.5 Sensitivity analysis

We conducted sensitivity analyses to test model uncertainty by varying the expected parameter values (Briggs, 2000). Parameter value uncertainty ranged within the reported 95% confidence interval or standard deviation. In rare circumstances where no uncertainty range was reported, we varied the parameter by ±25% of its mean/median in order to assess the impact on the model results. One-way sensitivity analyses were done first. This approach produced a tornado diagram to evaluate parameters that had the greatest univariate impact on model results (i.e., that a single parameter could change the ICER insofar as to adjust our reporting of overall findings between interventions as "cost-effective" or "cost-ineffective").

A Bayesian multivariate probabilistic sensitivity analysis was performed using 10,000 Monte Carlo simulations with no intervention as the baseline approach (Briggs, Goeree, Blackhouse, & O'Brien, 2002). The probabilistic sensitivity analysis applied a distribution for each variable to characterize the impact of uncertainty on all parameters simultaneously. We used beta distributions for variables with values ranging between 0.0 and 1.0 such as probabilities and utilities, and gamma distributions for positive values greater than 1.0, such as costs.

4.4.3 Results

4.4.3.1 Estimated costs of the pandemic

Using this economic model, we were able to estimate the economic impact of the COVID-19 pandemic across 330 million people in the US. The baseline approach, doing nothing, could be associated with about $699 billion in financial impact to healthcare and labor sectors based on a combination of direct medical costs and lost wages due to sick leave (Table 4.4.2). These costs were mostly represented by about 67 million hospital days and over 200,000 deaths.

By contrast, considering our early understanding of the impact of social distancing, COVID-19 would have a lessened economic impact of about $548.6 billion. Thus, social distancing presented a potential savings of nearly $150 billion. This approach reduced the number of simulated outcomes across sectors, including 14.5 million fewer hospital days and about 50,000 deaths averted.

4.4.3.2 Effect of treatments and vaccines

Both treatments and vaccines were associated with large reductions in expected morbidity and costs. For example, the availability of a treatment presented a total cost of only $66.6 billion, a 90% cost reduction compared with doing nothing. This approach was associated with 31 million hospital days, and about 106,000 deaths.

By contrast, the availability of a vaccine reduced societal costs to only $9.9 billion, a 98% cost reduction compared with doing nothing. The presence of a vaccine and herd immunity for many improved outcomes to only about 30 million hospital days, and 104,000 deaths.

4.4.4 Cost-effectiveness findings

Under the base-case findings of our cost-effectiveness analysis, each proposed intervention offered greater value to US society than the prospect of doing nothing. In particular, all three options (social distancing, treatment, and vaccination) dominated doing nothing by lowering societal costs and increasing QALYs. On an individual basis, treatment and vaccination were more efficient

Table 4.4.2 Cost-effectiveness analysis comparing mitigation interventions to no intervention to address US COVID-19 pandemic

Comparator	Economic impact					Program cost ($ billions)	Budget impact ($ per person per month)	Epidemiologic impact	
	Cost ($)	Δ cost ($)	Effectiveness (QALYs)	Δ effectiveness (QALYs)	ICER ($/QALY)			Hospital-days (N)	Deaths (N)
Do nothing	2,115		0.874			697.83	176.22	67,166,963	227,513
Social distancing	1,738	−377	0.875	0.001	Dominates	548.85	138.60	52,687,745	177,981
Treatment	1,299	−885	0.877	0.003	Dominates	66.56	16.81	31,349,944	106,186
Vaccination	999	−1115	0.892	0.019	Dominates	9.90	2.50	30,784,605	104,265

ICER, incremental cost-effectiveness ratio; QALY, quality-adjusted life year.

Dominates indicates that the alternative is preferred at a lower cost and higher effectiveness relative to "do nothing."

than social distancing alone, although a vaccination program would provide greater QALY gains and reduce costs further than a treatment option based on currently available data about COVID-19 outcomes.

In terms of budget impact, both treatment and vaccination represent lower-cost alternatives to US society and payers, who would have to front the initial costs of technologies compared with long-run costs of disease burden on health systems. If we assume that the costs of technology can be financed across a risk pool of 330 million Americans in a 12-month period, then doing nothing comes at a societal budget impact of $176 per person per month. By comparison, the budget impacts of treatment, $16.81 per person per month, and vaccination, $2.50 per person per month, are much more affordable.

4.4.5 Sensitivity analysis

In one-way sensitivity analysis, uncertainty intervals around parameter estimates did not change the results of the model from the main conclusions (Fig. 4.4.2). Parameters with the greatest impact on model results included *treatment efficacy, treatment cost, societal cost of social distancing, vaccination*

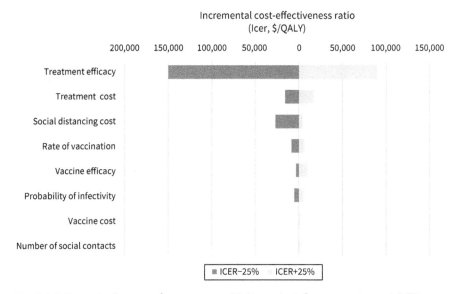

Fig. 4.4.2 Tornado diagram of one-way sensitivity analysis for parameter variabilities with greatest impact on study results.

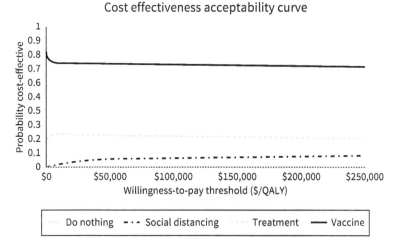

Fig. 4.4.3 Cost-effectiveness acceptability curve of the probability that a comparator is cost-effective at a given willingness-to-pay threshold, based on results of a probabilistic sensitivity analysis of 10,000 Monte Carlo simulations.

rate, and *vaccine efficacy*. The probabilistic sensitivity analysis confirmed findings from the base-case cost-effectiveness analysis. At a willingness-to-pay threshold of $100,000/QALY, the vaccination option was cost-effective in 71% of simulations (Fig. 4.4.3). Treatment was also cost-effective at this threshold in 21% of simulations. Social distancing was cost-effective in 8% of simulations.

4.4.6 Discussion

The COVID-19 pandemic has resulted in enormous morbidity, mortality, and societal upheaval worldwide. Given this, as well as uncertainty regarding the pandemic's future course, tremendous scientific effort was devoted to identifying treatments and vaccines that reduced the likelihood or consequences of coronavirus infection. We used economic modeling to explore the relative value of such technologies. We found that both alternatives offered more efficient options compared to doing nothing or social distancing.

While treatments represent efficient technology to address individual COVID-19 cases, a vaccination program comes at a lower cost, offers greater effectiveness, and averts more deaths and hospital days (Armstrong, 2007; Van Damme & Beutels, 1996). Perhaps these data imply the extended dominance of a vaccine over treatment for COVID-19 in particular. One reason for this is that treatments introduce additional burdens on the healthcare system since, presumably, payers would expect providers to conduct appropriate testing and write prescriptions for the treatment to authorize reimbursement. In addition, treatments do not minimize the asymptomatic spread of infection, which we now know represents a substantial proportion of infected cases; nor is it clear how treatments would impact people's behavior to self-isolate (Bai et al., 2020; Salathe et al., 2020). Furthermore, the treatment options do not sufficiently alleviate the disproportionate impact on the most vulnerable of our population, including the elderly, those who are chronically ill, and racial and ethnic minorities (Devakumar, Shannon, Bhopal, & Abubakar, 2020; Liu, Chen, Lin, & Han, 2020; McMichael et al., 2020). Thus, compared to vaccination, treatment would prove to be a much larger burden on the healthcare system in the long run if additional measures are not implemented to stop the spread of infection.

As with all models, ours had several limitations. First, our model did not completely demonstrate the time dependency of the COVID-19 epidemic based on a limited understanding of the virus at this time. Transition probabilities are usually regressed over several time periods of seasonal data, whereas our understanding of COVID-19 infection globally was based on a few short months of initial reports between March and September of 2020. That being said, we ranged all model parameters within credible uncertainty intervals for the sensitivity analysis to provide a realistic outlook for multiple scenarios. Second, our model presumes a static rather than dynamic population, and thus, we do not consider the entry or exit of individuals due to birth, or death from other causes. Third, our approach did not account for the different proportions and corresponding risks of age groups in the US population, yet the risks of COVID-19 infection may vary considerably by sociodemographic factors. As more data became available, this model provided a useful template for subgroup analyses. Fourth, our results varied depending on the actual costs and efficacies of treatments and vaccines that undergo development. Fifth, the model assumed availability of important resources that payers often leverage as gatekeepers to authorize treatments, such as diagnostic tests. We acknowledge that global shortages of COVID-19 diagnostic tests biased our estimates since the cost of disease management without technological intervention would be more efficient. Sixth, the health utilities for this study were based on values of previous studies about SARS infection. Finally, we did not capture complete information on the costs to payers and the healthcare system at this time.

In conclusion, this economic model represented an attempt to understand the burden of COVID-19 on the US economy, particularly on the healthcare and labor sectors. A treatment or vaccine for COVID-19 presented exceptional potential value to the US healthcare system and economy even early on in the outbreak before many other countries faced similarly concerning rates of infection and mortality. Vaccine-based COVID-19 control options likely could save 90% or more on COVID-19 costs to US society while significantly improving clinical benefit for millions of individuals. While many treatments and vaccines are undergoing clinical development, there are two practical issues that governments, health systems, and payers should begin to address now. One concern is the budget impact that a single technology could have if uptake is high. The other concern is that this demand will necessitate capacity building to properly allocate these technologies to the right individuals. Governments should begin mapping out policies for cross-subsidies and an expanded healthcare infrastructure with other healthcare stakeholders so that business transactions with manufacturers are not the hold up for patients to receive medically necessary and beneficial technology to address the COVID-19 pandemic.

References

Anderson, R. M., Heesterbeek, H., Klinkenberg, D., & Hollingsworth, T. D. (2020). How will country-based mitigation measures influence the course of the COVID-19 epidemic? *Lancet*, *395*(10228), 931–934.

Apuzzo, M., & Kirkpatrick DD. (2020, April 1). COVID-19 changed how the world does science, together. *New York Times*. https://www.nytimes.com/2020/04/01/world/europe/coronavirus-science-research-cooperation.html

Armstrong, E. P. (2007). Economic benefits and costs associated with target vaccinations. *Journal of Managed Care Pharmacy*, *13*(7 Suppl B), 12–15. doi:10.18553/jmcp.2007.13.s7-b.12

Bai, Y., Yao, L., Wei, T., Tian, F., Jin, D. Y., Chen, L., & Wang, M. (2020). Presumed asymptomatic carrier transmission of COVID-19. *JAMA*, *323*(14), 1406–1407. doi:10.1001/jama.2020.2565

Briggs, A. (2000). Handling uncertainty in cost-effectiveness models. *PharmacoEconomics*, *17*(5), 479–500. doi:10.2165/00019053-200017050-00006

Briggs, A., Goeree, R., Blackhouse, G., & O'Brien, B. J. (2002). Probabilistic analysis of cost-effectiveness models: Choosing between treatment strategies for gastroesophageal reflux disease. *Medical Decision Making*, *22*(4), 290–308. doi:10.1177/0272989x0202200408

Bureau of Labor Statistics. (2008). *Technical information about the BLS major sector productivity and costs measure. Major sector productivity and costs.* https://www.bls.gov/lpc/lpcmethods.pdf

Carvalho, N., Jit, M., Cox, S., Yoong, J., & Hutubessy, R. (2018). Capturing budget impact considerations within economic evaluations: A systematic review of economic evaluations of rotavirus vaccine in low- and middle-income countries and a proposed assessment framework. *PharmacoEconomics, 36*(1), 79–90. doi:10.1007/s40273-017-0569-2

Cascella, M., Rajnik, M., Cuomo, A., Dulebohn, S. C., & Di Napoli, R. (2020). *Features, evaluation and treatment coronavirus (COVID-19)*. Treasure Island, FL: StatPearls Publishing

Castlight Health. (2020). *The costs of COVID-19*. https://www.castlighthealth.com/wp-content/uploads/2020/03/Costs-of-COVID-19.pdf

Centers for Disease Control and Prevention. (2020). Severe outcomes among patients with coronavirus disease 2019 (COVID-19). *Morbidity and Mortality Weekly Report, 69*(12), 343–346. doi:10.15585/mmwr.mm6912e2

Chinese Center for Disease Control and Prevention. (2020). [The epidemiological characteristics of an outbreak of 2019 novel coronavirus diseases (COVID-19) in China.] *Zhonghua Liu Xing Bing Xue Za Zhi, 41*(2), 145–151. doi:10.3760/cma.j.issn.0254-6450.2020.02.003

Devakumar, D., Shannon, G., Bhopal, S. S., & Abubakar, I. (2020). Racism and discrimination in COVID-19 responses. *Lancet, 395*(10231), 1194. doi:10.1016/S0140-6736(20)30792-3

Drugs.com. (2020a). *Acetaminophen prices, coupons and patient assistance programs. Price guide.* https://www.drugs.com/price-guide/acetaminophen#oral-tablet-325-mg

Drugs.com. (2020b). *Benzonatate prices, coupons and patient assistance programs. Price guide.* https://www.drugs.com/price-guide/benzonatate

Drugs.com. (2020c). *Tussin expectorant. Price guide.* https://www.drugs.com/otc/102841/tussin-expectorant.html

Eames, K. T., Tilston, N. L., Brooks Pollock, E., & Edmunds, W. J. (2012). Measured dynamic social contact patterns explain the spread of H1N1v influenza. *PLoS Computational Biology, 8*(3), e1002425.

Fine, P., Eames, K., & Heymann, D. L. (2011). "Herd immunity": A rough guide. *Clinical Infectious Diseases, 52*(7), 911–916. doi:10.1093/cid/cir007

Gavi. (2020). *What is herd immunity?* https://www.gavi.org/vaccineswork/what-herd-immunity

Hou, C., Chen, J., Zhou, Y., Hua, L., Yuan, J., He, S.,... Jia, E. (2020). The effectiveness of the quarantine of Wuhan city against the corona virus disease 2019 (COVID-19): Well-mixed SEIR model analysis. *Journal of Medical Virology, 92*(7), 841–848. doi:10.1002/jmv.25827

Institute for Health Metrics & Evaluation. (2020). *COVID-19 projections assuming full social distancing through May 2020: Total deaths.* https://covid19.healthdata.org/

Iwata, K., & Miyakoshi, C. (2020). A simulation on potential secondary spread of novel coronavirus in an exported country using a stochastic epidemic SEIR model. *Journal of Clinical Medicine, 9*(4), 944. doi:10.3390/jcm9040944

Johns Hopkins Coronavirus Resource Center. (2020). *COVID-19 map. Coronavirus COVID-19 global cases by the Center for Systems Science and Engineering.* https://coronavirus.jhu.edu/

Khan, K., Muennig, P., Gardam, M., & Zivin, J. G. (2005). Managing febrile respiratory illnesses during a hypothetical SARS outbreak. *Emerging Infectious Diseases, 11*(2), 191–200. doi:10.3201/eid1102.040524

Lee, B. Y., Bartsch, S. M., Brown, S. T., Cooley, P., Wheaton, W. D., & Zimmerman, R. K. (2015). Quantifying the economic value and quality of life impact of earlier influenza vaccination. *Medical Care, 53*(3), 218–229. doi:10.1097/mlr.0000000000000302

Liu, K., Chen, Y., Lin, R., & Han, K. (2020). Clinical features of COVID-19 in elderly patients: A comparison with young and middle-aged patients. *Journal of Infection, 80*(6), e14–e18. doi:10.1016/j.jinf.2020.03.005

Mauskopf, J., Standaert, B., Connolly, M. P., Culyer, A. J., Garrison, L. P., Hutubessy, R.,... Severens, J. L. (2018). Economic analysis of vaccination programs: An ISPOR good practices for outcomes research task force report. *Value in Health, 21*(10), 1133–1149. doi:10.1016/j.jval.2018.08.005

McMichael, T. M., Currie, D. W., Clark, S., Pogosjans, S., Kay, M., Schwartz, N. G.,... Duchin, J. S. (2020). Epidemiology of Covid-19 in a long-term care facility in King County, Washington. *New England Journal of Medicine*, *382*(21), 2005–2011. doi:10.1056/NEJMoa2005412

Monto, A. S., Pichichero, M. E., Blanckenberg, S. J., Ruuskanen, O., Cooper, C., Fleming, D. M., & Kerr, C. (2002). Zanamivir prophylaxis: An effective strategy for the prevention of influenza types A and B within households. *Journal of Infectious Diseases*, *186*(11), 1582–1588. doi:10.1086/345722

Park, A. (2020, February 25). COVID-19 vaccine shipped, and drug trials start. *Time*. https://time.com/5790545/first-covid-19-vaccine/

Rae, M., Claxton, G., Kurani, N., McDermott, D., & Cox, C. (2020). *Potential costs of coronavirus treatment for people with employer coverage*. Health System Tracker. https://www.healthsystemtracker.org/brief/potential-costs-of-coronavirus-treatment-for-people-with-employer-coverage/

Salathe, M., Althaus, C. L., Neher, R., Stringhini, S., Hodcroft, E., Fellay, J.,... Low, N. (2020). COVID-19 epidemic in Switzerland: On the importance of testing, contact tracing and isolation. *Swiss Medical Weekly*, *150*, w20225. doi:10.4414/smw.2020.20225

Sanders, G. D., Neumann, P. J., Basu, A., Brock, D. W., Feeny, D., Krahn, M.,... Ganiats, T. G. (2016). Recommendations for conduct, methodological practices, and reporting of cost-effectiveness analyses: Second Panel on Cost-Effectiveness in Health and Medicine. *JAMA*, *316*(10), 1093–1103. doi:10.1001/jama.2016.12195

Sanders, J. M., Monogue, M. L., Jodlowski, T. Z., & Cutrell, J. B. (2020). Pharmacologic treatments for coronavirus disease 2019 (COVID-19): A review. *JAMA*, *323*(18), 1824–1836. doi:10.1001/jama.2020.6019

Shaw, J. W., Johnson, J. A., & Coons, S. J. (2005). US valuation of the EQ-5D health states: Development and testing of the D1 valuation model. *Medical Care*, *43*(3), 203–220.

Shi, Y., Wang, Y., Shao, C., Huang, J., Gan, J., Huang, X.,... Melino, G. (2020). COVID-19 infection: The perspectives on immune responses. *Cell Death & Differentiation*, *27*(5), 1451–1454. doi:10.1038/s41418-020-0530-3

Sullivan, P. W., & Ghushchyan, V. (2006). Preference-based EQ-5D index scores for chronic conditions in the United States. *Medical Decision Making*, *26*(4), 410–420. doi:10.1177/0272989x06290495

Sullivan, P. W., Lawrence, W. F., & Ghushchyan, V. (2005). A national catalog of preference-based scores for chronic conditions in the United States. *Medical Care*, *43*(7), 736–749. doi:10.1097/01.mlr.0000172050.67085.4f

Van Damme, P., & Beutels, P. (1996). Economic evaluation of vaccination. *PharmacoEconomics*, *9*(3), 8–15. doi:10.2165/00019053-199600093-00005

Wei, Y. Y., Lu, Z. Z., Du, Z. C., Zhang, Z. J., Zhao, Y., Shen, S. P.,... Chen, F. (2020). [Fitting and forecasting the trend of COVID-19 by SEIR(+ CAQ) dynamic model.] *Zhonghua Liu Xing Bing Xue Za Zhi*, *41*(4), 470–475. doi:10.3760/cma.j.cn112338-20200216-00106

Whitehead, S. (2020). *CDC director on models for the months to come: "This virus is going to be with us."* NPR. https://www.npr.org/sections/health-shots/2020/03/31/824155179/cdc-director-on-models-for-the-months-to-come-this-virus-is-going-to-be-with-us

World Health Organization. (2015). *WHO guideline on country pharmaceutical pricing policies*. https://apps.who.int/iris/bitstream/handle/10665/153920/9789241549035_eng.pdf

Xu, X., Grossetta Nardini, H. K., & Ruger, J. P. (2014). Micro-costing studies in the health and medical literature: Protocol for a systematic review. *Systematic Reviews*, *3*, 47. doi:10.1186/2046-4053-3-47

Yang, Z., Zeng, Z., Wang, K., Wong, S.-S., Liang, W., Zanin, M.,... He, J. (2020). Modified SEIR and AI prediction of the epidemics trend of COVID-19 in China under public health interventions. *Journal of Thoracic Disease*, *12*(3), 165–174. doi:10.21037/jtd.2020.02.64

5

FINANCING AND RESOURCE TRACKING OF VACCINATION PROGRAMS

Edited by Logan Brenzel and Shreena Malaviya

5.0

Section introduction: financing and resource tracking of vaccination programs

Logan Brenzel and Shreena Malaviya

The ability of national immunization programs to introduce and deliver new vaccines, and reach their target populations, particularly those children and communities who are hard to reach, is related to the resources available to provide services. Sustaining adequate financing is a critical function of immunization programs and is reflected as one of the pillars of the global Immunization Agenda 2030. This section of the handbook focuses on various dimensions of immunization financing. Chapter 5.1 examines historical immunization spending by governments, development partners, and households/private sector for the total program, and split between routine and campaign services, as well as vaccines and delivery. Chapter 5.2 elaborates on the current sources of financing, and how these might be better utilized to improve adequacy and sustainability of the program, particularly as coronavirus disease 2019 (COVID-19) has affected economies and health budgets. Finally, Chapter 5.3 explores the development partner landscape for immunization, particularly focusing on Gavi, the Vaccine Alliance and some of the innovative financing instruments that have been developed. Various resources exist that provide further details on health and immunization financing, and these are provided for readers.

Logan Brenzel and Shreena Malaviya, *Section introduction: financing and resource tracking of vaccination programs* In: *Handbook of Applied Health Economics in Vaccines*. Edited by: David Bishai, Logan Brenzel and William V. Padula, Oxford University Press.
© Oxford University Press 2023. DOI: 10.1093/oso/9780192896087.003.0026

5.1

Introduction to immunization financing and expenditure

Logan Brenzel and Shreena Malaviya

Immunization offers a first line of protection for households against imminent catastrophic direct and indirect costs in treating vaccine-preventable illnesses and infections. Immunization programs have been successful in reaching children worldwide. In 2018, 86% of children received all three doses of the diphtheria, pertussis, and tetanus (DPT3) vaccine. The high coverage of immunization programs forms a critical backbone of the universal health coverage expansion strategy.

Immunization programs need sustainable financing to remain effective and efficient. Each year a new cohort of children must be reached at high levels of coverage which requires reliable resources. Immunization programs must continue indefinitely to ensure a high coverage of vaccines, unless and until a disease is eradicated. Well-planned immunization programs have the potential to reach remote and geographically constrained settings that are less linked to the formal health system, offering opportunities to those communities to access basic and critical healthcare interventions. A drop in coverage could result in disease outbreaks that can undo all the years of investment. Moreover, in some countries, access to immunization is considered a basic health right and a public responsibility to be funded by the government. As a public good, governments have a unique role in funding vaccination programs. Trends in immunization expenditure highlight both the large financial requirement for the program and the challenges that remain to ensure sustainability.

A recent comprehensive review and analysis estimated government, private, and donor spending for immunization in 135 low- and middle-income countries (Ikilezi et al., 2021b). Data were also disaggregated between vaccine and delivery cost spending, as well as between routine immunization delivery and supplementary campaigns. Immunization spending increased threefold from $3.2 billion in 2000 to $10.2 billion in 2017, for a total of $112.4 billion over the period (Fig. 5.1.1). Increases in spending occurred in 90% of

Logan Brenzel and Shreena Malaviya, *Introduction to immunization financing and expenditure* In: *Handbook of Applied Health Economics in Vaccines.* Edited by: David Bishai, Logan Brenzel and William V. Padula, Oxford University Press.

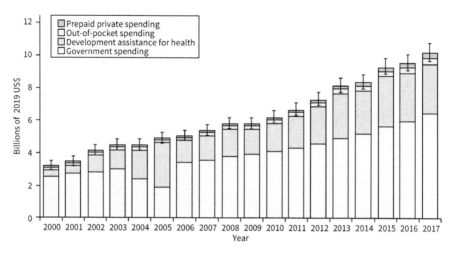

Fig. 5.1.1 Immunization spending by source (2000–2017).

Source: Ikilezi et al. (2021b).

countries, while eight countries with primarily fragile and conflict settings experienced declines.

Government spending accounted for the largest share of total spending on immunization throughout the period, ranging between 60% and 79% of total spending each year. Development assistance for health represented nearly a third of all spending at $31.7 billion (28%), with more than $13 billion channeled through Gavi, the Vaccine Alliance. Development assistance for health represented 49% and 48% of total immunization spending in sub-Saharan Africa and Asia, respectively. While immunization services are usually provided free of charge, the study estimated that $4 billion had been spent out of pocket over the period. Finally, spending on vaccines nearly tripled over this period, while actual spending on delivery remained relatively stable and accounted for 44% of total spending in 2017 (Fig. 5.1.2).

Nearly 90% of government spending was allocated to routine immunization. More than half of development assistance for health (58%) was allocated to routine immunization activities. Immunization spending averaged $40 per surviving infant in lower-income countries. Spending was highest in Latin America and the Caribbean at $208 per surviving infant. While higher DPT3 coverage was associated with increased government spending on immunization, there were exceptions.

Analysis of JRF data also shows expenditure per surviving infant varies by region and country income level. Two percent of global health expenditure is spent on immunization, ranging from 2.8% of current health spending in

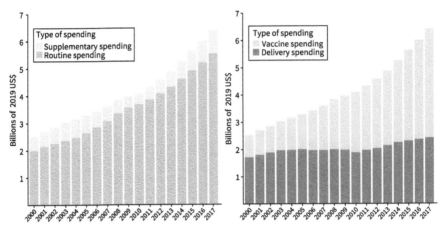

Fig. 5.1.2 Spending patterns on immunization (2000–2017).
Source: Ikilezi et al. (2021b).

low-income countries to 0.3% of current health spending in high-income countries. Higher income countries spent much more on immunization per surviving infant ($1,000) in 2017 than lower income countries ($29.50) according to the World Health Organization (WHO, 2020b).

Variation in expenditure levels between countries is related to some extent by unit price differences of vaccines in each country. Pooled procurement mechanisms tend to offer countries lower prices for a majority of vaccines. Self-procuring middle-income countries pay twice as much as countries that procure through UNICEF or the PAHO Revolving Fund. Longer contracts are also associated with lower vaccine unit prices, as well as higher volumes procured (WHO: Immunization Vaccines and Biologicals, 2019). Higher income countries, particularly those in the Region of the Americas and the European Region, represent the largest share of the global market value of vaccines (68%).

Gavi-eligible countries benefit from lower vaccine prices because of the larger volumes of doses. The WHO 2019 Global Vaccine Market Report high-income countries introduce more vaccines (74% more than low-income countries and 23% more than middle-income countries) in their routine immunization programs than lower-income countries (WHO, 2020b).

Lower income countries that are eligible for support from Gavi, the Vaccine Alliance may have a higher share of donor support for their immunization program because of the initial subsidy for each new vaccine introduced. Gavi support is tiered on the basis of the gross national income (GNI) of the country. For the lowest income countries, the subsidy level doesn't change until a country's GNI crosses a threshold, in which case the subsidy level is ramped down. Every time a new vaccine is introduced with Gavi support, the share of donor support would be expected to rise. Gavi's co-financing policy has so far been a successful strategy to build in sustainable financing for immunization (Gavi, 2019; Kallenberg et al., 2016).

An increase in government funding would be expected as countries increase their co-financing responsibilities and transition out of Gavi support. As countries transition from primarily external aid funded immunization programs to domestically-funded, they face a variety of financial and institutional challenges. Countries experience financial obstacles such as high total vaccine costs and the need to create additional fiscal space in government health budgets within a relatively short period of time. There are also programmatic and institutional challenges such as limited procurement and regulatory capacities. Of Gavi-transitioned countries (16) have experienced increases in domestic expenditures for vaccines up until 2018 (Ikilezi et al., 2021b).

Additional expenditures will be required to scale-up immunization coverage, add in new vaccines, technologies, or delivery strategies, and reach zero dose children and communities, Estimates suggest it could cost $54 USD on average to fully immunize a child against ten antigens at high coverage levels (Sim et al., 2020). An additional US $38.5 billion will be needed in 64 countries for child immunization between 2016 and 2030, representing 30% more than what these countries are currently spending (Stenberg et al., 2017). Countries will be challenged to fill the gap with domestic resources, which are at risk following COVID-19 health and economic impacts.

5.1.1 Benefits of resource tracking in immunization financing

The Immunization Agenda 2030—A Global Strategy to Leave No One Behind—encourages countries to consistently track and evaluate expenditures to achieve national immunization program goals (WHO, 2020a). The cornerstone of a robust immunization program is reliable and sustainable financing. The regular collection and analysis of immunization expenditure data can provide the necessary data for better planning and budgeting of the national program, and for advocating for additional resource mobilization. evidence required to plan and secure sufficient funding for immunization activities.

Resource tracking captures the sources and uses of resources (e.g. financial, material, and human) for the health sector and immunization programs. The types of policy questions that can be addressed with resource tracking include:

- How much do governments, households, partners spend per year on vaccines, routine services, campaigns?
- What percentage of spending for routine services comes from government (domestic) sources or external sources?
- What percentage of total and government health expenditure is spent on routine immunization?
- How have trends in 1-3 above changed over time and how do they compare to the aspirations of the country on sustainable financing?

5.1.2 Expenditure tracking for program planning and budgeting

Analyzing a country's immunization expenditure estimates over the years and comparing it to other countries, allows Expanded Program on Immunization managers and policymakers to gain insight into a number of critical issues (Abt Associates, 2018).

- Sustainability of immunization financing: Data on immunization expenditure by various sources—internal and external—can provide further insights into the government's contribution to immunization financing compared to that of donors. It is important to understand patterns of funding for different sources and how these relate to goals of self-sufficiency and transition from donor support.
- Equitable access to immunization services: Out-of-pocket immunization expenditure can be evaluated alongside income levels of households to understand the potential financial burden and impact on the access to immunization services (Abt Associates, 2018).
- Accountability of decision makers on spending: Actual spending on immunization from Health Accounts exercises can be compared to resource requirements as outlined in national plans, such as the Comprehensive Multi-Year Plan (cMYP), to understand any potential funding gaps (Abt Associates, 2018). These data, when accurately captured, can also be used to monitor the country's progress as well as to compare budgets against spending (budget execution rate).

- Efficiency of immunization spending: Comparing immunization spending per live birth between countries can provide insight into how their immunization spending and coverage compares to other programs (Abt Associates, 2018).
- Impact: comparing total spending for immunization with coverage levels and other measures of program output or outcomes can provide a measure of the performance of the program.

5.1.3 Types and sources of data

The main sources of cross-country and relatively comparable information on immunization expenditures are the Joint Reporting Form (JRF) and the National Health Accounts (NHA). The JRF was developed by the WHO and UNICEF and tracks self-reported spending information from countries on both government and total spending through seven indicators (WHO, 2020b). These expenditures pertain to immunization-specific, noncapital expenditures of the program. Hence, these data exclude spending on shared resources or large investments like cold chain. JRF expenditure data are reported and evaluated by WHO annually since 2010. Data can be obtained through a request to WHO.

The NHA is a robust expenditure tracking methodology that allows countries to evaluate and monitor total health spending across different disease classifications funded from various sources. This approach yields consistent and comprehensive data on health spending in a country. Within this system, countries can track changes in policy priorities and understand if the introduction of reforms and new programs resulted in changes in resource allocation and expenditure. In this methodology, immunization spending relates to the function of preventive services (Abt Associates, 2018; WHO, 2017). Data are posted in the public domain in the Global Health Expenditure Database (GHED) which currently contains estimates on immunization spending for nearly 60 countries, with half of those estimates from countries in sub-Saharan Africa (WHO, 2017). Higher-income countries may report data into the OECD Health Expenditure Database (Organization of Economic Cooperation and Development, 2021).

Gavi and UNICEF regularly monitor country-level procurement and spending on new and underused vaccines as part of co-financing of new vaccines. These data are updated at least twice per year and exclude data on vaccines administered during supplementary activities. These reports are used to assess the trajectories of Gavi countries in increasing the ownership of vaccine financing and sustainability.

The cMYP is a comprehensive planning framework developed by WHO and UNICEF for integrating immunization program strategies and identifying the resources required to implement and achieve them (WHO: Immunization Vaccines and Biologicals, 2014). An associated Excel-based tool is used to estimate the resource requirements and financing needed for a 5-year period, along with a funding gap. While the cMYP is a planning tool and not a costing study per se, estimates of the resources used in the first or year (baseline) has been used as a proxy for immunization program costs. WHO and UNICEF have developed a new strategic framework for national immunization planning (National Immunization Strategy) which builds off of the country experience with the cMYP.

Comparisons between various sources of immunization spending reveal data quality issues and inconsistencies though some improvements are occurring over time (Ikilezi et al., 2021b). Vaccine spending by governments is reported more completely than routine immunization spending. This may be due in part to the complexity of estimating immunization-specific routine program spending. Some consistency is observed in the various sources on vaccine spending. Based on cMYP data, routine immunization spending was nearly twice as much as that reported through the JRF, and almost four times higher than that reported through the NHA on average Both the JRF and cMYP reported higher spending than was reported through Gavi co-financing (Ikilezi et al., 2021a).

Thus, it is important to consider these factors when utilizing the data for immunization financing development and planning. All stakeholders should be encouraged to collaborate and work with the government to ensure better reporting of vaccine and immunization spending.

5.1.4 Conclusion

Immunization is a highly cost-effective intervention whose effectiveness and efficiency benefits from robust and sustainable financing. Resource tracking on a frequent basis is a powerful tool for understanding the sources and uses of funding, as well as to benchmark country immunization spending relative to neighboring countries achieving similar levels of performance. Expenditure data can be sourced from a variety of sources, and factors such as the completeness, reliability, and validity of expenditure data need to be considered when interpreting trends.

References

Abt Associates. (2018). *Understanding and using immunization expenditure data: A primer for immunization program managers.* https://www.abtassociates.com/insights/publications/report/understanding-and-using-immunization-expenditure-data-primer-for

Gavi. (2019). *Annual program report.* https://www.gavi.org/progress-report

Ikilezi, G., Bachmeier, S. D., Cogswell, I. E., Maddison, E. R., Stutzman, H. N., Tsakalos, G., . . . Micah, A. E. (2021a). Tracking government spending on immunization: The joint reporting forms, national health accounts, comprehensive multi-year plans and co-financing data. *Vaccine, 39*(25), 3410–3418. doi:10.1016/j.vaccine.2021.04.047

Ikilezi, G., Micah, A. E., Bachmeier, S. D., Cogswell, I. E., Maddison, E. R., Stutzman, H. N., . . . Dieleman, J. L. (2021b). Estimating total spending by source of funding on routine and supplementary immunisation activities in low- and middle-income countries, 2000–2017: A financial modelling study. *Lancet Global Health, 398*(10314), 1875–1893. doi:10.1016/S0140-6736(21)01591-9

Kallenberg, J., Mok, W., Newman, R., Nguyen, A., Ryckman, T., Saxenian, H., & Wilson, P. (2016). Gavi's transition policy: Moving from development assistance to domestic financing of immunization programs. *Health Affairs, 35*(2), 250–258. doi:10.1377/hlthaff.2015.1079

Organization of Economic Cooperation and Development. (2021). *OECD health expenditure database.* https://data.oecd.org/healthres/health-spending.htm

Sim, S. Y., Watts, E., Constenla, D., Brenzel, L., & Patenaude, B. N. (2020). Return on investment from immunization against 10 pathogens in 94 low-and middle-income countries, 2011–30. *Health Affairs, 39*(8), 1343–1353.

Stenberg, K., Hanssen, O., Edejer, T. T., Bertram, M., Brindley, C., Meshreky, A., . . . Soucat, A. (2017). Financing transformative health systems towards achievement of the health Sustainable Development Goals: A model for projected resource needs in 67 low-income and middle-income countries. *Lancet Global Health, 5*(9), e875–e887. doi:10.1016/s2214-109x(17)30263-2

World Health Organization. (2017). *Expenditure on prevention activities under SHA 2011—supplementary guidance.* https://apps.who.int/nha/database/DocumentationCentre/Index/en

World Health Organization. (2020a). *Immunization Agenda 2030: A global strategy to leave no one behind.* https://www.who.int/publications/m/item/immunization-agenda-2030-a-global-strategy-to-leave-no-one-behind

World Health Organization. (2020b). *Situation analysis of immunization expenditure.* https://www.who.int/docs/default-source/immunization/financing/situation-analysis-key-facts.pdf?sfvrsn=8c65d922_2

World Health Organization: Immunization Vaccines and Biologicals. (2014). *Comprehensive multi-year plan costing tool.* https://apps.who.int/iris/bitstream/handle/10665/128051/WHO_IVB_14.06_eng.pdf

World Health Organization: Immunization Vaccines and Biologicals. (2019). *MI4A: Market information for access to vaccines.* https://www.who.int/teams/immunization-vaccines-and-biologicals/vaccine-access/mi4a

5.2

Financing of immunization programs

Logan Brenzel

With a return on investment of $21 for every $1 invested, vaccination is a good investment in health (Ozawa et al., 2016). Because of the public goods nature of vaccination, governments have a significant role to play in financing services. However, many countries struggle to fully fund their programs to be able to reach 100% coverage. Global immunization coverage for the third dose of diphtheria, tetanus, and pertussis vaccine has hovered at 85% for several years and countries face challenges to fully reach their population with life-saving vaccines. More than 22 million children a year miss out on life-saving vaccines (World Health Organization, 2020b). The vision of the Immunization Agenda 2030—"a world where everyone, everywhere, at every age, fully benefits from vaccines for good health and well-being" (World Health Organization, 2020b)—requires adequate and sustainable financing for immunization.

5.2.1 Sources of financing for immunization

This chapter provides an overview of how countries are currently financing their national immunization programs. Prospects for sustainable financing cannot be disconnected from the reliability and adequacy of various sources of financing. A key message is that in fiscally constrained settings, resources available for the immunization program are a function of funding available for the entire health sector and how those resources are prioritized and allocated. Second, the mechanisms of health system financing can influence the availability and predictability of financing for immunization. The three main sources of immunization financing are (1) government, (2) private, and (3) external. The mechanisms for each are discussed in turn below. Several toolkits have been developed which describe country experiences with

Logan Brenzel, *Financing of immunization programs* In: *Handbook of Applied Health Economics in Vaccines.* Edited by: David Bishai, Logan Brenzel and William V. Padula, Oxford University Press. © Oxford University Press 2023. DOI: 10.1093/oso/9780192896087.003.0028 various sources of financing which will provide further details (Results for Development, 2017; World Bank & Gavi, 2010).

5.2.1.1 Government (domestic) financing for immunization

On average, $8.5 trillion, equivalent to 10% of global gross domestic product was spent on healthcare in 2019. Health spending in lower-income countries primarily came from out-of-pocket and external sources. Primary healthcare spending accounted for almost half of total spending, ranging from $12 in DR Congo to $3,800 in Switzerland, highlighting the huge disparities in health-care spending around the world. Cross-country inequality is rising over time. Government health financing accounted for less than 2% of gross domestic product in 2019 in lower-income countries (World Health Organization, 2020a, 2021).

While government allocations to health have generally grown over time, overall economic growth, rather than reallocation between sectors has driven this growth (Barroy & Gupta, 2020; Tandon, Cain, Kurowski, & Postolovska, 2018). The dependence upon economic growth means that government health sector financing is vulnerable to economic shocks, such as during the coronavirus 2019 (COVID-19) pandemic.

5.2.1.1.1 National level financing for immunization

Immunization should be a government financial responsibility as benefits ex-tend beyond the individuals vaccinated through herd immunity. Ensuring reliable, predictable funding to immunize all newborn children every year with the vaccines in the national schedule and with potentially new vaccines to be introduced requires considerable resources. Health services in most countries are a financed through tax and revenue collection from individuals, corporations, and other sources. These are pooled and allocated across sec-tors, including health, as part of the annual budget cycle and planning pro-cess. Government health spending compared to total government spending reflects the priority of health in the country. This estimate ranges from 5.6% in low-income countries, to 14.3% in high-income countries (World Health Organization, 2020).

Government health financing at the national level can be allocated directly from the national Treasury to the Ministry of Health which will allocate funds across preventive and promotive health programs and services, as well as to specific service providers, such as hospitals and clinics. Health funding allocated to the Ministry of Health may also be transferred to subnational units or programs. The Treasury may also direct health funding to subnational units through block grants, or to facilities through direct facility financing. Direct facility financing is an approach that attempts to solve the delays and bottlenecks in resources reaching frontline facilities.

The share of financing allocated for immunization from government budgets depends upon competing priorities for those resources. Often this share is based on historical budget levels rather than evidence of the cost of providing those services. Incorporating the actual costs of vaccine delivery into annual and multi-year health budget processes can improve the alignment of budgets to actual resource needs, and ensure greater predictability of allocations (Lydon et al., 2008). Having a line item for vaccines and immunization may assist in creating greater visibility for the recurrent needs of the program. A recent evaluation of African government budgets for immunization revealed that countries with input-based budgeting had several line items for vaccine purchase, vaccine co-financing, campaigns, and other immunization program inputs, with an average of nine line items, ranging from 0 to 42 (Griffiths et al., 2020).

Greater advocacy on the return on investment to immunization and the role of vaccination in reducing poverty and generating economic benefits may aide program manager and ministry staff in effectively garnering additional funding. Recent evidence suggests that vaccination can protect households in the poorest countries from slipping into poverty, due to the high costs of treating measles, pneumonia, and other illnesses (Chang et al., 2018). In Bangladesh, the average out-of-pocket cost to households for treating a case of childhood measles was $48 in public facilities and over $80 in private facilities (de Broucker, Ahmed, et al., 2020). In Uganda, caregivers were responsible for $23 in payments for measles treatment and paid the equivalent of 30% of the household's monthly income to treat it (De Broucker, Ssebagereka, et al., 2020).

Governments may allocate resources to immunization programs through earmarks which are guaranteed allocations. Earmarking, or setting aside either a specific amount or a proportion of health funding each budget cycle, for immunization may be mandated in public law. Nine countries in Asia, Africa, and Latin America have tried to institute or have such laws. Bolivia finances its program through allocation of a certain percentage of government health funding. While there are obvious short-term benefits, earmarking introduces rigidities in the government budget which may, in the long run, be detrimental to services. For instance, earmarks may cover the cost of procuring vaccines, but support for delivery and operating the program may be cut to accommodate increasing costs of vaccines. In economic shocks, if health budgets are cut, the proportion going to the program may also falter (Results for Development, 2017).

5.2.1.1.2 Subnational level financing

Government funding for healthcare is generated at subnational levels through local tax and revenue collection. Funds generated at the local level and those that are transferred from national sources through inter-fiscal transfers form the basis for government subnational financing. Allocation and use of locally generated and managed healthcare resources are critical to cover the operating costs of immunization programs. This requires working with local mayors and decision makers over how best to support service delivery. This source of financing is often overlooked in relation to mobilizing additional resources for the immunization program.

In a decentralized context, roles, responsibilities, and authority for immunization program functions are spread between the national and subnational level. Local government health officers may not report directly to the Ministry of Health, but to ministries of local government or other agencies. The national government is usually responsible for policy guidance, regulation, and vaccine procurement, while decentralized units must cover the cost of delivery, often based upon national recommendations and standards. In Indonesia, districts are fully responsible for implementing the immunization program and must finance key components. In Pakistan, the central level procures vaccines, but financing is supported by the provincial level as well (Learning Network for Countries in Transition, 2021). Immunization programs at subnational level face challenges with respect to coordination, budgeting, and management capacity. Managing and ensuring adequate subnational funding flows to facilities and frontline providers for immunization services is critical.

5.2.1.1.3 National health insurance

National government health financing may also be allocated to social insurance mechanisms that aim to cover the healthcare needs of the population. Many countries in Europe, Asia, the UK, and Canada provide health services to their population through a single-payer system (i.e., the government). Several lower-income countries also committed to national health insurance (NHI) as a mechanism for supporting universal health coverage such as such

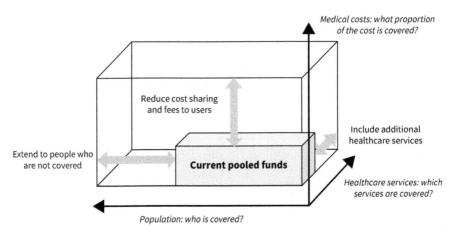

Fig. 5.2.1 Services and coverage for universal healthcare.
Source: Adapted from Maeda et al. (2014).

as Ghana (Grépin & Dionne, 2013), Kenya (Union for International Cancer Control, 2020), and Côte d'Ivoire (Dagnan, 2018).

Universal health coverage is based on three components as represented in Fig. 5.2.1): (1) service coverage (expanding scope and quality of essential services), (2) population coverage (expanding population groups that benefit from essential packages of services, and (3) financial risk protection (Maeda et al., 2014).

Making positive gains in these three domains may require countries to undertake significant reforms and policy choices related to the financing and delivery of health services. The additional cost of achieving universal health coverage and the Sustainable Development Goals targets by 2030 have been estimated to reach $371 billion annually or $58 per person (Stenberg et al., 2017). Prioritizing preventive health services can result in potential health systems savings from reduced utilization of expensive curative services and hospital care. NHI relies heavily on public/government financing and is a way of pooling different health risks and providing a benefits package of quality health services. A "health benefits package" is essentially a selection of services to be delivered to the covered population (Glassman, Giedion, & Smith, 2017).

A recent review found that maternal and child health services were the services most often included in the benefits packages of 26 countries. Nearly half of those specifically included immunization services, and 20% of them partially reflected immunization in their benefits packages (Regan, Wilson, Chalkidou, & Chi, 2021).

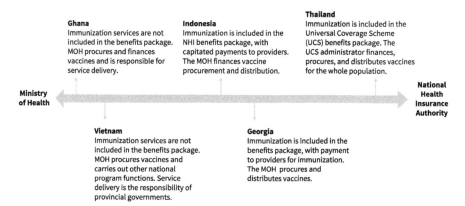

Ghana
Immunization services are not included in the benefits package. MOH procures and finances vaccines and is responsible for service delivery.

Indonesia
Immunization is included in the NHI benefits package, with capitated payments to providers. The MOH finances vaccine procurement and distribution.

Thailand
Immunization is included in the Universal Coverage Scheme (UCS) benefits package. The UCS administrator finances, procures, and distributes vaccines for the whole population.

Ministry of Health

National Health Insurance Authority

Vietnam
Immunization services are not included in the benefits package. MOH procures vaccines and carries out other national program functions. Service delivery is the responsibility of provincial governments.

Georgia
Immunization is included in the benefits package, with payment to providers for immunization. The MOH procures and distributes vaccines.

Fig. 5.2.2 Funding of vaccines and immunization through NHI schemes. MOH, Ministry of Health.
Source: Adapted from Learning Network for Countries in Transition (2020).

While including immunization in the benefits packages for NHI may bring benefits in terms of coverage, there may be some unanticipated impacts on the national immunization program that should be considered. NHI does not necessarily translate into additional resources for the health sector or for the immunization program, as reductions in allocations to other Ministry of Health programs and services may occur in order to finance NHI. NHI can coexist alongside Ministry of Health funding which may create fragmented funding flows to the program. NHIs may focus more on curative services, potentially crowding out the financing and provision of preventive services such as immunization. If NHI population coverage is limited, the immunization program may not be able to vaccinate newborns and infants at the same level of coverage. The cost of introducing new vaccines is higher than those currently in the program, and this may pose greater challenges for financing and sustaining NHI (Learning Network for Countries in Transition, 2020). Fig. 5.2.2 shows the range of country experiences with financing vaccines through NHI and other sources.

5.2.1.1.4 Health taxes
Taxes on alcohol, tobacco, and sugar have been a useful mechanism for raising additional revenues for public spending. Evidence suggests that these types of taxes also help to reduce the consumption of unhealthy commodities (Wright, Smith, & Hellowell, 2017). Health taxes have also been shown to raise a significant amount of revenue for additional resources for the health sector. A 50% increase in the prices of sugar-sweetened drinks, alcohol, and tobacco

can achieve $24.7 billion in 54 low- and middle-income countries (LMICs) by 2030 (Marquez & Dutta, 2020). There are a few instances of health taxes being used for immunization, including the Philippines. Ghana's NHI scheme is funded through a value-added tax, which also supports the country's co-financing requirements for Gavi (Results for Development, 2017). Health taxes may be one way of expanding budgetary space for health services in the future, given the impacts of COVID-19 vaccines on government budgets.

5.2.1.2 Private financing

The private sector may play a range of roles in the national immunization program by either extending service coverage in low-income countries or aiding the introduction of new vaccines in middle-income countries (Levin & Kaddar, 2011). Public and private sector collaboration is essential, aided by regulations and oversight to ensure quality vaccination (Ahmed, DeRoeck, & Sadr-Azodi, 2019; Mitrovich, Marti, Watkins, & Duclos, 2017).

Most LMICs have official policies to provide vaccination free of charge, though households may incur some costs related to seeking care. Country-level studies have shown a wide variation in both the volume of private sector immunization services as well as the cost to patients paying out of pocket for those services. For instance, in Benin, 64% of clients in facilities reported paying for vaccination, down to 14% in Malawi. Clients reported paying for vaccination cards, vaccination services, and syringes, among other services. The average out-of-pocket cost per vaccination was $0.50 in Malawi and up to $14 in Georgia (Levin et al., 2019).

There are very few health systems that are primarily financed from private sources and where vaccination services are financed 100% out of pocket. In mixed systems with public and private financing for health, private insurance may be a source of financing for vaccination and immunization services. This tends to be the case for higher-income countries. Private, voluntary insurance and employer-based insurance may cover most of the cost of vaccination, but households are responsible for monthly premiums, deductibles, and co-pays at the time of service. In the US, the Affordable Care Act mandated that priority preventive vaccinations must be covered by private insurance.

Trust funds may be financed through private donations and government allocations which are invested and managed to fund a share of the cost of running health and immunization programs. For instance, Bhutan has established a trust fund for health services which covers immunizations. This is a long-running trust fund with significant political commitment and support. Other countries have examined setting up trust funds, but the complexity and cost of operating and maintaining the fund may outweigh the additional resources generated (Results for Development, 2017).

Lotteries generated through out-of-pocket purchases of tickets may be another source of financing for immunization programs. For instance, the government of Costa Rica dedicates net funds from the November draw of the national lottery which covers approximately 1% of vaccine purchasing requirements (Results for Development, 2017; World Bank & Gavi, 2010).

5.2.1.3 External financing

External financing for immunization has been used for both procurement of vaccines as well as support for the delivery of immunization services in many LMICs. In general, the share of external financing is inversely related to the country's gross domestic product. Sustainable financing to meet immunization program needs is critical, particularly as countries transition away from donor support. Chapter 5.3 examines in greater depth the various external sources for immunization financing, which include subsidies for new vaccines and systems strengthening from Gavi, the Vaccine Alliance; bilateral development assistance; and foundation support.

5.2.2 Improving budgetary space for immunization

The level of funding available for the health sector can be increased through various mechanisms. Fiscal space is related to economic growth; allocating more resources to primary health care and immunization services; earmarking; utilizing immunization resources more effectively and efficiently; and funding through donor support (Tandon et al., 2018). However, expanding fiscal space is not the only approach for garnering more resources for health, and for primary health care and immunization programs by extension. Improving budgetary space through better public financial management (PFM) will likely lead to additional health sector outcomes. A study examining the relationship between PFM and child mortality found that a 1% improvement in PFM translated into a 14% reduction in child mortality (Piatti-Fünfkirchen & Smets, 2019). Four PFM interventions enhance budgetary space for health: (1) reducing unnecessary expenditures through more flexibility in budget structures, (2) a results-based approach to budgeting, (3) improving budget execution, and (4) influencing future allocations by good budget performance (Barroy & Gupta, 2020).

Improving budgetary space for health will have positive benefits for primary health care and immunization programs. There are specific actions that can be taken by programs themselves to further expand budgetary space. First, budgeting and planning should be related to achieving results both in the medium term and annually. The World Health Organization has recently launched the National Immunization Strategy (NIS) which aims to bring a greater strategic lens to planning and budgeting for the Immunization Agenda 2030 (World Health Organization: Immunization Vaccines and Biologicals, 2021). Second, immunization budgets need to be fully utilized and executed within the fiscal year. There are often challenges in full utilization of resources given delays in receipt of disbursements, particularly at the subnational level. Third, greater efficiency in the use of immunization resources, through lower-cost procurement options, better planning and organization of campaigns, reducing wastage, and using resources in more cost-effective ways, among others. These approaches can help to achieve greater performance and coverage of the program.

5.2.3 Conclusion

This chapter has explored the range of financing sources available for ensuring adequate and sustainable financing for immunization programs. Because of the public goods nature of vaccination, governments have a unique role in financing these programs, complemented by other sources. Providing vaccinations free of charge or at highly subsidized costs can ensure that no one is deterred from seeking immunization services if they want them. Government commitment is key to mobilizing resources. However, countries, particularly LMICs, face constraints and competing priorities for government spending. Greater attention to better financial management and use of program resources may provide additional budgetary space, particularly during economic crises.

References

Ahmed, N., DeRoeck, D., & Sadr-Azodi, N. (2019). Private sector engagement and contributions to immunisation service delivery and coverage in Sudan. *BMJ Global Health*, 4(2), e001414. doi:10.1136/bmjgh-2019-001414

Barroy, H., & Gupta, S. (2020). *From overall fiscal space to budgetary space for health: Connecting public financial management to resource mobilization in the era of COVID-19.* Center for Global Development. https://www.cgdev.org/sites/default/files/overall-fiscal-space-budget ary-space-health-connecting-public-financial-management.pdf

Chang, A. Y., Riumallo-Herl, C., Perales, N. A., Clark, S., Clark, A., Constenla, D., . . . Verguet, S. (2018). The equity impact vaccines may have on averting deaths and medical impoverishment in developing countries. *Health Affairs (Millwood), 37*(2), 316–324. doi:10.1377/hlthaff.2017.0861

Dagnan, S. (2018). Health system reforms to accelerate universal health coverage in Côte d'Ivoire. *Health Systems & Reform, 4*(2), 69–71. doi:10.1080/23288604.2018.1446123

de Broucker, G., Ahmed, S., Hasan, M. Z., Mehdi, G. G., Martin Del Campo, J., Ali, M. W., . . . Patenaude, B. (2020). The economic burden of measles in children under five in Bangladesh. *BMC Health Services Research, 20*(1), 1026. doi:10.1186/s12913-020-05880-5

De Broucker, G., Ssebagereka, A., Apolot, R. R., Aloysius, M., Ekirapa Kiracho, E., Patenaude, B., & Constenla, D. (2020). The economic burden of measles in children under five in Uganda. *Vaccine: X, 6*, 100077. doi:https://doi.org/10.1016/j.jvacx.2020.100077

Glassman, A., Giedion, U., & Smith, P. C. (2017). *What's in, what's out? Designing benefits for universal health coverage.* Center for Global Development. https://www.cgdev.org/sites/defa ult/files/whats-in-whats-out-designing-benefits-final.pdf

Grépin, K. A., & Dionne, K. Y. (2013). Democratization and universal health coverage: A case comparison of Ghana, Kenya, and Senegal. *Global Health Governance, VI*(2). http://blogs. shu.edu/ghg/files/2014/02/GHGJ-Volume-V1-No.-2-Summer-2013.pdf#page=5

Griffiths, U. K., Asman, J., Adjagba, A., Yo, M., Oguta, J. O., & Cho, C. (2020). Budget line items for immunization in 33 African countries. *Health Policy and Planning, 35*(7), 753–764. doi:10.1093/heapol/czaa040

Learning Network for Countries in Transition. (2020). *LNCT brief: Considerations for managing immunization programs within national health insurance.* https://lnct.global/wp-content/uploads/2020/02/Considerations-for-Immunization-Programs-within-NHI_FI NAL.pdf

Learning Network for Countries in Transition. (2021). *Mobilizing resources in decentralized health systems: A desk review of LNCT country experiences.* https://lnct.global/wp-content/uploads/2021/03/Decentralization-resource-doc-formatted-FINAL.pdf

Levin, A., & Kaddar, M. (2011). Role of the private sector in the provision of immunization services in low- and middle-income countries. *Health Policy and Planning, 26*(Suppl 1), i4–i12. doi:10.1093/heapol/czr037

Levin, A., Munthali, S., Vodungbo, V., Rukhadze, N., Maitra, K., Ashagari, T., & Brenzel, L. (2019). Scope and magnitude of private sector financing and provision of immunization in Benin, Malawi and Georgia. *Vaccine, 37*(27), 3568–3575. doi:https://doi.org/10.1016/j.vacc ine.2019.05.023

Lydon, P., Levine, R., Makinen, M., Brenzel, L., Mitchell, V., Milstien, J. B., . . . Landry, S. (2008). Introducing new vaccines in the poorest countries: What did we learn from the GAVI experience with financial sustainability? *Vaccine, 26*(51), 6706–6716. doi:10.1016/j.vaccine.2008.10.015

Maeda, A., Araujo, E., Cashin, C., Harris, J., Ikegami, N., & Reich, M. R. (2014). *Universal health coverage for inclusive and sustainable development: A synthesis of 11 country case studies.* Washington, DC: World Bank.

Marquez, P. V., & Dutta, S. (2020). *Taxes on tobacco, alcohol, and sugar-sweetened beverages reduce health risks and expand fiscal space for universal health coverage post-COVID 19.* World Bank. https://blogs.worldbank.org/health/taxes-tobacco-alcohol-and-sugar-sweetened-beverages-reduce-health-risks-and-expand-fiscal

Mitrovich, R., Marti, M., Watkins, M., & Duclos, P. (2017). *A review of the private sector's contribution to immunization service delivery in low, middle, and high-income countries.* World

Health Organization. https://www.who.int/immunization/sage/meetings/2017/april/2_Review_private_sector_engagement_Mitrovich_et_al.pdf?ua=1

Ozawa, S., Clark, S., Portnoy, A., Grewal, S., Brenzel, L., & Walker, D. G. (2016). Return on investment from childhood immunization in low- and middle-income countries, 2011–20. *Health Affairs, 35*(2), 199–207. doi:10.1377/hlthaff.2015.1086

Piatti-Fünfkirchen, M., & Smets, L. (2019). *Public financial management, health financing and under-five mortality: A comparative empirical analysis.* Washington, DC: Inter-American Development Bank.

Regan, L., Wilson, D., Chalkidou, K., & Chi, Y. L. (2021). The journey to UHC: How well are vertical programmes integrated in the health benefits package? A scoping review. *BMJ Global Health, 6*(8), e005842. doi:10.1136/bmjgh-2021-005842

Results for Development. (2017). *Immunization financing: A resource guide for advocates, policymakers, and program managers.* https://r4d.org/resources/immunization-financing-resource-guide-advocates-policymakers-program-managers/

Stenberg, K., Hanssen, O., Edejer, T. T., Bertram, M., Brindley, C., Meshreky, A., . . . Soucat, A. (2017). Financing transformative health systems towards achievement of the health Sustainable Development Goals: a model for projected resource needs in 67 low-income and middle-income countries. *Lancet Global Health, 5*(9), e875–e887. doi:10.1016/s2214-109x(17)30263-2

Tandon, A., Cain, J., Kurowski, C., & Postolovska, I. (2018). *Intertemporal dynamics of public financing for universal health coverage: Accounting for fiscal space across countries.* World Bank. https://documents1.worldbank.org/curated/en/639541545281356938/pdf/133115-19-12-2018-14-44-10-AccountingforFiscalSpaceinHealthFINAL.pdf

Union for International Cancer Control. (2020). *Kicking off UHC in Kenya.* https://www.uicc.org/case-studies/kicking-uhc-kenya

World Bank, & Gavi. (2010). *Immunization finance toolkit: A resource for policy-makers and program managers.* http://hdl.handle.net/10986/20784

World Health Organization. (2020a). *Global spending on health: Weathering the storm.* https://www.who.int/publications/i/item/9789240017788

World Health Organization. (2020b). *Immunization Agenda 2030: A global strategy to leave no one behind.* https://www.who.int/publications/m/item/immunization-agenda-2030-a-global-strategy-to-leave-no-one-behind

World Health Organization. (2021). *Global expenditure on health: Public spending on the rise?* https://www.who.int/publications/i/item/9789240041219

World Health Organization: Immunization Vaccines and Biologicals. (2021). *National immunization strategy (NIS).* https://www.who.int/teams/immunization-vaccines-and-biologicals/vaccine-access/planning-and-financing/nis-(national-immunization-strategy)

Wright, A., Smith, K. E., & Hellowell, M. (2017). Policy lessons from health taxes: A systematic review of empirical studies. *BMC Public Health, 17*(1), 583. doi:10.1186/s12889-017-4497-z

5.3

Donor architecture for immunization financing

Grace Chee, George Pariyo, and Shreena Malaviya

5.3.1 The role of Gavi and other institutions in immunization financing

5.3.1.1 Origins and structure of Gavi, the Vaccine Alliance

Building on the successful eradication of smallpox, the Expanded Program on Immunization was launched by the World Health Organization (WHO) in 1974 targeting six diseases—diphtheria, tetanus, whooping cough, polio, measles, and tuberculosis. The program achieved a significant increase in immunization rates up to 60% in the lowest income countries (Zerhouni, 2019). In 1984, a collaboration with UNICEF initiated the Universal Childhood Immunization by 1990 initiative to help countries reach 80% immunization coverage. In 1990, UNICEF declared that the target of the initiative had been achieved (Hardon & Blume, 2005).

During the 1990s, as donor financing waned, progress in immunization rates stagnated and declined in some countries (Clemens, Holmgren, Kaufmann, & Mantovani, 2010; Muraskin, 2005). To counter this, the Children's Vaccine Initiative was launched in 1990, led by UNICEF, the United Nations (UN) Development Programme, WHO, the World Bank, and the Rockefeller Foundation. The Children's Vaccine Initiative's aims were to develop new vaccines to improve performance of the Expanded Program on Immunization, such as combination and heat-stable vaccines, as well as to ensure an adequate supply of vaccines in lower-income countries. Despite some initial success, the Children's Vaccine Initiative was unable to mobilize enough resources to fulfill its goals (Clemens et al., 2010; Muraskin, 2005; Zerhouni, 2019). By the late 1990s, it had become clear that despite these efforts, there were still many childhood deaths from vaccine-preventable diseases. For instance, measles outbreaks were still commonplace even though a highly effective measles

Grace Chee, George Pariyo, and Shreena Malaviya, *Donor architecture for immunization financing* In: *Handbook of Applied Health Economics in Vaccines.* Edited by: David Bishai, Logan Brenzel and William V. Padula, Oxford University Press. © Oxford University Press 2023. DOI: 10.1093/oso/9780192896087.003.0029 vaccine had been around for decades (Zerhouni, 2019). Additionally, vaccines that were routinely used in high-income countries, most notably hepatitis B, were not widely provided in low-income countries.

The Global Alliance for Vaccines and Immunization (GAVI) was formed on January 31, 2000, at the World Economic Forum in Davos. GAVI's focus was to improve the disparities in access to life-saving vaccines between wealthy and lower-income countries. GAVI aimed to increase the availability and affordability of new and underused vaccines, building on a partnership between countries, donors, the private sector, and multilateral and civil society organizations (Zerhouni, 2019). GAVI's founding partners include UNICEF, WHO, the World Bank, and the Bill & Melinda Gates Foundation.

The first phase of GAVI (2000–2005) focused on introducing new and underused vaccines in the poorest countries. GAVI's second phase (2006–2010) included a new focus on strengthening health systems to sustainably deliver immunization and other services, accelerating the uptake of new and underused vaccines, and promoting sustainable financing for immunization. With the progress made previously, GAVI's third strategy (2011–2015) continued to focus on increasing the use of new vaccines and strengthening of health systems, and added a focus on market shaping to increase the supply of high-quality and affordable vaccines. GAVI 4.0 (2016–2020), built on the success of previous periods, with renewed focus on sustainability. Over this period, GAVI's name changed to Gavi, the Vaccine Alliance (Gavi). Gavi's current Phase (2021–2025), Gavi 5.0, has a new orientation toward reducing the number of zero-dose and under-immunized children.

Gavi is governed by a Board responsible for strategic direction and policies. The Board is comprised of recipient country governments, donor agencies, vaccine industry and pharmaceutical company representatives, civil society, research and health institutes, and independent individuals (Zerhouni, 2019). The four founding partners hold permanent seats on Gavi's Board while other partners rotate on a time-limited basis. Each partner brings a complementary perspective and expertise to the complex multifaceted field of vaccines and immunization, as well as well representing the interests of their respective constituencies, and providing technical support This complex partnership and governing arrangement has stood the test of time and ensures that all key players have an opportunity to express their concerns and priorities.

The Gavi Secretariat is based in Geneva, with an office in Washington, DC. The Secretariat is responsible for the operation of Gavi. Gavi has an international institution status in Geneva, Switzerland, and a public charity status in the US. Gavi has no in-country presence and relies on its core partners (WHO, UNICEF, and the World Bank) as well as extended partners, for technical support.

WHO is the UN agency charged with normative functions such as setting standards for healthcare practices, products, and safety, and pre-certification of healthcare and pharmaceutical products. The Department of Immunization, Vaccines and Biologicals (IVB) plays a key role in ensuring state-of-the art scientific practices and safety of vaccines supported by Gavi. The agency also plays an important role in advising Ministries of Health of member states, and through the World Health Assembly developing global consensus through resolutions on pressing health matters such as immunization.

UNICEF is the UN agency charged with protecting the health of women and children. Through its country offices in every member state, UNICEF provides critical programmatic and funding support to countries on implementing immunization programs. UNICEF Supply Division acts as the main procurement agency for vaccines and immunization cold chain logistics and equipment for Gavi-eligible countries. This function is particularly important in helping Gavi-eligible countries procure quality and effective vaccines efficiently and at subsidized prices.

The *World Bank* is an international institution that provides financial assistance, such as loans and grants, to governments of low- and middle-income countries for development projects. The Bank was involved in the development of two innovative financing mechanisms—the International Finance Facility for Immunization (IFFIm) and the Advance Market Commitment (AMC)—that raise additional resources for vaccines. The Bank acts as a steward for the IFFIm program and manages the AMC, while serving as a development partner to Gavi (World Bank, 2015).

Extended partners include international and country-level civil society organizations and consulting firms with expertise and experience in providing technical support.

5.3.1.2 Donor funding to Gavi

Every 5 years, Gavi holds a donor pledging conference and raises funds to finance a new phase of Gavi with a 5-year strategy. By March 2021, Gavi had received nearly US $21 billion through donor contributions (Table 5.3.1). Approximately 57% of the contributions are from direct donations provided by governments. The UK, the US, and Norway are the top three donors, followed

Table 5.3.1 Donor contributions to Gavi, 2000–March 2021

Donors	Contributions (in US $, millions)	% of total contributions
Government contributions	12,018	57.3
UK	3,000	14.3
US	2,760	13.2
Norway	1,908	9.1
Germany	876	4.2
Canada	681	3.2
Netherlands	606	2.9
Sweden	587	2.8
Others	1,600	7.6
Private contributions	4,300	20.5
Bill & Melinda Gates Foundation	4,051	19.3
Others	249	1.2
Innovative financing mechanisms	4,661	22.2
International Finance Facility for Immunization (IFFIm)	3,348	16.0
Advance Market Commitment (AMC)	1,313	6.3
Total	20,979	100.0

by Germany. Private donations account for 24% of total contributions, with the Bill & Melinda Gates Foundation accounting for 19% of total donations to Gavi. Other notable private donors include TikTok, Mastercard, Comic Relief, and the International Federation of Pharmaceutical Wholesalers. Around 22% of the funding comes from the proceeds of IFFIm and AMC. IFFIm is projected to ramp up significantly in the 2021–2037 period.

For the next phase of Gavi from 2021 to 2025, an additional US $8.8 billion was pledged by world leaders at the Global Vaccine Summit 2020, surpassing the target of US $7.4 billion (Gavi 2021a). This included US $2 billion from the UK, US $1.6 billion from the Bill & Melinda Gates Foundation, and US $1 billion from Norway (Gavi, 2020d).

5.3.1.3 Bilateral donors

In addition to the main central donor funds that support Gavi's strategy and vaccine and programmatic grants to countries outlined above, other funding for countries' immunization activities comes in the form of bilateral donor support provided for immunization or to the broader health sector directly in-country through development cooperation agencies. Some of this support, for instance, to strengthen health workforce, infrastructure, information systems, or transport and logistics, ends up also benefitting or strengthening immunization activities. Some of the agencies that have historically provided direct in-country support to Gavi-eligible countries in the form of bilateral aid to governments or through nongovernmental organizations include USAID, the Japan International Cooperation Agency, and the UK Department for International Development. For example, USAID investments help build and sustain routine immunization systems to deliver Gavi-supported vaccines. In Tanzania, USAID supported the pilot of an innovative Vaccine Information Management System to improve access and use of data at all levels and to drive improvements in routine immunization, which is now being supported with resources from Gavi (USAID, 2018). In Mozambique, USAID funded health worker training, supply chain procurement, and system strengthening to support the distribution of new vaccines (USAID, 2020).

5.3.2 Gavi policies and support to countries

5.3.2.1 Types of Gavi support

Gavi offers two main types of support to eligible countries:

1. **New vaccine support.** This is support for new and underutilized vaccines. As of 2020, Gavi supports vaccines that protect against 17 infectious diseases.
2. **Health system and immunization strengthening (HSIS) support.** This support bundles several types of cash support to countries. HSIS grants support priorities to improve delivery of immunization services. New vaccine introduction grants support some of the introduction activities for new vaccine introduction. Gavi supports vaccines and operational costs of immunization campaigns. Beginning in 2021, support for cold chain equipment previously provided through the Cold Chain Equipment Optimization Platform was rolled into HSIS support.

Additionally, Gavi supports immunization partners to provide targeted technical assistance at country level to improve coverage rates and reduce equity barriers.

Since its inception through July 2019 (last data available), Gavi has disbursed over US $1.6 billion to support 76 low- and middle-income

Table 5.3.2 Gavi country support by type, 2000–July 2019 (latest available data)

Types of support	Funding in US $ millions (percentage)
New and under-utilized vaccines	10,432.93 (70.9)
Health system and immunization strengthening (HSIS)	2,156.8 (14.7)
Vaccine introduction grants	196.0 (1.3)
Other cash support	121.7 (0.8)
Operational costs for immunization campaigns	642.9 (4.4)
Outbreak support and response	1.055.16 (7.2)
Other programs	99.4 (0.7)
Total	14,704.89

countries (Table 5.3.2). About 67% of the disbursements were towards new and underutilized vaccines, followed by cash support including HSIS, introduction grants, and other (16.9%). HSIS alone accounted for 14.7% of Gavi disbursements (Gavi 2021c).

To support countries during the coronavirus disease 2019 (COVID-19) pandemic, Gavi provided new flexibility to allow up to 20% of HSIS funding to be reallocated to the COVID-19 response, and to repurpose technical assistance implemented by partners to the COVID-19 response.

5.3.2.2 Gavi eligibility and transition policy

Since its creation, Gavi has been committed to working with countries to achieve financial sustainability of their immunization programs. Through its eligibility and transition policy and its co-financing policy, Gavi aims to encourage countries to expand their immunization programs with vaccines of public health importance, increase domestic ownership of vaccine financing, and fully self-finance vaccines when Gavi support ends. As of the end of 2019, 16 countries have successfully transitioned from Gavi support (Gavi, 2019a).

In the beginning, Gavi aimed to support the world's poorest countries, and selected 75 countries with gross national income (GNI) per capita below US $1,000 as the focus for eligibility. In 2011, Gavi's GNI per capita eligibility threshold was reset at US $1,500, with the threshold updated annually to account for inflation. In 2015, the eligibility policy was revised to determine eligibility based on average GNI per capita over a 3-year period, with some adjustments for large single-year increases in GNI per capita, in order to smooth out annual fluctuations. As of 2019, the threshold stood at US $1,580, with 58 countries eligible for Gavi support (Gavi, 2018). Once a country's GNI per capita exceeds the eligibility threshold, it begins a transition process, during which Gavi support is phased out over 5 years.

Due to disruptions caused by COVID-19, Gavi announced that countries would retain their eligibility status from 2020 to 2021. Vaccine co-financing in 2021 would also remain at the 2020 levels.

In 2020, the Gavi Board approved an approach for engaging with former and never-eligible middle-income countries, with GNI per capita up to US $4,000.

5.3.2.3 Gavi co-financing policy

To help countries on a pathway to financial sustainability for new vaccines, Gavi developed the concept of co-financing in 2006. This was a novel co-procurement mechanism whereby a country, depending upon its GNI per capita, would be responsible for procuring a complementary portion of vaccine doses to those procured by Gavi. Country contributions are phased over time based on national income. For countries whose GNI per capita is below the World Bank threshold for a low-income country, their initial co-financing was set at US $0.20 per dose for all new vaccines (Gavi, 2016). These countries

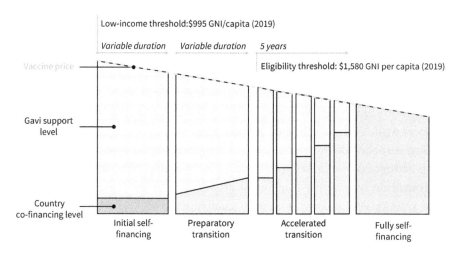

Fig. 5.3.1 How the Gavi co-financing model works.

Source: Adapted from https://www.gavi.org/vaccineswork/how-gavis-co-financing-model-works

are in Gavi's initial phase of transition. Once a country's income surpasses this threshold, its co-financing obligation on a per dose basis increases by 15% per year—this is referred to as the preparatory transition phase. The duration of this phase is entirely dependent on the country's income growth rate. Once its income exceeds the Gavi eligibility threshold, a country enters accelerated transition. During this period, co-financing obligations are increase linearly each year, in order to reach full self-financing at the end of 5 years. If a country's GNI per capita falls below the threshold amount after it enters accelerated transition, it would regain its eligibility status.

A Board-approved modification to Gavi's co-financing policy aims to simplify the calculation of co-financing requirements to a percentage of doses. Operationalization of this policy decision is still under development (Gavi, 2019b).

5.3.3 Transition from Gavi support

5.3.3.1 Transition planning

The Gavi Secretariat and partners work with countries to plan for both the financial and programmatic aspects of transition from support. Transition assessments were conducted and plans were developed approximately 2–3 years before a country was projected to enter accelerated transition. Based on the transition plan, Gavi supported activities deemed critical for successful transition.

Unlike the preparatory transition phase, which is not time-bound, the accelerated transition phase is limited to a 5-year period. During the accelerated transition phase, Gavi continues to support already introduced vaccines and maintains its existing commitments for HSIS support. In 2018, Gavi revised its eligibility and transition policy to allow countries to apply for new vaccine support while in the accelerated transition phase.

Gavi launched the Learning Network for Countries in Transition in 2017 to support successful country transitions. The Learning Network for Countries in Transition uses a peer-learning approach to provide countries with practical solutions to address transition challenges. The Learning Network for Countries in Transition facilitates access to peer countries' experiences, technical resources, and global expertise to support countries to develop solutions to transition challenges (Learning Network for Countries in Transition, 2021). Currently, the peer learning platform has been renamed to the Linked Learning Action Network.

5.3.3.2 Transition challenges

The highest priorities for most countries as they prepare for transition are often domestic resource mobilization and vaccine procurement. In addition to securing adequate funding for vaccines, countries must decide how best to manage vaccine procurement. While countries have the option of procuring through UNICEF Supply Division, which manages procurement of Gavi-supported vaccines, conflicts between domestic procurement regulations and UNICEF procedures can be challenging to overcome. Some countries with small populations face challenges securing competitive pricing with independent procurement.

Transitioning countries also face challenges to their immunization programs posed by the broader health financing context. Countries that are expanding social health insurance are in the midst of decisions regarding whether immunization and other preventative services are included as part of insurance benefits or funded separately. If immunization is funded through health insurance, key program functions may need to be transferred to the insurance administrator. Countries with decentralized health systems may need to mobilize funding from multiple entities, including subnational governments or subnational health offices, in order to fund necessary immunization functions. Transitioning countries may also face growing vaccine hesitancy among their population that threatens the achievements of the immunization program.

Some countries face more significant programmatic and institutional challenges to scaling-up and sustaining immunization coverage, even as they prepare for transition away from Gavi support. For the countries that have more deep-rooted obstacles to achieving high coverage, Gavi works with the country to develop tailored plans to support successful transition. In rare cases where a country faces a high risk of unsuccessful transition, specific flexibilities, including time-limited extension of the accelerated transition phase, may be approved (Gavi, 2019b).

5.3.3.3 Post-transition engagement

Gavi continues to engage with countries after they transition away from Gavi support, including monitoring vaccine coverage rates and new vaccine introduction. Immunization program sustainability is facilitated by affordable vaccine prices. Gavi has negotiated with vaccine manufacturers to secure pricing commitments so that transitioned countries can access prices for pentavalent, pneumococcal, rotavirus, and human papillomavirus vaccines at prices similar to those paid by Gavi for 5–10 years after transition (Gavi, 2020c).

In addition, the Gavi Board allocated US $30 million to mitigate any risks for successful transition (Gavi, 2020c). These risks include those related to supply chain and data system weaknesses, as well as leadership, management, and coordination. This post-transition support has encouraged government commitment to long-term financial sustainability and innovation of the program (Gavi, 2020c).

5.3.3.4 Middle-income country engagement

In December 2020, the Gavi Board approved engagement with middle-income countries, including former-Gavi (transitioned) countries and never Gavi-eligible (previously ineligible) countries with per capita GNI under US $4,000. The objectives of the engagement are to prevent backsliding in former Gavi countries and to drive the sustainable introduction of key missing vaccines in former and select never Gavi-eligible countries.

The primary focus over the first 18 months is to prevent and mitigate backsliding in former-Gavi countries, prioritizing those countries with large numbers of children who have received no vaccine doses. Gavi engagement will focus on building political will and advocating for improving equity in routine immunization, proving technical assistance to re-establish routine immunization services, targeted interventions to restore coverage and catch up missed children, and fostering peer-to-peer learning for disseminating best practices. Gavi will lay the groundwork for future introductions of pneumococcal conjugate, rotavirus, and human papillomavirus vaccines by leveraging its country-level engagement with COVID-19 vaccines (Gavi, 2020a). More guidance from Gavi on the practical implementation of this decision will be needed, particularly as it relates to countries that are currently in accelerated transition.

5.3.4 Innovations for immunization financing

5.3.4.1 Advance market commitments

AMCs have been shown to be an effective mechanism for mobilizing resources and incentivizing development of new vaccines for lower-income markets. By announcing a donor commitment to purchase vaccines at a set price with predetermined specifications and level of demand, this would incentivize manufacturers' and producers' interest in developing a vaccine. Greater reliability and certainty around price and demand would motivate vaccine manufacturers to invest in development. Based on the initial concept developed by the Center for Global Development, the World Bank and Gavi convened experts in public health, health economics, and contract law to develop key terms and structure of a pilot AMC (Levine, Kremer, & Albright, 2005).

The pilot AMC for pneumococcal vaccine was announced in February 2007. The Governments of Italy, the UK, the Russian Federation, Canada, Norway, and the Bill & Melinda Gates Foundation pledged a total of US $1.5 billion to fund the AMC. By March 2010, GlaxoSmithKline and Pfizer both agreed to provide 30 million doses per year for up to 10 years. While both the GlaxoSmithKline and Pfizer vaccines were already in advanced stages of development when the AMC was announced, the long-term demand stimulated by the AMC led to investments to expand capacity and to create presentations specifically for Gavi countries. The AMC also contributed to bringing in two donors who had previously not provided funding to Gavi.

In June 2020, Gavi launched the COVAX AMC led by Gavi, the Coalition for Epidemic Preparedness (CEPI), and WHO. The Facility is designed to guarantee rapid, fair, and equitable access to COVID-19 vaccines for 92 low- and middle-income countries. Another 81 self-financing countries have also indicated interest in COVAX. The Facility pools resources from many countries, shares risks by investing in a portfolio of vaccine candidates, and will provide vaccines for low-income countries. The AMC was established to mobilize resources from Organisation for Economic Co-operation and Development countries with a goal of providing 2 billion doses of COVID-19 vaccine by the end of 2021 to low- and middle-income countries. The AMC enters advanced purchase agreements with suppliers prior to vaccine licensure and WHO prequalification. As of May 10, 2021, COVAX has shipped 58 million doses of COVID-19 vaccine to 122 countries (Gavi, 2021b).

5.3.4.2 International Finance Facility for Immunization vaccine bonds

The IFFIm is a global development finance tool launched by Gavi in 2006. Based on a concept developed by the UK Treasury and Goldman Sachs, pledges from donor governments are used to issue bonds, often referred to as "vaccine bonds," on capital markets around the world to finance immunization programs. IFFIm bonds are backed by irrevocable, legally binding funding pledges from ten sovereign governments, including the UK, France, the US, and Norway. More information is available at https://iffim.org/donors. Since its inception, IFFIm has attracted more than US $6.5 billion in sovereign pledges and disbursed US $2.6 billion (as of October 2018) to support immunization, or approximately one-quarter of Gavi's program funding since 2006. The World Bank acts as the treasury manager for IFFIm.

In July 2020, IFFIm issued NOK 2 billion (US $224 million) in vaccine bonds to finance COVID-19 vaccine research and development, against a 10-year commitment from the Kingdom of Norway. The IFFIm mechanism allowed a 10-year pledge to be converted into cash in order to maximize urgent investments in vaccine candidates and vaccine trials.

5.3.5 Partnerships with private sector

Since its inception, private sector partners have played a key role in supporting Gavi's mission. Gavi has mobilized the private sector to contribute both financially and technically to improve immunization program operations. Gavi continues to seek new private sector partnerships, aiming to drive innovation, cut costs, and increase operational efficiency to achieve its goals.

With the UPS Foundation, Gavi engaged in a vaccine delivery network innovation in three districts of Uganda reaching more than 150 clinics that serve 3 million people. The pilot employed a range of supply chain tools and innovations. A stock management system was used to help reduce vaccine stock-outs. A "Strategic Training Executive Program" leadership development program helped build management supply capacity.

Deutsche Post DHL Group was another Gavi partner whose expertise in transportation and logistics was applied to immunization. Using DHL's global network, the Ministry of Health of Kenya, DHL, and Gavi developed a transportation management innovation. A transport support hub coordinated third-party transport carriers to improve the reliability and speed of vaccine deliveries to points of service delivery.

The Zipline drone network in Ghana works with the national supply chain to prevent vaccine stockouts in facilities and for campaigns. The current service of 30 drones covers 2,000 health facilities. UPS also provides technical guidance and consultancy services as needed. Zipline drones are also used in delivery of COVID-19 vaccines to the hardest-to-reach areas of Ghana. The drone vaccine network builds on Zipline's experience in Rwanda to provide blood products to remote clinics in Rwanda.

To identify and fund potential innovations, Gavi established the INFUSE platform (Innovation for uptake, scale and equity in immunization) to connect private sector partners and funders with high-tech innovators (Gavi, 2020b). One innovation to improve cold chain performance relies on Nexleaf sensor technology to provide real-time data paired with targeted analytics to analyze the root causes of cold chain failures in the field, which allows for prioritization of resources, efficient repairs, and informed procurement. Also identified through INFUSE, Zenysis provides its software platform, analytical training, and IT skills development to integrate data from their fragmented information systems and help decision makers see where children are not receiving vaccines. Advanced analytics will then help countries decide how to target their limited resources for maximum impact.

Gavi is also collaborating with Airtel to improve the quality of reporting on immunization coverage through the E-Reporting Project through the digitization of paper-based reports, and provision of digital tools to primary healthcare workers across Nigeria.

These advanced logistics, transport, and technology are innovations that have potential to strengthen vaccine supply chains, identify under-immunized children, and improve immunization data. Whether they are true breakthroughs in resolving longstanding challenges will depend on whether they can be implemented sustainability at scale.

5.3.6 Conclusion

This chapter provides an overview of the various public–private partnerships that have served to support immunization coverage, new vaccine introduction, and strengthened immunization systems since the 1980s. Gavi has and continues to provide a significant level of funding and technical support to countries, as well as to lead on innovations related to financing and sustainability of the program. It was one of the first partnerships that developed a cost-sharing/co-procurement relationship with countries and was the basis for innovations such as the AMC and IFFIm which are being explored for other life-saving commodities. Innovative partnerships with the private sector on data and supply chain can promote delivery of life-saving vaccines to the remotest populations.

References

Clemens, J., Holmgren, J., Kaufmann, S., & Mantovani, A. (2010). Ten years of the Global Alliance for Vaccines and Immunization: Challenges and progress. *Nature Immunology, 11*, 1069–1072. doi:10.1038/ni1210-1069

Gavi. (2016). *Gavi, the Vaccine Alliance co-financing policy.* https://www.gavi.org/sites/default/files/document/gavi-co-financing-policypdf.pdf

Gavi. (2018). *Eligibility and transition policy.* https://www.gavi.org/programmes-impact/programmatic-policies/eligibility-and-transitioning-policy

Gavi. (2019a). *Annual program report.* https://www.gavi.org/sites/default/files/programmes-impact/our-impact/apr/Gavi-Progress-Report-2019_1.pdf

Gavi. (2019b). *Gavi 5.0: Funding policy review.* https://www.gavi.org/sites/default/files/board/minutes/2019/4-dec/09%20-%20Gavi%205.0%20Funding%20Policy%20Review.pdf

Gavi. (2020a). *Gavi's approach to engagement with former and never-eligible middle-income countries (MICs).* https://www.gavi.org/sites/default/files/board/minutes/2020/15-dec/07%20-%20Gavi%27s%20approach%20to%20engagement%20with%20former%20and%20never-eligible%20MICs.pdf

Gavi. (2020b). *INFUSE.* https://www.gavi.org/investing-gavi/infuse

Gavi. (2020c). *Transitioning out of Gavi support.* https://www.gavi.org/types-support/sustainability/transition

Gavi. (2020d). *World leaders make historic commitments to provide equal access to vaccines for all.* https://www.gavi.org/news/media-room/world-leaders-make-historic-commitments-provide-equal-access-vaccines-all

Gavi. (2021a, March 31). *Cash receipts 31 March 2021.* https://www.gavi.org/news/document-library/cash-receipts-31-march-2021

Gavi. (2021b). *COVAX.* https://www.gavi.org/covax-facility

Gavi. (2021c). *Disbursements and commitments.* https://www.gavi.org/programmes-impact/our-impact/disbursements-and-commitments

Hardon, A., & Blume, S. (2005). Shifts in global immunisation goals (1984–2004): Unfinished agendas and mixed results. *Social Science & Medicine, 60*(2), 345–356. doi:10.1016/j.socscimed.2004.05.008

Learning Network for Countries in Transition. (2021). *Homepage.* https://lnct.global/

Levine, R., Kremer, M., & Albright, A. (2005). *Making markets for vaccines: Ideas to action.* https://www.cgdev.org/sites/default/files/archive/doc/books/vaccine/MakingMarkets-complete.pdf

Muraskin, W. (2005). *Crusade to immunize the world's children.* Durham, NC: Lulu.com.

USAID. (2018). *USAID's investment to Gavi, the Vaccine Alliance.* https://www.usaid.gov/sites/default/files/documents/1864/GAVI_factsheet_4_16-508.pdf

USAID. (2020). *Support community health interventions to address neonatal and child health—UNICEF.* https://www.usaid.gov/mozambique/fact-sheets/support-community-health-interventions-address-neonatal-and-child

World Bank. (2015). *Global program review: The World Bank's partnership with the GAVI Alliance.* https://openknowledge.worldbank.org/bitstream/handle/10986/23612/The0World0Bank0th0the0GAVI0alliance.pdf

Zerhouni, E. (2019). GAVI, the Vaccine Alliance. *Cell, 179*(1), 13–17. doi:10.1016/j.cell.2019.08.026

Exercise: a case study on estimating the total and unit routine immunization costs from the facility to the national level

Ijeoma Edoka[1]

A.1.1 Background

The objectives of the exercise are to:

- Identify recurrent and capital cost components of an immunization program.
- Calculate average total costs at facility level using sampling weights.
- Generate a weighted national estimate of total and unit costs using the averaging method.

Accurate data on the costs of routine and new vaccines immunization can improve country-level planning and financing for immunization. These data can build a base of evidence to provide inputs for policy and resource mobilization domestically and externally. Applying standardized methods to analyze facility-based data will make it easier to compare and apply results more widely.

The Expanded Program on Immunization Costing and Financing (EPIC) project was an initiative that collected facility-based data on the costs of immunization across six countries. The study used an approach which applied a bottom-up, ingredients-based costing methodology from the perspective of a health service provider. The study created a unique pooled dataset of 316 sites to explore cross-country determinants of costs (Brenzel, Young, & Walker, 2015). This exercise below will focus on the data collected from the Uganda EPIC study.

Uganda had a population of approximately 34.5 million people in 2011. The types of health facility in Uganda are health centers (HC; level II, III, and IV) and hospitals (general, regional, and national hospitals). An estimated 72% of the population lived within 5 km of a health facility in 2010, and coverage with most vaccines has remained above 80% but with variations between districts (Guthrie et al., 2014).

The Uganda study applied a multistage, purposive, and stratified random sampling approach (Brenzel et al., 2015). All ten regions were represented and one or two districts per region were purposively sampled to represent a range of typical service contexts. Fifty-two health facilities were randomly sampled from the strata of health facilities in these districts (general hospitals and HC II, III, and IV) and 49 of them were included in the study (Guthrie et al., 2014). The costs were estimated retrospectively for 2011 and were captured in Ugandan shillings (UGX).

1. Open the excel document named "Costing Exercise". 🔵 Additional content on (Costing Exercise) is available online, 10.1093/oso/9780192896087.012.0001. In Sheet A, you have been provided with the raw data collected during the Uganda study. In the subsequent sheets, you will be analyzing the data.

---

[1] 'Teaching Vaccine Economics Everywhere' materials: https://immunizationeconomics.org/

2. Go to Sheet A and briefly go through the data provided. You will notice that column B contains the cost and output items, and columns C–AY contain the values of the items corresponding to each facility. Hover on the cells in column B to see a more detailed definition of the item.

A.1.2 Categorize cost items and complete the cost table

3. Cells B7–B27 contain cost line items. In column A (the red box), mark the items with a 'C' if they are capital costs, or with a 'R' if they are recurrent costs.
4. Go to Sheet B and you will find Table B-1, the cost table for the HC III facility Kiswa.
5. Complete column B of the table by filling in the values for the cost items. Column C will automatically be filled in with the USD values. The values for Kiswa will be found in Sheet A, column AA.
6. Calculate the total capital cost (cell B6), the total recurrent cost (cell B17), and the overall total cost (cell B19) for Kiswa.
7. Complete column D of the table in Sheet B by calculating the share of the total cost for each item.
8. What are your observations about the costs of the Kiswa facility?

A.1.3 Sampling weights

Analysts use sampling weights to get nationally representative value estimates of average weighted facility costs. The sampling weights for each facility's costs were calculated separately based on inverse probabilities of sampling at each sampling stage.

- A sample of I regions was selected from a total of L regions in the country, and their probability of selection was = I × L (IL).
- A sample of n districts was selected from a total of N districts in a region, and their probability of selection was thus = n × N (nN).
- A sample of m facilities have the probability of being selected from a total of Mi similar health units in the same district (i) was equal to m × Mi (mMi).

The overall probability of selection of a specific health unit in a district is therefore = IL × nN × mMi.

The weight of a sampled health unit was the reciprocal of its probability of being selected:

$$1/IL \times nN \times mMi = LNMilnm$$

In Uganda, there ten regions and 112 districts. All regions were included in the study and so IL = 1, and that simplifies the sample weights to NMinm.

9. Lira is one of the two districts sampled from the region mid-north of Uganda. This region has 15 districts in total. Assuming Lira has been selected at random and that Lira is representative of mid-north Uganda, how much weight do we need to give to observations from Lira when we include them in estimates that are intended to be nationally representative of Uganda?
10. Ober is one of the two HC III facilities sampled in Lira. There are 14 HC III facilities in this district. Let us assume that Ober has been selected at random and that Ober is a representative HC III facility in Lira.
    a. How much weight do we need to give to observations from Ober when we include them in estimates that are intended to be representative of Lira district?

b. What weight should we apply to make Ober's contribution appropriate for a nationally representative estimate?

A.1.4 Weighted estimate of total immunization costs at facilities

We want to calculate the total cost of carrying out immunization at facilities in Uganda and to break this total cost down by the different types of facilities from HC II, HC III, all the way to regional hospitals.

11. Go to Sheet C. Here you will find data on the facility name, facility type, total facility cost, and the adjusted sample weights of all facilities. In Sheet D, calculate the weighted estimate of total cost for each health facility type that is nationally representative.

a. For each facility, multiply the total cost with their sample weight in column E to obtain the weighted facility total cost.

b. Select row 1. Click on Sort & Filter button in the toolbar (on the right-hand side). Select Filter.

c. Click on the drop-down button on the column B header, cell B1. Select Sort A to Z.

d. Go to Sheet D, where you will Table D-1 set up to calculate average total cost by facility type.

e. In cell B2 of Sheet D, sum all the weighted total costs for HC II.

f. Similarly, in cell B3 of Sheet D, sum all the facility weights for HC II.

g. In cell B4 of Sheet D, divide the weighted total costs by the sum of the facility weights to obtain the weighted average facility cost for HC II facilities.

h. Repeat steps e–g for other facility types.

A.1.5 Total costs and unit costs of Ugandan routine immunization

The handbook describes various options for aggregating costing data from a sample into a total national estimate. These options vary by how much bias they introduce into the total cost estimate for the country (Clarke-Deelder, Vassall, & Menzies, 2019).

A relatively simple approach to aggregating costs is presented below. The total national cost of routine immunization in Uganda can be calculated as:

Equation A.1.1:

$$T_{country} = T_{HF} + T_{District} + T_{National}$$

In the previous step, we calculated a weighted estimate of the total cost (including vaccines) for each facility type. We apply this to all of the same type of facilities in the country. The average total cost of the sampled districts, excluding vaccines, was then applied to all the districts in the country. These aggregated facility- and district-level estimates were then added to the national-level spending (after excluding the national-level vaccine costs).

To calculate nationally representative estimates of average cost, we simply divide the total national cost by a denominator. Commonly used denominators are doses, infant population, three-dose diphtheria, tetanus, and pertussis (DTP3)-vaccinated children yielding costs per dose, cost per infant, and cost per DTP3.

12. Go to Sheet E. Table E-1 is set up to calculate total national routine immunization cost. Table E-2 is set up to calculate unit costs of national routine immunization.

From prior calculations we happen to know that average cost per district-level facility is 29,923 USD and that total central facility cost is 4,511,957 USD. We also know that there are 2215 HC II facilities, 1180 HC III facilities, 185 HC IV facilities, 127 general hospitals, and 112 district-level facilities.

13. Complete column B for the facilities section using the values calculated in the previous step.
14. In column C, calculate the total facility cost for each row in the facility and district sections. (Multiply the weighted average total costs with the number of facilities of the same type present in Uganda.)
15. Calculate the total immunization costs in cell D12 ($T_{country} = T_{HF} + T_{District} + T_{National}$).
16. Calculate the share of total cost for each row.
17. What do you observe?

The population of Uganda in 2011 was 32,939,800 and the infant population was 1,476,164. The total child doses administered was 11,964,835 and the total DTP3 vaccinated children were 1,219,455 (estimates derived from the Comprehensive Multi-Year Plan 2011).

18. Complete the table (Table E-2) below the total cost table in Sheet D with the above estimates.
19. Calculate the cost per dose, cost per infant, and cost per DTP3-vaccinated child.

A.1.6 Analyzing the relationship between unit costs and output

20. Go to Sheet F. For each facility, you are given the total facility cost, total doses administered, and total DTP3-vaccinated children.
21. In Table F-1, calculate the cost/dose for each facility. (Tip: enter the formula in cell B7, select the cell, and drag it horizontally to autofill the formula in the row.)

The graph below the table will plot each data point. To see the facilities corresponding to the data point:
   a. Click on the green cross and left click on "Add Data Labels."
   b. Click on the arrow and select click "More Options."
   c. A new window appears to the right, deselect X and Y Value.
   d. Enable "Value from cells."
   e. Select cell range B3:AY3.
   f. Click OK.

The graph next to the main graph provides a zoomed-in look at the data points.

22. Can you locate the outliers? What do you observe?
23. In Table E-2, calculate the cost/DTP3-vaccinated child. Repeat step 21.
24. Can you locate the outliers? What do you observe?
25. What can you say about the relationship between unit costs and output volume?

A.1.7 Discussion prompt

26. Carmen has analyzed the graphs of unit costs versus output, and she decided to close down all clinics that have very high unit costs and minimal output. Would you and your team advise Carmen to proceed with her decision? Explain your reasoning.

References

Brenzel, L., Young, D., & Walker, D. G. (2015). Costs and financing of routine immunization: Approach and selected findings of a multi-country study (EPIC). *Vaccine, 33,* A13–A20. doi:10.1016/j.vaccine.2014.12.066

Clarke-Deelder, E., Vassall, A., & Menzies, N. A. (2019). Estimators used in multisite healthcare costing studies in low- and middle-income countries: A systematic review and simulation study. *Value in Health, 22*(10), 1146–1153. doi:10.1016/j.jval.2019.05.007

Guthrie, T., Zikusooka, C., Kwesiga, B., Abewe, C., Lagony, S., Schutte, C.,... Kinghorn, A. (2014). *Costing and financing analyses of routine immunization in Uganda.* Health & Development Africa. https://static1.squarespace.com/static/556deb8ee4b08a534b8360e7/t/5596fa4ae4b07b7dda4dd04d/1435957834829/UGANDA+Immunization+Costing+Report+1+December+14+submitted+FINAL+update+15+12+14+errors.pdf

Exercise: estimating new vaccine introduction costs

Susmita Chatterjee[1]

A.2.1 Introduction

Information on the cost of procuring vaccines and of running a national immunization program is a key factor in planning and managing an effective immunization program. This information is also needed to conduct a cost-effectiveness analysis of a new vaccine.

Vaccine program costs are context specific and not generalizable from one country to another—vaccination schedules, target populations, vaccine introduction strategies, and prices may vary.

In this exercise, you will be given a scenario and asked to estimate how much it would cost to introduce a new vaccine into routine immunization, to produce information that can be used as input into a cost-effectiveness assessment, or to assist with planning and budgeting. The exercise provides a practical demonstration on the application of concepts introduced throughout this appendix.

Specific objectives of the exercise are to:

- Gain deeper understanding on the cost components of a cost-effectiveness analysis and the types and sources of data required.
- Practice some of the basic processes and logic of estimating immunization program costs.
- Learn some ways to generate cost estimates that can inform decisions about the adoption of a new vaccine or a change in vaccine program strategies.
- To interpret cost data, and understand their usefulness, challenges, and limitations.

A.2.2 Case scenario

A ministry of health planner has been asked to investigate the introduction of pneumococcal conjugate vaccine (PCV) into the national routine immunization program in the lower middle-income country Contagia. The country has a total population of 14,752,000 and a crude birth rate of 38/1000. An estimated 81% of children are fully immunized. The country is a lower middle-income country which has been receiving Gavi support but expects to have to fund more of its immunization program over the next few years. The current routine childhood immunization schedule is given in Table A.2.1.

PCV will be in single-dose vials and administered by injection at the same time as the diphtheria, tetanus, and pertussis (DTP) vaccine at 6, 10, and 14 weeks of age. Using the information provided, please answer the following questions:

---

[1] 'Teaching Vaccine Economics Everywhere' materials: www.immunizationeconomics.org

Table A.2.1 Current routine immunization schedule

Antigen	Age of administration
OPV0	At birth up to 13 days
BCG	At birth or first contact
OPV1, DTP–HepB–Hib1	6 weeks of age
OPV2, DTP–HepB–Hib2	10 weeks of age
OPV3, DTP–HepB–Hib3	14 weeks of age
Measles—MCV1	9 months of age
Measles—MCV2	18 months of age

BCG, bacillus Calmette–Guérin; HepB, hepatitis B; Hib, *Haemophilus influenzae* type B; MCV, measles-containing-vaccine; OPV, oral polio vaccine.

A.2.3 Exercise: part 1

1. Using the routine immunization schedule (Table A.2.1), calculate the total number of doses administered in Contagia per annum.
2. What do you think the percent wastage of the PCV vaccine should be based on? How could you more accurately estimate the potential wastage of the PCV?
3. The cost of PCV, under an agreement with manufacturers to incentivize the development of vaccines, is expected to be $7 per dose for the first 3 years. During this time, the vaccine will be donor funded. After 3 years, the cost is expected to decline to $3.50 per dose and will be funded by the country. What cost would you use when completing your total vaccine cost calculation and why?
4. Use your estimates of vaccine price from question 3 and wastage from question 2 to calculate total PCV costs.

A.2.4 Exercise: part 2

5. Table A.2.2 shows the total costs of delivering all vaccines in the country's routine immunization program before PCV introduction. How are the results useful from a program planning and management perspective?
6. What are the major cost drivers of the existing immunization program in this country?
7. Which costs of introducing PCV will be most important to estimate accurately for a cost-effectiveness analysis? Would any of these be less important for program budgeting?
8. For national programs, an important estimate is the cost per fully immunized child. The simplest way to estimate this is to divide the total costs of the program by the number of children with a complete vaccine schedule.
   a. Using information from Table A.4.2, what is the cost per fully vaccinated child in this country?
   b. List one or two limitations on using estimates of the cost per fully immunized child.
9. Using information provided in Tables A.2.1 and A.2.2:
   a. Estimate the total cost per dose of all vaccines currently in the immunization schedule where total cost is cost of vaccine plus non-vaccine (or delivery) costs. (For the two vaccines given at birth, OPV0 and BCG, assume 100% coverage. For the other vaccines in the schedule, assume 81% coverage.)

Table A.2.2 Total costs of routine immunization program in Contagia before PCV introduction (2016)

	Cost ($, 000)	% of cost
Capital costs		
Cold chain	570	1.5
Vehicles	2,000	5.2
Buildings	1,085	2.8
Other	557	1.5
Subtotal	4,212	11.0
Recurrent costs		
Vaccine and supplies	6,168	16.2
Vaccine injection and safety supplies	186	0.5
Paid labor	18,130	47.5
Volunteers/community health workers	730	1.9
Allowances for travel/subsistence	4,390	11.5
Cold chain (energy)	120	0.3
Vehicles (maintenance, fuel)	2,770	7.3
Communications	725	1.9
Building maintenance, utilities	350	0.9
Other supplies and printing	372	1.0
Subtotal	33,941	89.0
Total	38,153	100

    b. Estimate the service delivery cost per dose, that is, non-vaccine cost in the current immunization schedule.

    c. Estimate the total cost per dose of PCV. Note any limitations of your estimate.

10. Do you think that the total cost per dose estimated in question 9 will vary within a country? Where would you expect total cost per dose to be higher or lower?

11. PCV is usually administered alongside the DTP vaccine at 2, 4, and 6 months. Some countries now use a "2 + 1" schedule (i.e. two doses alongside the DTP series plus one booster later—usually around 12 months). What would be the implications (financial and logistical) of implementing the new schedule?

12. What are the most important components that need to be taken into consideration to calculate the cost of introducing PCV into your own country's routine immunization program? List up to five major inputs of this program.

Further reading

Griffiths, U. K., Bozzani, F. M., Chansa, C., Kinghorn, A., Kalesha-Masumbu, P., Rudd, C.,... Schutte, C. (2016). Costs of introducing pneumococcal, rotavirus and second dose measles vaccine into the Zambian immunization program: are expansions sustainable? *Vaccine, 34*(35), 4213–4220. doi:10.1016/j.vaccine.2016.06.050

Immunization activities and line item costs

Logan Brenzel

Table A.3.1 illustrates a crosswalk between immunization line items (cost elements) and activities (Brenzel, 2014). When analyzing immunization service costs, analysis can be done to represent costs in these different ways.

Table A.3.1 Immunization activities and line item crosswalk for routine immunization

Line item	Immunization activities									Program management	Other
	Routine facility-based service delivery	Record keeping & HMIS	Supervision	Outreach service delivery	Training	Social mobilization & advocacy	Surveillance	Cold chain maintenance	Vaccine collection, distribution, storage		
Salaried labor											
Volunteer labor											
Per diem & travel allowances											
Vaccines											
Vaccine injection & safety supplies											
Other supplies											
Transport/fuel											
Vehicle maintenance											
Cold chain energy costs											
Printing											

Building overhead, utilities, communication								
Other recurrent								
Cold chain equipment								
Vehicles								
Lab equipment								
Other equipment								
Other capital								
Buildings								
TOTAL								

Source: Brenzel (2013).

Reference

Brenzel, L. (2014). Working Paper: Common approach for the costing and financing analyses of routine immunization and new vaccine introduction costs (EPIC). Mimeograph. Bill & Melinda Gates Foundation. www.immunizationeconomics.org/epic-info

Markov decision processes

Emmanuel F. Drabo and William V. Padula

A.4.1 Designing a Markov decision process

A Markov model of the type described in Chapter 4.1 typically assumes that only one decision is made, at the start of the model. From that point forward, a sequence of events unfolds according to state-dependent transition probabilities.

A Markov decision process (MDP) extends a simple Markov model by allowing for multiple decision points over time. Each decision period is defined by a set of possible health states, S, a set of possible actions, A, a probability matrix, T_a, and a reward matrix, R_a. The probability of transitioning from state s to s' if action a is taken at time t is then defined as $T_a(s, s') = \Pr(s_{t+1} = s' \mid s_t = s, a_t = a)$; the corresponding immediate reward associated with transitioning from state s to s' if action a is taken at time t is $R_a(s, s')$.

The solution to the MDP is calculated recursively and is defined by an optimal policy π, and value function V, defined as follows:

Equation A.4.1:

$$\pi(s) = \operatorname*{argmax}_a \sum_{s'} P_a(s, s') V(s') \, st$$

Equation A.4.2:

$$V(s) = R(s) + \beta \sum_{s'} P_{\pi(s)}(s, s') V(s')$$

where β denotes the one-period discount factor. It should be noted that MDPs optimize in one dimension (i.e., minimize costs or maximize health benefits), and can thus be unattractive in cost-effectiveness analysis. In MDPs, an optimal policy is first determined, and the value function associated with that optimal policy is calculated. Once these are determined, then the costs and benefits of different optimal policies with different objective functions are compared using cost-effectiveness analysis.

A.4.2 Additional considerations about using Markov models

At this juncture, it is worthwhile asking when is using Markov model appropriate? As we have noted at the start of this appendix, Markov models are most useful for representing events that are recurrent, when we want to model the "natural history" of a disease, when the time horizon is long, and when the quantity and quality of time spent in different health states are outcomes of interest, as they are in cost-effectiveness analysis.

One additional important consideration when developing Markov models is the choice of computational tool to implement the model. Most Markov models are developed using basic spreadsheet software such as Microsoft Excel, as illustrated in our example above, or commercial packages such as TreeAge. For simple processes and most vaccine economics problems, these tools will be sufficient. However, for more complex processes, these tools may prove inadequate (Filipović-Pierucci, Zarca, & Durand-Zaleski, 2017; Williams, Lewsey, Briggs, & Mackay, 2017).

References

Filipović-Pierucci, A., Zarca, K., & Durand-Zaleski, I. (2017). Markov models for health economic evaluations: The R package heemod. *ArXiv*. https://arxiv.org/pdf/1702.03252.pdf

Williams, C., Lewsey, J. D., Briggs, A. H., & Mackay, D. F. (2017). Cost-effectiveness analysis in R using a multi-state modeling survival analysis framework: A tutorial. *Medical Decision Making*, *37*(4), 340–352. doi:10.1177/0272989X16651869

Derivation of the annual expected costs associated with the Infected state

Emmanuel F. Drabo and William V. Padula

We calculated the annual expected cost of an acute hepatitis B infection to be $1,481. This expected annual cost is the weighted average cost of outpatient care for acute symptomatic infection, the cost of hospitalization for those with acute fulminant hepatitis B infection, and the cost of hospitalization for non-fulminant cases, as calculated below:

$$C_{Acute} = p_A \times C_A + (1-p_A) \times \left\{ (1-p_H) \times C_O + p_H \times \left[p_F \times C_F + (1-p_F) \times C_H \right] \right\}$$

where C denotes costs, and p denotes the probabilities of each event. Specifically, C_{Acute} represents the annual cost per capita of an acute infection, C_A denotes the cost of an asymptomatic infection (assumed to be zero), C_O is the outpatient costs for symptomatic patients, C_F represents the annual hospitalization cost for fulminant cases, and C_H denotes the annual hospitalization cost for non-fulminant cases. Similarly, p_A is the proportion of asymptomatic cases among individuals with an acute infection, p_H is the hospitalization risk among symptomatic patients, and p_F denotes the proportion of hospitalized patients that are fulminant cases. Substituting the values of each parameter into the equation, we calculate the health-related quality of life (HRQoL) weight for acute infections as:

$$C_{Acute} = 0.70 \times \$0 + (0-0.70) \times \{(1-0.38) \times \$402 + 0.38$$
$$\times [0.04 \times \$19,481 + (1-0.04) \times \$12,034]\} = \$1,481.$$

The HRQoL utility weight associated with the Infected state is calculated in a similar fashion as costs:

$$HRQoL_{Acute} = p_A \times HRQoL_A + (1-p_A) \times \{(1-p_H) \times HRQoL_O + P_H$$
$$\times [p_F \times HRQoL_F + (1-p_F) \times HRQoL_H]\}$$

where C denotes costs, and P denotes the probabilities of each event, as defined above. Specifically, C_{Acute} represents the annual cost per capita of an acute infection, C_O is the outpatient costs for symptomatic patients, C_F represents the annual hospitalization cost for fulminant cases, and C_H denotes the annual hospitalization cost for non-fulminant cases. Substituting the values of each parameter into the equation, we calculate the HRQoL weight for acute infections as:

$$HRQoL_{Acute} = 0.70 \times 1.00 + (1-0.70) \times \{(1-0.38) \times 0.99 + 0.38$$
$$\times [0.04 \times 0.94 + (1-0.04) \times 0.99]\} = 0.997.$$

The derivation of the annual expected cost and HRQoL utility weights associated with a chronic infection from the data in Hoerger, Young, and Walker (2013) requires a slightly more complex analysis. The mathematical derivation of these expected costs goes beyond the scope of this handbook. But it is enough for the reader to know that these costs are calculated by accumulating the expected lifetime medical costs of an individual with a chronic hepatitis B infection, as they cycle through various stages of chronic hepatitis B disease progression, including chronic hepatitis, inactive carrier, compensated cirrhosis, decompensated cirrhosis, hepatocellular carcinoma, liver transplantation, and death (see Figure 1.b in the Supplementary Data of Hoerger et al. (2013)). From that model, we estimated the expected annual cost of chronic hepatitis B infection to be approximately $4,688; the expected HRQoL utility weight for chronic hepatitis B is approximately 0.939.

With these annual estimates, we are nearly ready to calculate the expected cost of spending a year in the Infected state. But we need one more parameter, the prevalence of chronic (or acute) hepatitis B infection in the population, so that we can calculate the proportions of the Infected population who have acute and chronic hepatitis B infections. Fortunately, data from the epidemiological literature allow us to calculate such a parameter. Data from 1999 to 2010 from the National Health and Nutrition Examination Survey reported that the relative risk of chronic hepatitis B infection for diabetes patients in the US was 60% higher than the risk for individuals without diabetes, with odds ratios (OR) of 1.7 (95% confidence interval (CI) 1.3–2.2) for persons aged 18 through 59 years, and 1.3 (95% CI 1.0–1.6) for persons aged 60 years and older. The reported prevalence of chronic hepatitis B infection among diabetics in the sample was 8.2% (95% CI 6.8–9.8) (Schillie, Xing, Murphy, & Hu, 2012). We will use this prevalence estimate in our model. Applying this prevalence and its complement as weights to the annual costs and HRQoL utility weights of acute and chronic hepatitis B infection, we estimate an expected cost and HRQoL utility weight of $1,744 (i.e., 0.082 × $4,688 + (1 − 0.082) × $1,481) and 0.992 (i.e., 0.082 × 0.939 + (1 − 0.082) × 0.997), respectively, for spending a year in the Infected state. These are the cost and HRQoL utility weight estimates that we use in the simplified Markov model that was introduced in Chapter 4.1.

References

Hoerger, T. J., Schillie, S., Wittenborn, J. S., Bradley, C. L., Zhou, F., Byrd, K., & Murphy, T. V. (2013). Cost-effectiveness of hepatitis B vaccination in adults with diagnosed diabetes. *Diabetes Care, 36*(1), 63–69. doi:10.2337/dc12-0759

Schillie, S. F., Xing, J., Murphy, T. V., & Hu, D. J. (2012). Prevalence of hepatitis B virus infection among persons with diagnosed diabetes mellitus in the United States, 1999–2010. *Journal of Viral Hepatitis, 19*(9), 674–676. doi:10.1111/j.1365-2893.2012.01616.x

Making models probabilistic and estimating the value of information

Ciaran N. Kohli-Lynch

A.6.1 Making models probabilistic

The core parameters in most decision models relate to costs, utilities, probabilities, and treatment effect sizes. Below is a list of candidate distributions for these data types and information on how these distributions are constructed. Non-normal distributions accept parameters as inputs which help determine the shape and size of their curves. Using the *method of moments*, these can be derived from sample statistics like the mean and standard error of a dataset. When a random variable has more than one candidate distribution, sensitivity analysis and goodness-of-fit tests can be conducted to determine which distribution is most suitable (Nixon & Thompson, 2004).

A.6.1.1 Costs

Healthcare costs are typically calculated as the product of resource counts and unit costs. Uncertainty may exist in both these parameters. The distributions used to represent count and cost data are both defined by the fact that values less than 0 are impossible. For count data, a discrete probability distribution which can only assume whole numbers. Cost data are typically represented by continuous probability distributions that can take on any value greater than or equal to 0.

The unit cost of a healthcare resource can vary anywhere from 0 to positive infinity. Negative unit costs are not possible. Cost data also tend to be highly skewed. Unlike the normal distribution, they do not tend to be symmetrically distributed around a peak value. Typically, costs are very low in a large proportion of observations but the mean is "skewed" higher by a small number of very high costs in a dataset (Malehi, Pourmotahari, & Angali, 2015).

One candidate distribution to represent cost data is the gamma distribution. This distribution is constrained on the range 0 to positive infinity and can be highly skewed. If α and β are parameters which describe the shape and scale of gamma distribution, then the expected value and variance of the distribution are defined by the following equations:

Equation A.6.1:

$$EVSI = E\left[NMB_{si}\right] - E\left[NMB_{ci}\right]$$

Equation A.6.2:

$$var[X] = \alpha\beta^2$$

To produce a distribution which fits observed data, we substitute the expected value and variance of the distribution for the sample mean and variance, respectively. After setting $E(X) = \bar{x}$ and $\mathrm{var}(X) = s^2$ and rearranging the above equations, the following equations are derived:

Equation A.6.3:

$$\alpha = \frac{\bar{x}^2}{s^2}$$

Equation A.6.4:

$$\beta = \frac{s^2}{\bar{x}}$$

The gamma distribution may provide a reasonable fit for the seasonal influenza vaccine cost data. We know that we need a distribution that is bounded by 0 and positive infinity. We have additional information from our cost study: the arithmetic mean was \$3.00 and the standard error was \$2.34. We require a probability distribution that exists on the domain 0 to positive infinity and maintains these attributes. It is therefore reasonable to assume that the vaccine cost data are gamma(α, β) distributed, where $a = \dfrac{\bar{x}^2}{s^2} = \dfrac{3.00^2}{2.34^2} \approx 1.68$ and $\beta = \dfrac{s^2}{\bar{x}} = \dfrac{2.34^2}{3.00} \approx 1.81$.

The blue curve in Fig. 4.3.4 shows a gamma distribution of the vaccine data which evidently provides a better fit for the data than the red normal distribution.

The log-normal distribution may also be assigned to costs in probabilistic sensitivity analysis (PSA). Like the gamma distribution, it is constrained on the interval 0 to positive infinity and can be skewed. The log-normal distribution assumes that the logarithm of a random variable is normally distributed. In statistical software it is often parameterized as log-normal(μ, s), where μ and s are the mean and standard deviation of the log-transformed dataset, respectively.

A.6.1.2   Utilities

The utility associated with a health state (also known as the quality or disability weight) is usually bounded between 0 and 1. A candidate distribution for data that exist in this domain is the beta distribution. If α and β are parameters which describe the shape and scale of beta distribution, then the expected value and variance of the beta distribution are defined by the following equations:

Equation A.6.5:

$$E[X] = \frac{\alpha}{\alpha + \beta}$$

Equation A.6.6:

$$\mathrm{var}[X] = \frac{\alpha\beta}{(\alpha + \beta)^2 (\alpha + \beta + 1)}$$

As above, we set we $E[X] = \bar{x}$ and $var[X] = s^2$ and rearrange the equations. After rearrangement, we arrive at the following equations:

Equation A.6.7:

$$\alpha = \bar{x}\left[\frac{\bar{x}(1-\bar{x})}{s^2} - 1\right]$$

Equation A.6.8:

$$\beta = \alpha\frac{(1-\bar{x})}{\bar{x}}$$

Disability-adjusted life years are always constrained between 0 and 1 (Burstein et al. 2015). Therefore, the beta distribution should always be considered as a candidate to represent disability weights. For quality-adjusted life years (QALYs), almost all health states have values between 0 and 1. In rare circumstances, health states can have a QALY value less than 0 (Lamers, 2007). A QALY less than 1 represents a health state deemed "worse than death." In this situation, we need to use a distribution which is bounded by negative infinity and 1. A simple workaround involves modelling health state utility as decrements to perfect health. Health state utility, U, for health state, s, is now calculated using the function: $U_s = 1 - D_s$. The random variable D_s is the deviation of U_s from full health. Since it is defined on the domain 0 to infinity, we can represent it using the gamma and log-normal distributions.

A.6.1.3 Probabilities

A clear constraint for probabilities is that they can only assume values in the domain 0 to 1. If we have estimates for the mean and variance of a probability, we can use the methods described for utilities to define an appropriate beta distribution.

In studies which produce binomial event data (i.e., event or no event), a beta distribution can be constructed to predict the likelihood of an event occurring. Consider a study with n observations. Each observation records whether or not an event of interest occurs. If r events occur, the beta(α, β) distribution with $\alpha = r$ and $\beta = n - r$ will produce a distribution representative of the observed data.

An additional constraint should be considered when we model probabilities for multiple mutually exclusive events. The probabilities of a set of mutually exclusive events must sum to 1. When there are only two possible events at some point in a decision model, we can easily code the probability of one event as the probabilistic complement to the other. Hence, including one event probability as a distribution will inevitably alter rates of the complementary event. Uncertainty for more than two mutually exclusive events can be represented with a Dirichlet distribution. The Dirichlet distribution is the multivariate generalization of beta distribution. Instead of outputting a single value, it accepts k parameters and outputs k values.

Consider a clinical study of patients at risk of three mutually exclusive events: Event A, Event B, and No Event. Five hundred patients are observed for the entirety of the study. At the end of follow-up, 300 patients have experienced Event A, 150 have experienced Event B, and 50 did not have an event. The *Dirichlet* (300,150,50) distribution describes the range of probabilities that can be assigned to these events. Its output is a vector of three values which align with each of the study endpoints. More generally, the *Dirichlet* $(\alpha_1, \alpha_2, ..., \alpha_n)$ distribution can be employed to predict the respective probabilities of n mutually exclusive events.

A.6.1.4 Treatment effects

Treatment effects are a key source of uncertainty in decision modelling studies. It is important to consider specific constraints on a treatment effect before assigning a distribution. Some treatments can be modeled through absolute changes in risk factor values. For example, antihypertensive medications tends to drop blood pressure by a fixed amount (Ogden, He, Lydick, & Whelton, 2000). As blood pressure can either increase or decrease after a treatment, positive and negative treatment effects are possible. The treatment effect exists on the domain negative infinity to positive infinity and could be modeled with a normal distribution.

Often, treatments lead to a relative reduction in an individual's likelihood of experiencing an event. We represent such treatment effects with statistical measures like the hazard ratio, odds ratio, and relative risk. The lowest possible value for this parameter is 0 which occurs when no events are observed in the treatment arm of a study. It is also possible that a treatment will cause a large increase in events. Hence, the domain for this parameter is 0 to positive infinity. It is commonly assumed that relative measures of event probability are log-normally distributed (Barendregt, 2010).

A.6.1.5 Defining distributions in Excel and running Monte Carlo simulations

Distributions can be defined in many ways. Sometimes they are defined with the mean and variance from a dataset, sometimes with descriptive statistics of transformed data, and sometimes with shape and scale parameters. The parameters we use to define a distribution depends on the type of distribution and the statistical software being used. The exercises in this handbook use a Microsoft Excel model. Hence, the description of distributions and key parameters included above generally align with the way that distributions are defined in Excel.

When conducting a PSA in Excel, we want to draw a value from each parametric distribution employed in our decision model. Many distributions are available for use in Excel. We must pull randomly selected values from these distributions, using inverse distribution functions.

In Fig 4.3.4, we fitted a *gamma*$(1.68, 1.81)$ distribution to approximate the unit cost of vaccines in South Africa. In Excel, the function $GAMMA.DIST(x, alpha, beta, FALSE)$ can model this distribution if one sets alpha = 1.68 and beta = 1.81. When function type "cumulative" is declared FALSE, the output of this function is the probability density function and can be described mathematically as $GAMMA.DIST(x, alpha, beta, FALSE) = P(X = x)$. When cumulative is declared TRUE, the output is the probability that the true value is less than or equal to x. This is the cumulative density function and can be presented mathematically as $GAMMA.DIST(x, alpha, beta, TRUE) = P(X \leq x)$.

When conducting a PSA in Excel, we wish to draw a number randomly from a predefined distribution. To do so we use inverse cumulative density functions. Alongside parameters like *alpha* and *beta* which describe the form of a distribution, inverse cumulative density functions accept a probability, L, as input. They output a value, x, such that the probability of random variable X is less than or equal to x equals L. Mathematically, $GAMMA.INV(L, alpha, beta) = x; x : P(X \leq x) = L$.

In Fig. A.6.2, it appears that approximately 50% of the gamma distribution lies between $2.00 and $3.00. In Excel, the function *GAMMA.INV* (0.50,1.68,1.81) predicts that the median cost in the dataset is $2.46. This means that if we were to randomly select an observation from the *gamma*(1.68,1.81) distribution, there is a 50% chance it would be less than $2.46.

In the PSA process, we randomly select parameters from a distribution multiple times. In Excel, the function *RAND()* randomly selects a value between 0 and 1. Hence, it can be used in the inverse cumulative density function to randomly select a value from a distribution. For example, *GAMMA.INV(RAND(),1.68,1.81)* will select a random value from the vaccine cost distribution. When repeated multiple times, this process will draw a range of plausible values from across the entirety of the *gamma*(1.68,1.81) distribution.

Once distributions have been defined for each parameter in a decision model, a set of parameter values are randomly selected, the model is run with these parameter values, and outcomes are re-corded. At this point, this first iteration of the PSA is complete. Parameter values are subsequently redrawn from their respective distributions and model outcomes are recorded again. This process is repeated until the total number of desired iterations have been completed. These steps are outlined below. In Excel, this process can be automated using Visual Basic for Applications (VBA) macros.

Steps to conduct a PSA in Excel for a decision model with random variables X and Y:

1. Select a random value L between 0 and 1 using *RAND()* function. Example: *RAND()* selects 0.60 from the range of possible values (Fig A.6.1).
2. Draw value from distribution of X such that $P(X \leq x)$ equals random value drawn in step 1, using function *GAMMAINV(RAND(),alpha,beta)*. Example: 60th percentile of X's *gamma*(1.68,1.81) distribution is drawn. As shown, this value equals approximately $3.03.
3. Repeat Steps 1–2 for random variable Y, selecting a random value from its distribution.
4. Compute and record model outcomes with inputs derived from Steps 1–3.
5. Repeat Steps 1–4 multiple times, using different values for random variables X and Y each time to inform model parameters.
6. Average over results from all model iterations to obtain central cost-effectiveness es-timate. Range of observed results can be used to determine confidence interval for estimate.

A.6.2 Value of information analysis

The processes required to estimate expected value of perfect information (EVPI), expected value of perfect parameter information (EVPPI), and expected value of sample information (EVSI) are described below. A summary of the subscripts and terms used henceforth to de-scribe value of information calculations is provided in Table A.6.1.

A.6.2.1 Calculating expected value of perfect information

Let $NMB_{x,j}$ equal net monetary benefit (NMB) for eventuality x and treatment j. Each eventu-ality occurs with probability $p(x)$. The expected NMB for strategy j is calculated by averaging across all possible eventualities:

Equation A.6.9:

$$E_x[NMB_j] = \sum_x p(x) * NMB_{x,j}$$

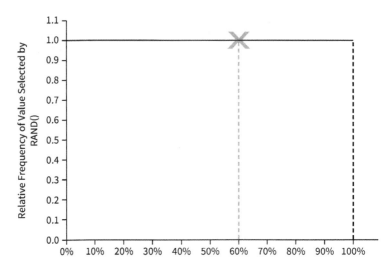

Fig. A.6.1 Relative frequency of value selected by RAND().

When estimating the expected NMB of a treatment using PSA results, we assume that a discrete number of eventualities are possible (i.e., x is a discrete random variable). In reality, many sources of parametric uncertainty are continuous random variables, and it would be mathematically more correct to estimate their expected value using integration. Here, the process is discretized to help illustrate the processes involved in value of information analysis. In addition, most decision models are too complex to easily evaluate using integration. Monte Carlo simulation uses a discrete approach to simulate the process of integration.

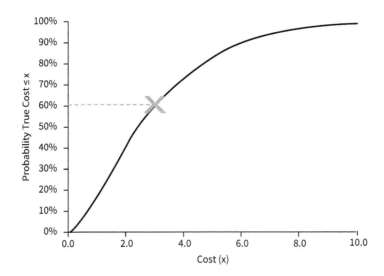

Fig. A.6.2 Probability that the true cost is ≤x.

To maximize health benefits with current levels of information, a decision maker will fund the intervention with the highest expected NMB. The expected NMB achieved by a decision maker with current information (ci) can therefore be calculated as follows:
Equation A.6.10:

$$E[NMB_{ci}] = \max_{j}(E_{x}[NMB_{j}])$$

A decision maker with perfect information knows which eventuality will occur and will choose the intervention with the highest NMB in this situation. Based on current information, we do not know which eventuality will occur; the uncertainty in the decision is not resolved. We simply know that some theoretical perfectly informed decision maker would have this information. The various eventualities still have $p(x)$ probability of occurring. Hence, the expected NMB *with* perfect information (pi) equals the probability-weighted sum of the maximum NMB across each eventuality:
Equation A.6.11:

$$E[NMB_{pi}] = E_{x}[\max_{j}(NMB_{x,j})] = \sum_{x} p(x) \times \max_{j}(NMB_{x,j})$$

Finally, the expected value of perfect information equals the expected gains that would be achieved by obtaining perfect information compared to current information. This is the difference between the expected NMB with perfect information and the expected NMB with current information:
Equation A.6.12:

$$EVPI = [ENMB_{pi}] - E[NMB_{ci}]$$

The following steps describe how to calculate EVPI using Monte Carlo simulation with a decision-analytic model and predefined probability distributions for parameters:

1. Simulate the "true value" of random variable x by randomly drawing a value, x_{s}, from its distribution S times.
2. Estimate $E[NMB_{ci}]$ by computing the treatment strategy with maximum $E_{x}[NMB_{j}]$ averaged across the S simulations of x.
3. Estimate $E[NMB_{pi}]$ by computing the treatment strategy with maximum $NMB_{x,j}$ in each of the S simulations of x then averaging across all S results.
4. Calculate EVPI by subtracting $E[NMB_{ci}]$ from $E[NMB_{pi}]$.

A.6.2.2 Calculating expected value of perfect parameter information

The EVPPI is calculated in a similar way to EVPI. To calculate EVPPI, we must consider the range of uncertain parameters in a decision problem. Let us denote the parameter of interest as x_{ref} and the remaining sources of parametric uncertainty as $x_{o}th$. For simplicity, the following example assumes that x_{ref} and $x_{o}th$ are independent. This means that eliminating uncertainty regarding one parameter provides no information on the true value of the other. We will also assume that x_{ref} is a single parameter. Neither of these assumptions is fundamental to the estimation approach for EVPPI presented below.

Table A.6.1 Parameters for value of information analysis

Value	Definition
ci	Current information
$E[NMB_{ci}]$	Expected net monetary benefit with current information
$E[NMB_{pi}]$	Expected net monetary benefit with perfect information
$E[NMB_{ppi}]$	Expected net monetary benefit with perfect parameter information
$E[NMB_{si}]$	Expected net monetary benefit with sample information
$E_x[\ldots]$	Expected value across all possible values of x
j	Treatment under consideration
$\max_j(NMB_{x,j})$	Value of NMB$_{x,j}$ with for treatment with the highest net monetary benefit among a set of alternative options under eventuality x
$NMB_{x,j}$	Net monetary benefit of intervention j under eventuality x
$p(x)$	Likelihood that a given value of x is the true state of the world
pi	Perfect information
ppi	Perfect parameter information
si	Sample information
x	Eventuality, or state of the world, represented by parameter or set of parameters in a decision model
x_{oth}	Remaining parameter(s) in EVPPI analysis
x_{ref}	Parameter(s) of interest in EVPPI analysis
z	Summary statistics obtained from new sample information

Now, consider a decision maker who has perfect information regarding the true value of x_{ref}. Each possible value of x_{ref} occurs with probability $p(x_{ref})$. Let $NMB_{x_{ref},x_{oth},j}$ equal the NMB for treatment j with parameters x_{ref} and x_oth. To estimate the expected NMB for strategy j when we know the value of x_{ref}, we must average over all remaining sources of decision uncertainty (see Equation A.6.13).

Equation A.6.13:

$$E_{x_{oth}}[NMB_j \mid x_{ref}] = \sum_{x_{oth}} p(x_{oth}) * NMB_{x_{oth},x_{ref},j}$$

The decision maker with perfect parameter information will know the true value of x_{ref}. At this value, they will choose to implement the treatment with the highest value of $E_{x_{oth}}[NMB_j \mid x_{ref}]$. With current information, the true value of x_{ref} is unknown. To calculate the expected NMB given perfect parameter information, we must average across all possible values of x_{ref} (see Equation A.6.14).

Equation A.6.14:

$$E[NMB_{ppi}] = E_{x_{ref}}[\max_j(E_{x_{oth}}[NMB_j \mid x_{ref}])] = \sum_{x_{ref}} p(x_{ref}) \times \max_j(E_{x_{oth}}[NMB_j \mid x_{ref}])$$

To calculate EVPPI, we subtract the expected NMB given current information from the expected NMB with perfect parameter information (see Equation A.6.15).
Equation A.6.15:

$$EVPPI = E[NMB_{ppi}][-E[NMB_{ci}]$$

When estimating $E[NMB_{ppi}]$ with a decision model, it is necessary to conduct a PSA with two loops. The outer loop randomly samples the parameter of interest, x_{ref}. The inner loop samples all remaining parameters, $x_o th$. An additional PSA is required to estimate $E[NMB_{ci}]$.
The following steps describe how to calculate EVPPI using Monte Carlo simulation with a decision-analytic model and predefined probability distributions for parameters:

1. Simulate a set of random variables $x = \{x_{ref}, x_{oth}\}$ by randomly drawing two values, $x_s = \{x_{ref,s}, x_{oth,s}\}$, from their distributions S times.
2. Estimate $E[NMB_{ci}]$ by computing the treatment strategy with maximum $E_x[NMB_j]$ averaged across the S simulations of x.
3. *Outer loop*: simulate x_{ref} by randomly drawing a value, $x_{ref,o}$, from its distribution O times. *Inner loop*: for each value of $x_{ref,o} = \{x_{ref,1},...,x_{ref,O}\}$, simulate $x_o th$ by randomly drawing a value, $x_o th_i$, from its distribution I times.
   a. ... compute $NMB_{x_{oth,i},x_{ref,o},j}$ for each combination of value values $x_{ref,o}$ and $x_o th_i$.
   b. ... estimate $E_{x_{oth}}[NMB_j \mid x_{ref,o}]$ for each of $x_{ref,o}$ by averaging $NMB_{x_{oth,i},x_{ref,o},j}$ across the I simulations of $x_o th$.
4. Estimate $E[NMB_{ppi}]$ by recording the treatment strategy with maximum $E_{x_{oth}}[NMB_j \mid x_{ref,o}]$ in each of the O simulations of $x_o th$ and averaging across all O results.
5. Calculate EVPPI by subtracting $E[NMB_{ci}]$ from $E[NMB_{ppi}]$.

It may be desirable to relax the assumptions required for the above framework. In some cases, we cannot assume independence between x_{ref} and $x_o th$. Without this assumption we must account for the conditional distribution of $x_o th$ dependent on x_{ref} (Brennan, Kharroubi, O'Hagan, & Chilcott, 2007). Theoretically this involves replacing $p(x_{oth})$ with a probability distribution which conditions $x_o th$ on x_{ref}. Similarly, the simulation of $x_o th$ in Step 3a of the Monte Carlo simulation would be drawn from a conditional probability distribution of $x_o th$ dependent on $x_{ref,o}$. We may also wish to estimate the value of reducing uncertainty in multiple parameters concurrently. In this situation, x_{ref} can be replaced by a vector of parameters, with x_{oth} representing all remaining sources of parametric uncertainty in the decision.
The extensive process required to estimate EVPPI with Monte Carlo simulation can be computationally demanding. Dependent on the complexity of a decision model, traditional PSAs may take multiple days to complete. As technology develops, it will be possible for most researchers to quickly run these analyses. In the meantime, computational limitations will continue to inhibit the widespread use of EVPPI analysis. Algorithms have been developed which reduce the computational burden of EVPPI analysis (Brennan et al., 2007; Sadatsafavi, Bansback, Zafari, Najafzadeh, & Marra, 2013).

A.6.2.3 Calculating expected value of sample information

Any future research will be conducted in a sample of size n, which predicts a new state of the world $z \in Z$, where z represents summary statistics taken from the new sample and Z represents the set of all possible samples of size n in the population of interest. If the population of interest is of size N, there are $\dfrac{N!}{(N-n)!n!}$ such samples of size n. This new sample enables us to update our *prior belief*, $p(x)$, for each value x. The updated or *joint posterior* distribution, $p(x\,|\,z)$, assigns a likelihood to each eventuality x influenced by both our prior belief and the sample information provided by z. The degree to which sample information updates our prior belief depends on the type of data being observed, the effect size, and the variability of the observed effect in the sample.

Expected NMB with a new sample z is constructed in a similar fashion to $E[NMB_{ci}]$, with beliefs about the true value of x updated based on the information provided by z.

Equation A.6.16:

$$E[NMB\,|\,z] = \max_j (E_x[NMB_{x|z,j}]) = \max_j \left(\sum_x p(x\,|\,z) \times NMB_{x,j} \right)$$

Some samples will produce estimates of $p(x)$ similar to our prior belief and some will vary. Before conducting a study, we do not know which sample will be observed. Therefore, we must average across all possible samples when estimating the expected NMB with sample information. This is similar to the estimation approach required for EVPPI, where the true value of x_{ref} is unknown.

Equation A.6.17:

$$E[NMB_{si}] = \sum_z p(z) \times E[NMB\,|\,z]$$

To estimate Equation A.6.17, we need information on the distribution of z. This distribution is defined by the relationship $p(z,x) = p(x) \times p(z\,|\,x)$. The function $p(x)$ represents our prior belief about the value of x. The function $p(z\,|\,x)$ is called the *sampling distribution* of the data. The structure of this function is determined by the type of data being collected (Kunst et al., 2019).

Finally, we calculate EVSI by subtracting expected NMB given current information from expected NMB with sample information.

Equation A.6.18:

$$EVSI = E[NMB_{si}] - E[NMB_{ci}]$$

The following steps describe how to calculate EVSI using Monte Carlo simulation with a decision-analytic model and predefined probability distributions for parameters:

1. *Outer loop*: simulate the "true value" of random variable x by randomly drawing a value, x_s from its distribution S times. *Inner loop*: for each value $x_s = \{x_1, \ldots, x_S\}$, simulate a sample of n estimates $z_s = \{x_{s,1}, \ldots, x_{s,n}\}$. The sampling distribution of $z_{s,n}$ will depend on the structure of the parameter being analyzed and the sample size.
   a. ... estimate $E_x[NMB_{x|z,j}]$ for each sample z_s. This will involve updating the base estimate of x with the sample information provided by z_s.
   b. ... record $E[NMB\,|\,z_s]$, the maximum $E_{x|z_s}[NMB_j]$ for each sample z_s.

2. Estimate $E[NMB_{ci}]$ by computing the maximum $E_x[NMB_j]$, averaged across the S simulations of x.

3. Estimate $E[NMB_{si}]$ by computing the average value of $E[NMB|z_s]$ across the S simulations.

4. Calculate EVSI by subtracting $E[NMB_{ci}]$ from $E[NMB_{si}]$.

The framework above assumes we are only interested in one value of n. If we are only considering one sample size, a proposed study which recruits n patients and costs less than EVSI should be funded. To estimate the optimal sample size for a study, EVSI could be estimated for multiple different values of n. Intuitively, as n increases, we get closer to sampling the entire population and sample information tends towards perfect information. Hence, the upper bound for EVSI is EVPI.

For illustrative purposes, the example above did not disaggregate parameters into those being studied and those which will maintain existing levels of uncertainty. As with EVPPI, the framework can be extended to distinguish between sources of parametric uncertainty that will be studied and others which will remain unexamined. When a proposed study will focus on a limited set of model parameters, the upper bound for its EVSI is the corresponding EVPPI.

References

Barendregt, J. J. (2010). The effect size in uncertainty analysis. *Value in Health*, *13*(4), 388–391. doi:10.1111/j.1524-4733.2009.00686.x

Brennan, A., Kharroubi, S., O'Hagan, A., & Chilcott, J. (2007). Calculating partial expected value of perfect information via Monte Carlo sampling algorithms. *Medical Decision Making*, *27*(4), 448–470. doi:10.1177/0272989X07302555

Burstein, Roy, Tom Fleming, Juanita Haagsma, Joshua A. Salomon, Theo Vos, and Christopher JL. Murray. (2015). Estimating distributions of health state severity for the global burden of disease study. *Population Health Metrics*, *13*(1), 31. https://doi.org/10.1186/s12 963-015-0064-y

Kunst, N., Wilson, E., Alarid-Escudero, F., Baio, G., Brennan, A., Fairley, M., . . . Heath, A. (2019). *Computing the expected value of sample information efficiently: Expertise and skills required for four model-based methods*. ArXiv. https://arxiv.org/ftp/arxiv/papers/1910/1910.03368.pdf

Lamers, L. M. (2007). The transformation of utilities for health states worse than death: Consequences for the estimation of EQ-5D value sets. *Medical Care*, *45*(3), 238–244. doi:10.1097/01.mlr.0000252166.76255.68

Malehi, A. S., Pourmotahari, F., & Angali, K. A. (2015). Statistical models for the analysis of skewed healthcare cost data: A simulation study. *Health Economics Reviews*, *5*, 11. doi:10.1186/s13561-015-0045-7

Nixon, R. M., & Thompson, S. G. (2004). Parametric modelling of cost data in medical studies. *Statistics in Medicine*, *23*(8), 1311–1331. doi:10.1002/sim.1744

Ogden, L. G., He, J., Lydick, E., & Whelton, P. K. (2000). Long-term absolute benefit of lowering blood pressure in hypertensive patients according to the JNC VI risk stratification. *Hypertension*, *35*(2), 539–543. doi:10.1161/01.HYP.35.2.539

Sadatsafavi, M., Bansback, N., Zafari, Z., Najafzadeh, M., & Marra, C. (2013). Need for speed: An efficient algorithm for calculation of single-parameter expected value of partial perfect information. *Value in Health*, *16*(2), 438–448. doi:10.1016/j.jval.2012.10.018

Decision model

HepB_CEA-Tree_PartA

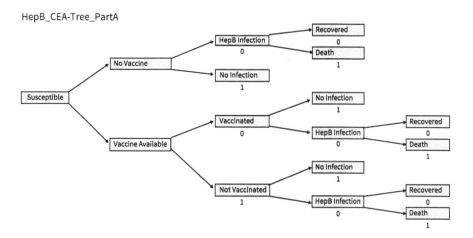

HepB_CEA-Tree_PartB

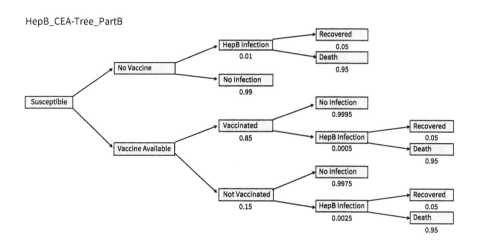

HepB_CEA-Tree_PartC

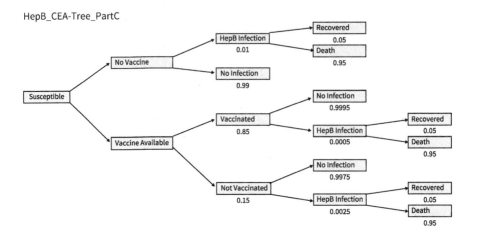

HepB_CEA-Tree_PartD

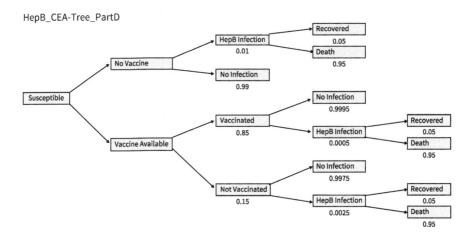

HepB_CEA-Tree_PartE

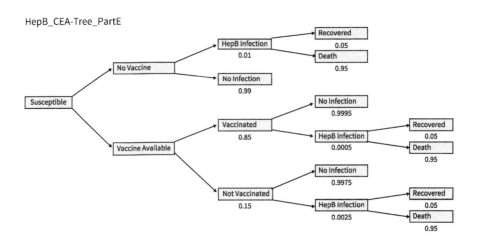

Index

For the benefit of digital users, indexed terms that span two pages (e.g., 52–53) may, on occasion, appear on only one of those pages.

Tables, figures, and boxes are indicated by *t*, *f*, and *b* following the page number